# Health Promotion
## and Aging

## Practical Applications for Health Professionals

### *Third Edition*

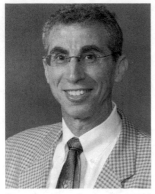

**David Haber, PhD,** is the John and Janice Fisher Distinguished Professor of Wellness and Gerontology at Ball State University in Muncie, Indiana. Dr. Haber was a professor at the University of Texas Medical Branch in Galveston, Texas, and before that served as the director of Creighton University's shopping mall-based Center for Healthy Aging in Omaha, Nebraska. He is a fellow in the Gerontological Society of America, and recognized for two Best Practice Awards from the National Council on the Aging, the Distinguished Teacher Award from the Association for Gerontology in Higher Education, and the Molly Mettler Award for Leadership in Health Promotion from the National Council on Aging. In addition to this third edition of *Health Promotion and Aging*, Dr. Haber authored *Health Care for an Aging Society*. He has been Project Director or Principal Investigator of 20 research or demonstration projects related to health and aging. Typically, these projects involve health profession students leading community health promotion projects with older adults, and contributing to the evaluation of these programs. He is currently working with health contract/calendars to help sedentary older adults become more physically active. Dr. Haber received his PhD in sociology from the Andrus Gerontology Center at the University of Southern California, Los Angeles.

# Health Promotion
## and Aging

## Practical Applications for
## Health Professionals

### *Third Edition*

**David Haber,** PhD

 **Springer Publishing Company**

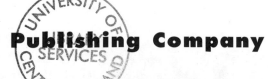

Springer Publishing Company, Inc.
536 Broadway
New York, NY 10012-3955

*Acquisitions Editor: Helvi Gold*
*Production Editor: Sara Yoo*
*Cover design by Joanne Honigman*

04 05 06 07 / 5 4 3 2

**Library of Congress Cataloging-in-Publication Data**

Haber, David, 1944–
    Health promotion and aging : practical applications for health
professionals / David Haber. — 3rd ed.
        p.   cm.
    Includes bibliographical references and index.
    ISBN 0-8261-8462-6
    1. Preventive health services for the aged—United States. 2. Health
promotion—United States. 3. Health education—United States. I. Title.

RA564.8.H33  2004
362.198'97'00973—dc22

                                                          2004061041

Printed in the United States of America by Maple-Vail Book
Manufacturing Group.

# Contents

# List of Figures

# List of Tables

# Foreword

## THE CHALLENGES AND OPPORTUNITIES OF POPULATION AGING

As an American population, we have experienced several dramatic trends over the 20th century including: 1) an unprecedented aging of the population with approximately 1 in 8 Americans now 65 years of age or older and many more people than ever before living into their 80s, 90s, or even 100s (Federal Interagency Forum, 2000; AOA, 2000); and 2) an unparalled improvement in health and functioning across the life span, with decreases in disability rates reported even among the oldest population (Manton et al., 2001; NCHS, 2001). With the aging of the baby boomers, population aging is expected to accelerate even faster in the first part of the 21st century (RWJF, 2001).

These demographic trends are now well documented with a growing knowledge base about the characteristics of the older population and the challenges facing older adults, their families, and society as a whole (NCHS, 1999; NCOA, 2002). Population aging has generally been viewed with a crisis mentality, but it can also signal an opportunity for action depending upon our understanding of factors associated with these trends and the identification of responses to enhance public health and quality of life in our aging society (NRC, 2001). This underscores the need to focus attention on how clinical, behavioral and social factors affect and are affected by the aging of the population.

## BRIDGING AGING AND HEALTH PROMOTION

Progress in understanding the utility of health promotion across the full life-course has been impeded by earlier stereotypes of the older population as frail and infirm combined with erroneous notions of health promotion as too late for older populations who were unable or unwilling to change their behaviors and situations (Ory, Hoffman, Hawkins, et al., 2003; Rowe & Kahn, 1998). In the past two decades there has been a welcomed convergence of research and practice around two previously distinct areas of study: aging and health promotion.

In my twenty years at the National Institute on Aging, I was privileged to be in the position to help spur the development of research on aging, health and behavior, with increased emphasis on understanding the multifaceted determinants of behavior and developing theory-based intervention strategies for enhancing health and functioning in the middle and later years (Ory, Abeles, & Lipman, 1992; Ory & DeFriese, 2000; Ory & Chesney, 2002). During that time I came to understand that the principles of aging were inextricable linked with health promotion processes.

Twenty years of research provides indisputable support for the vision of aging, first articulated eloquently by my colleague and dear friend, Matilda White Riley in the 1980s. These principles of aging serve as a harbinger of malleability of aging processes and the importance of disease prevention/disability prevention efforts in avoiding or delaying the onset and progression of typical age-related conditions and/or helping older adults manage their daily lives and health situations:

- Aging is multifaceted, consisting of social and psychological as well as biological processes;
- Aging is not entirely fixed for all time, but varies with social structure and social change;
- And, as a corollary, because aging is not immutable, it is subject to a degree of social and behavioral as well as biomedical modification and intervention (Riley, 1987, p. 2).

## TRANSLATION OF RESEARCH TO PRACTICE

In my new post-NIA role, I am fortunate to have the opportunity to forge new territory in understanding how to translate research into practice at the community level through the Active for Life™ Program, which is part of the Active Living Network funded by the Robert Wood Johnson Program (www.activeforlife.info). This activity represents the next frontier of aging research. Drawing on evidence-based intervention programs, Active for Life™ will examine the ways in which efficacy-based activity programs may need to be adapted in order to be widely disseminated, sustained, and replicated by a variety of community organizations in multiple settings—and responses that will also be required by our community partners.

The success of this project will undoubtedly be based, in part, on the implementation of what we have learned about behavioral change strategies (Coon, Ory, & Lipman, 2003; Ory, Jordan, & Bazzarre, 2002). The following represents a summarization of behavioral change principles culled from successful interventions in the lifestyle arena:

- Identify Multiple Opportunities for Intervention. Behavior change occurs within broader sociocultural contexts where initiating and maintaining healthy behaviors is best accomplished by taking advantage of the multiple opportunities for change in people's physical and social environments.
- Mechanisms of Change. Interventionists need to better understand and consider mechanisms of change including why people change (mediators) and, in turn, evaluate the ability of an intervention to optimize change among relevant mediators of change.
- Collaborative and Concrete Goals. The goals of healthy behavior change are more successful when they are collaborative in nature, reflecting a partnership between the participant as an active agent and the provider; collaborative goals must then be concretely stated.
- Goals as Moving Targets. The goals of behavior change should be conceptualized as moving targets impacted by multiple levels of sociocultural influence including personal, interpersonal, systemic or organizational, community and policy influences.
- Skills Training for the Real World. The adoption and maintenance of healthy behaviors requires basic skills that can be taught, practiced and used effectively in "real world" contexts. These skills need to be both generalizable as well as flexible enough to adapt to shifts in the target population's sociocultural contexts.
- Intervention Follow-up and Boosters. The adherence to and maintenance of healthy behaviors also requires consideration of sociocultural influences as well as the need for planned follow-up and "boosters."
- Variety. Sustained change in target populations requires the development of a variety of interventions aimed either singularly or in combination at multiple levels of influence. (Coon, Ory, & Lipman, 2003)

# DAVID HABER AS A PIONEER IN HEALTH PROMOTION AND AGING

David Haber is one of the true pioneers in the aging and health promotion field. This third volume of his classic text is the most comprehensive text on what is currently known about aging and health promotion. What makes this text especially useful is that it is research-based (with over 1,200 citations), but it is more than just an excellent research synthesis on key areas such as lifestyle behaviors, social supports, health care interactions; community and public health approaches. The text provides ample illustration of model health promotion programs and offers practical advice for implementing and evaluating model programs. So in this vein, Haber is one of those rare scholars who have already made a significant contribution to the translation of research to practice.

There are several nice touches that make this book especially useful for researchers, practitioners, and policymakers alike. This text has been updated to include breaking news about controversial issues in the recommendation of lifestyle behaviors as well as the diagnosis and treatment of age-related conditions (e.g., what are the relative advantages of mammograms or HRT for older women?). Theories and mechanisms of behavioral change are well documented, and definitional clarity is provided for key concepts (e.g., differences between health promotion, health protection, and disease prevention). In addition to being conceptually grounded and empirically based, there is also the inclusion of very practical and useable tips for conducting different types of health promotion programs (e.g., for exercise and nutrition programs). Seeing ordinary older people doing ordinary things helps visualize older adults in positive ways, and referral to easy-to-use assessment tools is helpful for those working with older adults.

The importance of having an armamentarium of different intervention strategies to address the multiple determinants of health and behavior is emphasized. Haber's philosophy regarding the desirability of collaboration in the health care setting, and in other interactions with older adults is critical for maximizing health promotion opportunities. There is both breathe and depth—for example, we learn about the advantages (and potential disadvantages) of many different types of social supports. Also included are topics such as e-health information that are on the cutting edge of health promotion efforts in the 21st century.

Moreover, there is appreciation of diversity of the aging population, and the influence of sociodemographic, cultural and environmental factors. Although Haber doesn't emphasize his social ecological approach, this text is a living embodiment of a social ecological model—and an excellent resource for understanding the intersection of public health and aging issues.

Refreshingly, Haber does not shy away from controversial issues. He provides latest on many controversial issues (e.g., recommendations about medical screening and preferred treatment options). Not only does the document policy and advocacy efforts by others, his concluding chapter provides a clear accounting of specific research and policy recommendations that he personally favors. While challenges and problems of aging are well documented, the overall flavor of the text is optimistic—with the take home message emphasizing multilevel strategies for helping assure the full vitality of individuals as they age.

While any text will inevitably suffer from datedness in this area of rapidly evolving information, the inclusion of contact information and website urls will be useful in helping the reader to stay up-to-date with key statistics and breaking news. Another useful component are the discussion questions which are thought-provoking, and will be a valuable stimulus for collegial or class discussion.

## SUMMARY

This text illustrates the challenges and the opportunities that await researchers, practitioners and policymakers focused on understanding the aging process, determinants of behavioral change, and the best interventions for enhancing the health and quality of life of Americans as they age. The important, and indeed, urgency, of health promotion efforts will only increase in the coming years as the advances in medicine, public health and technology being unveiled every day converge with unprecedented growth of the aging population. This text will serve as a road map for translating research into practice, and designing effective health promotion interventions that can reach large numbers of adults in settings where they live, work and play.

MARCIA G. ORY, PHD, MPH

## REFERENCES

Administration on Aging. (2000). *A profile of older Americans: 2000.* Washington, DC: HHS.

Coon, D. W., Lipman, P. D., & Ory, M. G. (in press). Designing effective HIV/AIDS social and behavioral interventions for the 50 plus population. *Journal of AIDS Research*.

Interagency Forum on Aging Related Statistics. (2000). *Older Americans 2000: Key indicators of well-being*. Washington, DC: DHHS.

Manton, K. G., & XiLiang, G. (2000). Changes in the prevalence of chronic disability in the United States black and nonblack population above age 65 from 1982 to 1999. *Proceedings of the National Academy of Sciences USA, 98*(11), 6354–6359.

National Center for Health Statistics. (1999). *Health, United States, 1999. With health and aging chartbook*. Hyattsville, MD: DHHS.

National Center for Health Statistics. (2000). *Healthy people 2000 final review*. Hyattsville, MD: Public Health Service.

National Council on the Aging. (2002). *American perceptions of aging in the 21st Century*. Sampling, Interviewing and Data Preparation by Harris Interactive, Inc. 2002. Retrieved from www.ncoa.org.

National Research Council. (2000). New horizons in health: An integrative approach. In B. H. Singer & C. D. Ryff (Eds.), *Committee on future directions for behavioral and social sciences research at the National Institutes of Health*. Washington, DC: National Academy Press.

National Research Council. (2001). *Preparing for an aging world: The case for cross-national research*. Panel on a Research Agenda and New Data for an Aging World, Committee on Population, Committee on National Statistics. Washington, DC: National Academy Press.

Ory, M. G., Abeles, R. P., & Lipman, P. D. (Eds.). (1992). *Aging, health and behavior*. Newbury Park, CA: Sage.

Ory, M. G., & Chesney, M. (2002). Aging and the life-course: Advancing psychosomatic medicine research. *Journal of Psychosomatic Medicine, 64*, 367–369.

Ory, M. G., & DeFriese, G. H. (Eds.) (1998). *Self care in later life*. New York: Springer Publishing.

Ory, M. G., Hoffman, M., Hawkins, M., Sanner, B., & Mockenhaupt, R. (in press). Challenging aging stereotypes: Designing and evaluating physical activity programs. *American Journal of Preventive Medicine*.

Ory, M. G., Jordan, P., & Bazzarre, T. (2002). Behavioral change consortium: Setting the stage for a new century of health behavior change research. *Health Education Research, 17*(5), 500–511.

Riley, M. W., Matarazzo, J. D., & Baum, A. (1987). *Perspectives in behavioral medicine: The aging dimension*. Hillsdale, NJ, Lawrence Erlbaum.

Robert Wood Johnson Foundation. (2000). National blueprint for increasing physical activity among adults 50 and older: Creating a strategic framework and enhancing organizational capacity for change. *Journal of Aging and Physical Activity, 9*(suppl.), S5–S28.

Rowe, J. W., & Kahn, R. L. (1998). *Successful aging*. New York: Pantheon Books.

U.S. Department of Health and Human Services. (2000). *Healthy People 2010: Understanding and improving health* (Conference Edition, in two volumes). Washington, DC: Government Printing Office.

# Preface

I was trained at the University of Southern California as a sociologist specializing in gerontology, but spent my career implementing and evaluating health promotion projects in the local community. This contradiction between training and practice has informed me on why promoting health is possible, but difficult.

From a sociological perspective it is clear to me that American society is not particularly health-promoting. For example, computers are increasingly promoting sedentary behavior, both at work and at play. A fast-paced society encourages us to seek convenient food and drink, and ubiquitous advertising—to the tune of tens of billions of dollars per year—promotes brand names over good nutrition. And the considerable stress engendered by a dynamic society leads to smoking, drinking excess alcohol, or engaging in other risky behaviors.

At the same time, however, we are becoming increasingly well educated on health matters, and eager to learn more from research findings that quickly reach Web sites, books, magazines, newspapers, and television programs. Primarily through public education we were able to reduce smoking rates in half between 1965 and 1990, and perhaps we can do the same with obesity and inactivity if we direct similar attention to these problems.

So while sociological truths are not to be denied, there is still considerable potential to empower individuals to live a healthy lifestyle. And while there is a vacuum of leadership created by a mostly hands-off federal government, there are an increasing number of local organizations taking the initiative in health promotion: religious institutions, businesses, community centers, hospitals, medical clinics, educational institutions, shopping malls, and city governments.

As we begin our journey in the new millennium, research is providing convincing evidence that health promotion works—no matter what our age and even after decades of practicing unhealthy habits. The findings are also providing specific ideas on what we need to do and how we ought to go about doing it. In some areas the strategies for improving health are a lot less onerous than we thought they had to be. For example, progressing from a sedentary lifestyle to brisk walking for up to a half hour most days of the week can do our health a world of good.

And even the dreadful piece of legislation enacted in 1994, the Dietary Supplement Health and Education Act, may have some value in spite of the plethora of worthless and sometimes harmful products that it now allows to be promoted over-the-counter with ridiculous claims, such as "reverses aging." Perhaps it is helping an American public become a bit more judicious in the evaluation of claims about what swallowing a pill can accomplish.

I would also like to note that the terms in the title of this book, *Health Promotion and Aging,* are not as straightforward as they might seem. Matters relating to health, for instance, are often dominated by medical issues. And it is not clear which terms are most salient to aging people: health promotion, disease prevention, management of chronic disease, health education, or other expressions.

And when does aging start: at the AARP eligible age of 50, the traditional retirement age of 65, or the eligibility age of 75 at some geriatric clinics? And how should we feel about the antiaging movement that urges us to defy or deny the aging process? This antiaging perspective has an appeal to many who have a vision of living vigorously and looking youthful for as long as possible. But what about us proagers who embrace the aging process, accept its deficits, and who creatively uncover its strengths?

The third edition of *Health Promotion and Aging* has several new or substantially revamped chapters, including the ones on health behavior, complementary and alternative medicine, mental health, diversity, and public health. It is focused on current research findings and practical applications. The content of the book is evidence-based and up-to-date, with 450 citations between the years 2000 and 2003.

This edition also includes detailed descriptions of two of my programs that have been recognized by the National Council on the Aging's Best Practices in Health Promotion and Aging: an exercise program in the community that includes aerobics, strength building, flexibility and balance, and health education; and a health contract/calendar to help older adults change health behaviors.

Much has happened since the second edition, many questions have been raised, and a good many questions have been answered, temporary though that may be. Perhaps the best way to preface this book is to select a few of those questions in each of the chapters.

Chapter 1—Introduction.   What are older adults doing and not doing in the way of health promotion? How can society reach its Healthy People 2010 objectives? What are several different ways to define healthy aging? Why do we call medical care, health care? Can we compress morbidity?

Chapter 2—Health Professionals and Older Clients.   Are health education materials effective? Which communication skills prevent lawsuits? How do you convert passive patients into empowered clients? Should you convert them? What are the best Web sites for health promotion and aging?

Chapter 3—Clinical Preventive Services.   Which 15 medical screenings should you know about? Why are mammograms, prostate cancer screening, and hormone replacement therapy so controversial? Should all older adults be on a statin? Who doesn't do immunizations, and why not? Medicare prevention: what is it, what should it be.

Chapter 4—Health Behavior.   How can you assess the health needs of older adults? What are 10 tips to get older adults to change a health behavior? Why is the author not excited about stages of change? Which health behavior theories are helpful?

Chapter 5—Exercise.   What is the latest research on exercise for preventing different types of diseases and improving function? Exactly what goes on in the author's exercise class? Where to exercise: home, health club, or religious setting? Is brisk walking enough?

Chapter 6—Nutrition.   How should the food guide pyramid be modified for older adults? Why is the personalized nutrition bull's-eye a better educational tool? How much should older adults know about the different kinds of fats? What are the latest cholesterol guidelines? What do we need to know about sugar and salt? Which is more of a problem for older adults, obesity or malnutrition? How could nutrition labeling be improved?

Chapter 7—Weight Management.   What is the major contributor to excess weight: genetics, lifestyle, or environment? What should we do, and what should society do about it? High protein/low carb diet: what does the research tell us? Should we gain weight with age? How should we measure body composition? Should churches promote weight loss?

Chapter 8—Complementary and Alternative Medicine.   Is CAM a crock? How prevalent is it? What is its relationship to medical education?

Which 12 CAM techniques do I describe? Which dietary supplements should older adults take? What is the story with vitamin E? What do older adults need to know about eight popular herbs?

Chapter 9—Other Health Education Topics.   Which older adults quit smoking? How well do we assess alcohol problems with older adults? What can health professionals and older adults do to reduce medication misuse? What can older adults do to prevent falls? When should older adults stop driving? Can pedestrian safety be improved? What can be done to improve sleep?

Chapter 10—Social Support.   How effective is pet support on mental health? Why are there two sides to the question of whether religious or spiritual support promotes health or extends longevity? What do you need to know about peer support? What is happening with hospice support?

Chapter 11—Mental Health.   What are the problems with identifying and treating depression? Can we improve cognitive fitness and stave off Alzheimer's? What are the insurance inequities with mental disorders? How do older adults deal with stress? Can we manipulate a positive attitude to extend longevity? How well do placebos work? Which mental health resources do older adults need to know about? Have you conducted a life review?

Chapter 12—Community Health.   What is going on in churches, hospitals, educational institutions, and shopping malls? Do you know about Healthwise, the Chronic Disease Self-Management Program, the Senior Wellness Project, the Ornish Program for Reversing Heart Disease, Community-Oriented Primary Care, and other model health promotion programs? What do you need to know about health professional associations, community volunteering, and health advocacy opportunities for older adults?

Chapter 13—Diversity.   Is it helpful to differentiate older adults by age? How does the aging of women differ from men? What do you need to know about racial and ethnic differences? Is socioeconomic status more important than race? What are the problems associated with rural aging? What can developed and developing countries learn from each other?

Chapter 14—Public Health.   How should we remake American society to promote healthy aging?

I have attempted to make the book practical by including health-promoting tools, resource lists, assessment tools, illustrations, checklists, and tables; thoughtful by raising issues in each chapter and posing additional questions at the end; and humorous because humor is essential to health promotion.

# Acknowledgments

I would like to thank the people who provided inspiration and support for my career in gerontology and health promotion: Jeanne St. Pierre, Stephen McConnell, Maggie Kuhn, Clavin Fields, Eugene Barone, David Chiriboga, and David Gobble.

# 1

# Introduction

D id you know that the federal government establishes goals for healthy aging? In 1990, for instance, the U.S. Public Health Service established the goal of increasing years of healthy life remaining at age 65 from the 11.8 years that it was in 1990, to 14 years by 2000. It turned out, however, that this goal for the decade was not met, though minority elders made substantially more progress than nonminority elders. Although healthy life remaining at age 65 had increased only .4 years, to 12.2 years, the data indicated an additional 1.3 years for Blacks and 1.8 years for Hispanics during this decade (From *Healthy People 2000 Final Review*, U.S. Public Health Service, 2000).

This, of course, raises the questions: How long has the federal government been doing this? Are they still doing it? Is it helping to promote healthy aging? For those readers who are impatient, the three answers are: about 25 years; yes; and, sorry, you will have to read on to find out about the third answer.

## HEALTHY PEOPLE INITIATIVES

In 1979, an influential document, *Healthy People: The Surgeon General's Report on Health Promotion and Disease Prevention*, was published (U.S. Department of Health and Human Services [USDHHS], 1979). Over the years, this report was widely cited by the popular media as well as in professional journals and at health conferences. Many attribute to it a seminal role in fostering health-promoting initiatives throughout the nation. It was followed by another report by the U.S. Public Health

Service in 1980, *Promoting Health/Preventing Disease: Objectives for the Nation,* which outlined 226 objectives for the nation to achieve over the following 10 years.

A decade later, in 1990, another national effort, Healthy People 2000, was initiated by the U.S. Public Health Service in an effort to reduce preventable death and disability for Americans by the year 2000. The Healthy People 2000 initiative focused on three broad public health goals for Americans: a) to increase the span of healthy life, b) to reduce health disparities, and c) to achieve access to preventive services.

In 2000, the Healthy People 2010 initiative was launched, with the number of objectives increased to 467, distributed over 28 priority areas. An interagency work group with the U.S. Department of Health and Human Services, however, pared this list to 10 leading health indicators (Table 1.1).

As you can observe, the table does not refer to an age-specific list of health indicators. Sexual irresponsibility and smoking, for instance, are much more prevalent problems among younger adults than among older adults. And access to health care is primarily an issue for younger persons without health insurance. Another limitation, unrelated to age, is that there are few federal funds earmarked specifically to accomplish improvement among these 10 health indicators.

On the positive side, setting health care priorities is no longer a simple matter of tabulating the number of deaths from a few diseases and then organizing a campaign against the most prevalent ones, like heart disease and cancer. The Healthy People Initiatives are health oriented, not disease oriented, and as such they recognize the complexity of the socioeconomic, lifestyle, and other nonmedical influences that impact our ability to attain and maintain health.

A second major benefit of the initiative is that they are focused on documenting baselines, setting objectives, and monitoring progress. According to the 1998-1999 Healthy People 2000 Progress Report (National Center for Health Statistics [NCHS], 1999), 15% of the objectives for the year 2000 were met, and 44% demonstrated movement toward the target. However, since the initiative relied mostly on data monitoring and a small amount of publicity—and very little financial support—it is unclear whether Healthy People 2000 contributed directly to this progress.

For example, in an area where there was no financial support for encouraging change—being overweight or obese—the trend in America for adults between the ages of 20 and 74 has been in the opposite direction. There has been a steady increase in weight gain for Americans over the decade (NCHS, 1999). There has been a similar result with sedentary

## TABLE 1.1   Healthy People 2010: Leading Health Indicators

1. Physical Activity
2. Overweight and Obesity
3. Tobacco Use
4. Substance Abuse
5. Responsible Sexual Behavior
6. Mental Health
7. Injury and Violence
8. Environmental Quality
9. Immunization
10. Access to Health Care

From "Healthy People 2010," U.S. Department of Health and Human Services. Healthy People 2010, January 2000, Volume I, Washington, DC, p. 24.

behavior among Americans. In the absence of financial support for encouraging change in this area, light to moderate physical activity on a near-daily basis between the ages of 18 and 74 has not improved over the decade (NCHS, 1999).

Focusing on those aged 65 and over, the Merck Institute on Aging & Health (go to www.miahonline.org) came out with a report card on the Healthy People 2000 Initiative and it revealed many failing grades. Older Americans did not reach the 2000 target goals, in fact fell far short of them, for physical activity, overweight, and eating fruits and vegetables. Additional failing grades were assigned to the target goals of reducing hip fractures for persons aged 65 and over, and fall-related deaths for persons aged 85 and over.

In contrast to the mere monitoring of *most* Healthy People 2000 target goals, financial assistance was provided to older adults through Medicare during the decade for mammogram coverage, pneumococcal vaccination, and influenza vaccination. With this financial support, the percentage of compliance in these three areas doubled among older adults during the decade (Haber, 2002a). Consequently, the Healthy People 2000 target goals were met for mammogram screening and influenza vaccination, and fell just short of being met for pneumococcal vaccination.

This raises the question of whether the federal government should be doing more than monitoring data changes when it comes to promoting healthy aging. A comparable question can be asked of state governments. The Healthy People initiatives are supposed to have a counterpart initiative at each of the state health departments. In my experience with several states, however, this initiative has been ignored or the state health department conducted a modest project that was accomplished several years ago, but did not follow-up with additional activity.

I will come back to this issue of whether the federal government should be doing more than monitoring data changes, in the last chapter of this book. In the meantime, to find out more about the Healthy People 2010 initiative, go to www.health.gov/healthypeople/state/toolkit. And, finally, back to the question "Does establishing goals help to promote healthy aging?" The answer is what you might expect: not if you are merely monitoring.

## SOCIODEMOGRAPHIC TRENDS

It has seemed almost obligatory to begin a gerontological article or book with comments about the rapid aging of society over the past quarter century. Around 1985, we began to see a slight variation of the ritual; many writings began with comments about the aging of the aged. About 10 years later, an additional spate of writings appeared on the coming onslaught of 50 year olds, i.e., the aging baby boomers born between 1946 and 1964.

Around the year 2005, when the vanguard of baby boomers contemplate becoming sexagenarians, both ends of the older age spectrum command our attention. The robust baby boomers-cum-gerontology boomers will make it obvious to all but the most ageist of younger persons that the vitality of the majority of aging persons remains strong. The stereotype of aging as a process synonymous with physical and mental deterioration will be tarnished even more.

At the other end of the age spectrum, among persons aged 85 and older, the growth in the percentage of the very old will continue to startle—about a 40% growth per decade. In 1980, there were 2.2 million Americans aged 85 and over; in 1990, 3 million; in 2000, 4.3 million; and in 2010, there will be 6 million.

Along with the increasing breadth of aging Americans comes increasing complexity. Fifty-year-olds are eligible for membership in AARP (formerly the American Association of Retired Persons), but they are quite different from 70-year-olds, who in turn are significantly different than 90-year-olds. Moreover, 90-year-olds are different from one another. A few of them are pumping iron and throwing away their canes (Fiatarone et al., 1990), while others are waiting to die.

What aging Americans have in common, be they 50 or 90, robust or frail, is a future with an intensified demand for medical care (euphemistically referred to in America as health care) and the ongoing escalation of medical care costs. Driving these demands and costs are the increasing numbers of aging persons with both chronic and acute medical conditions and an expensive, high-tech, acute care-oriented medical system.

As we entered the third millennium, this demand for costly and sophisticated medical care collided with an unpredictable federal budget. In less than 6 month's time during the year 2001, we went from a record-breaking and astoundingly huge budget surplus to budget deficits of uncertain duration—thanks to the one-two punch of legislation to launch a 10-year tax cut and the surging costs of a war on terrorism.

Matching the uncertainty of our economic future is our uncertainty over whether disease prevention and health promotion can help control the American public's voracious appetite for medical care. On an optimistic note, the media has allocated considerable time and space to the merits of promoting good health practices, including its potential for cost savings.

Joining the media are the federal and state governments, which have strongly endorsed disease prevention and health promotion; the health professions, which have proclaimed its importance in education and training; the business community, which has firmly supported it for employees; and individuals who often discuss their attempts at it, both successful and otherwise.

If disease prevention and health promotion have been vying for center stage in society, though, it has been the stage of a not very prosperous community theater. The federal government plays a limited role in disease prevention and will not subsidize health promotion. State governments have been more concerned about the expenditures that the federal government continues to pass along to them (welfare reform and antiterrorist measures among the more recent), rather than on new health initiatives that need funding.

Health professionals, too, have provided mostly lip service to health promotion because they have not been reimbursed for it. Health science students have received only a modicum of health promotion knowledge and skills, and infrequent experience in applying it (Haber & Looney, 2000; Haber et al., 2000, 1997). The business community has devoted resources to health promotion (often calling it worksite wellness) but has stopped short of focusing on the employees who need it most—older and more sedentary employees.

And last but not least, individuals have spent more time and money on health promotion. But they also have spent more time and money at restaurants, eating larger portions of food with higher fat content; and on computers, in front of which they have sat for an increasing number of hours.

Perhaps the disparity between the promise of health promotion and the attention shown it, and the allocation of inadequate resources toward supporting it, originates in the American value of individual responsibility. Unlike medicine, where we know we are not responsible for prescribing drugs or conducting surgery on ourselves and family members, we feel capable of walking briskly and eating healthfully—if we choose—without the necessity of experts, health programs, and taxpayer financial support. Thus, though most people are not doing as good a job as they would like at promoting their health, many believe it is up to the individual to take responsibility for it.

Individual responsibility is an important American value, but human beings are imperfect and need help. If that support can be provided by government, business, the media, the community, health professionals, religious institutions, family, and friends, we are going to do much better at promoting our own health and those of the people we love.

I hope the subsequent chapters of this book provide the reader with ample ideas and data on health promotion and aging to justify some degree of optimism and to inspire additional initiatives—from the individual level to all the major institutions of society, including family, work, government, religion, and education.

What follows are cautionary as well as hopeful sociodemographical data to suggest that aging adults may not only lead the way in escalating medical costs, but also have the potential to lead the way in the implementation of creative and cost-effective health promoting strategies. In this latter regard, the data reveal that the educational level of aging Americans has risen, that they are increasingly health-conscious, and that they are active in community health-promoting endeavors.

Much of the information in the next section is taken from summaries of data provided from the U.S. Bureau of the Census (www.census.gov), particularly the Administration on Aging's *A Profile of Older Americans: 2000*. The profile can be accessed through www.aoa.dhhs.gov/aoa/ stats/profile/default.htm. The National Center for Health Statistics has also provided data for this section through its *New Series of Reports to Monitor Health of Older Americans,* available through www.cdc.gov/nchs/releases/01facts/olderame.htm. Additional data were obtained from the National Council on the Aging's (2002) American's Perceptions of Aging in the 21st Century, accessible through www.ncoa.org.

## Population Growth Over Age 65

By now, all but the most uninformed know that the American population has been aging dramatically. Since 1900, the percentage of Americans aged 65 and over has more than tripled, from 4% in 1900 to about 13% in 2000, and the number has increased about 11-fold, from 3 million to almost 35 million. This trend will continue for several decades. Between 1995 and 2030, the number of people who are 65 and older is expected to more than double, from about 35 million to over 70 million, and the percentage to be almost doubled from 12% to 22%.

The figures in Table 1.2 show why the population "age pyramid"—a few older adults at the top and many children at the bottom—is rapidly becoming a population "age rectangle."

## The Baby Boomers

The baby boomers are the 76 million persons born between 1946 and 1964. Most were conceived when the millions of soldiers, sailors, and marines returned home from World War II and created a baby boom that started quickly—there were fewer than 2.8 million births in 1945, but more than 3.4 million in 1946—and lasted 18 years. The boomers challenged our hospital capacity when they were born, the school system a few years later, and society in general when they reached draft age and many did not agree with the politicians who wanted to expand the Vietnam War.

The baby boomer's impact as middle-aged persons is uncertain, despite their numbers. By the year 2010, the number of persons between ages 45 and 64 is projected to be twice that of those aged 65 and over: 79 million versus 39.4 million. Their influence on society, however, is not as clear as it will be when they become retirees.

As eloquently stated by Frank Whittington, director of Georgia State's Gerontology Center, (and I paraphrase): On January 2, 2008, shortly after 9 a.m., a simple bureaucratic event will harbinger a fundamental change in American society. Someone, probably a woman, will walk into the district office of the Social Security Administration and apply for retirement benefits. She will celebrate her 62nd birthday that day and will be the first baby boomer to apply for social security benefits. Over the next couple of decades over 70 million of her peers will follow suit. We must not doubt that when that woman strides up to the counter to ask for her benefits, all of our lives will begin to change.

When boomers retire they will make enormous demands on both the Social Security and Medicare programs, which, at the same time, will be

TABLE 1.2   Becoming an Age Rectangle

| Year | Under Age 18 | Over Age 65 |
|------|--------------|-------------|
| 1900 | 40% | 4% |
| 1980 | 28% | 11% |
| 2030 | 21% | 22% |

supported by a shrinking taxpaying workforce. By the time the last boomer turns 65 in the year 2029, the retirees drawing Social Security and Medicare benefits will include one in five Americans.

## THE OLDER OLD

The older population itself is getting older. The percentage of persons aged 85 and over is growing faster than any other age group. There was a 36% increase among Americans aged 85 and over from 1980 to 1990 (from 2.2 million to 3 million); a 43% increase from 1990 to 2000 (from 3 million to 4.3 million); and a 40% increase projected from 2000 to 2010 (from 4.3 million to 6 million). Every decade there is another 40% increase in the number of persons aged 85 and over.

This demographic trend is significant for two reasons. On the positive side, the rapid growth of this segment of the population converts this previously uncommon event into an increasingly likely stage of the life cycle. Moreover, the percentage of older adults aged 75 and over who report good health or better is 66%.

Experts believe that today's 70-year-old is more like the 60-year-old in previous generations (Trafford, 2000). Older adults have the same perception about themselves. The National Council on the Aging (2002) together with the Harris National Survey reported that 51% of persons between the ages of 65 and 74 and 33% of persons aged 75 and over perceive themselves as middle aged or younger! This certainly is evidence that many older adults are redefining old age as beginning later in the life cycle.

On the challenging side, for both individuals and society, is that the ability of this age group to function fully is significantly less than the younger old. Whereas only 6% of persons aged 65 to 69 reported difficulties with at least one activity of daily living task, 35% of persons aged 85-plus had such difficulties. Similarly, only 1% of persons aged 65 were residents of nursing homes, but 22% of persons aged 85-plus were residents. The older old person places more demands on family caregivers and societal resources.

## CHRONIC CONDITIONS AND DISABILITY

The leading chronic conditions among those aged 70-plus in 1996 were arthritis (58%), hypertension (45%), hearing impairments (30%), heart disease (21%), cataracts (17%), orthopedic impairments (16%), and diabetes (12%). The prevalence of each condition increases in old age, and many persons over age 80 have multiple chronic conditions and multiple physical impairments.

By age 65, approximately 14% have difficulty performing an activity of daily living (ADL) like bathing, transferring, dressing, toileting, or eating; or difficulty with walking. And about 21% have difficulty with an instrumental activity of daily living (IADL) like shopping, preparing meals, managing money, light housework, and getting around the community. By age 80-plus, however, the percentage having difficulty with ADLs (28%) and IADLs (40%) is double that of the younger old.

Although chronic conditions increase with age, disability rates for older Americans have been declining. In 1982, the disabled older population in the United States totaled 6.4 million. If the 1982 rate had continued, the number of disabled would have climbed to about 9.3 million in 1999. Instead, it rose to only 7 million—less than a quarter of the increase that might have been expected.

## CENTENARIANS

The world's oldest person in the year 2002, Maud Farris-Luse, turned 115 on January 21. As a centenarian, however, she had a lot of company. In the year 2002 there were more than 50,000 people aged 100 or older, an increase of 35% over the previous decade. Some census projections forecast as many as 1 million centenarians by the year 2050, when the baby boomers begin reaching age 100.

## HOSPITAL STAYS

In 1964 the average length of a hospital stay for an older patient was more than 12 days. By 1986 it was reduced to 8.5 days, and then to 6.5 days in 1996. Hospital expenses no longer account for the largest percentage of health expenditures for older persons, falling slightly behind medical/outpatient costs in 1996 (29% vs. 30%). In 1996, older adults accounted for 38% of all hospital stays, with persons aged 85 and over having twice the hospitalization rate of those between 65 and 74 years of age.

## VISITS TO HEALTH CARE PRACTITIONERS

In 1998, the average Medicare beneficiary visited or consulted with a physician 13 times during the year (Federal Interagency Forum on Aging-Related Statistics, 2000). It is estimated that older patients occupy almost 50% of the time of health care practitioners, and it is predicted that the percentage of time that health care practitioners will spend with older patients will continue to increase.

## MEDICATIONS

In 1995, older adults constituted 12% of the population but consumed 32% of all prescription drugs and 40% of over-the-counter drugs. Added to the frequency of drug consumption among older adults has been the burden of rising prescription drug expenditures over the past several years. The growth in prescription drug expenditures has been double-digit every year from 1994 to 2001. The growth reached an astonishing 19.7% in 1999, though it declined some in 2000 (16.4%) and 2001 (15.7%) as employers raised copayments.

By 2001, prescription drugs accounted for 9.9% of all health expenditures, due to higher-priced new drugs, advertising of prescription drugs on television, and an increase in the number of prescriptions written by physicians.

## HEALTH HABITS

On the brighter side, the health habits of older adults may, on balance, be slightly superior to those of younger adults. People aged 65 and over, for instance, are less likely to smoke, drink alcohol, be obese, or report high stress. They eat more sensibly than do younger adults, are as likely to walk for exercise, and are more likely to check their blood pressure regularly. Older adults over the past decade improved their participation in medical screenings and immunizations, and adults in general increased their seat belt use (D. Nelson et al., 2002).

## PERCEPTIONS OF HEALTH

Most people who are elderly tend to view their health positively. Seventy-six percent of the younger old, aged 65 to 74, rate their health as being good, very good, or excellent. Among those aged 75 and over, 66% report good, very good, or excellent health. This percentage declines to

56% among older adults 65 and over without a high school diploma, and to 52% among minorities who are aged 75 and older.

## VOLUNTEERING AND WORK

Many older adults are active and productive, choosing to engage in volunteer opportunities and work. In any given year, almost one out of every five older Americans engage in unpaid volunteer work for organizations like churches, schools, or civic organizations. In addition, an unknown additional percentage of older adults do other types of volunteer work, like helping the sick or disabled, or helping out with grandchildren.

Surprisingly, those who continue to work after age 65 are *not* less likely to volunteer than those older adults who retire (Caro & Morris, 2001). Researchers believe that the potential for increasing volunteerism among retired older adults is significant, and that "in the period immediately after retirement there is a heightened receptivity to volunteerism" (Caro & Morris, 2001, p. 349).

Participation in the labor force after age 65 rose in the United States between 1995 and 2000. In 2000, 19% of older adults were in the labor force, the highest percentage since 1979. Labor force participation is also higher in the United States than in most other countries (e.g., France, Germany, Italy, Sweden, United Kingdom, and Canada; although it is considerably lower than the rate in Japan—36% for men and 16% for women).

Labor force participation among older persons is expected to climb higher in the coming years, thanks to the bear market and weak economy that took hold in 2001. Labor force participation by workers aged 55 to 64 jumped 2% in 2002, an unprecedented increase in post-World War II economic history. And a study by AARP reported that 70% of workers ages 45 and older plan to work in some capacity in their retirement years, primarily due to economic reasons.

## EDUCATIONAL STATUS

Between 1960 and 1989, the median level of education among older adults increased from 8.3 to 12.1 years. Between 1970 and 2000, the percentage of older adults who had completed high school rose from 28% to 70%.

By the year 2000, the median number of years of education of people who had reached age 65 was equivalent to that of all adults age 25 and over (almost 13 years). However, the percentage who had completed high school varied considerably by race and ethnic origin among older persons in 2000: 74% of Whites, 63% of Asians and Pacific Islanders, 46% of Blacks, and 37% of Hispanics.

About 16% of older adults in 2000 had a bachelor's degree or more. As the formal educational level of older adults continues to rise, this may well correlate with an increase in their interest in seeking out health information and engaging in health-promoting activities in their communities.

## POLITICAL POWER

The Federal Election Commission reports that older adults are disproportionately likely to vote. Moreover, the percentage of voting elders has increased over the past 20 years. In 1978, older adults generated 19% of all votes cast; in 1986, 21%; and in 1998, 23%. Yet older adults in 1998 constituted only 13% of the population.

## INTERNET ACCESS

Half of American households had a computer in 2000, about twice the percentage of households of persons aged 65 or older. Internet access was 42% in general, versus 18% in households of persons aged 65 or older. These percentage differences between younger and older adults, however, are expected to close rapidly in the coming years.

## POVERTY

The poverty rate among older persons continued to fall slightly in 2000. About 3.4 million, or 10.2%, of older adults were below the poverty level in 2000, slightly less than the 11.4% rate for persons aged 18 to 64. Another 2.2 million, or 7%, were near-poor (up to 125% of poverty level), resulting in 17% of the older population's being poor or near-poor in 2000. The major source of income for older persons was Social Security (42%), public and private pensions (19%), earnings (18%), asset income (18%), and other (3%).

The poverty rate was almost three times higher for older Blacks and Hispanics than for older Whites, and more than twice as high for older women than older men.

## RACIAL AND ETHNIC COMPOSITION

In 2000, 16% of persons aged 65 and over were either African American (8%), Hispanic (6%), Asian or Pacific Islander (2%) and American Indian or Native Alaskan (less than 1%). Minority populations are projected to increase to 25% of the older adult population in the year 2030, and to 36% in the year 2050. Between 1990 and 2030, older Whites are projected to increase 91%, older Blacks 159% and older Hispanics 570%.

# DEFINITIONS OF HEALTHY AGING

## THE FEDERAL GOVERNMENT

Through its 1990 Health Objectives for the Nation, the federal government's Public Health Service encouraged a broad, and rather dry, definition of health. It included the following three components:

1. Disease prevention, which comprises strategies to maintain and to improve health through medical care, such as high blood pressure control and immunization.
2. Health protection, which includes strategies for modifying environmental and social structural health risks, such as toxic agent and radiation control, and accident prevention and injury control.
3. Health promotion, which includes strategies for reducing lifestyle risk factors, such as avoiding smoking and the misuse of alcohol and drugs, and adopting good nutritional habits and a proper and adequate exercise regimen.

## EXTRAORDINARY ACCOMPLISHMENT

The definition of healthy aging can be reframed substantially by viewing it from the unique perspective of extraordinary accomplishment. At age 99, Mieczyslaw Horszowski, a classical pianist, recorded a new album, and twin sisters Kin Narita and Gin Kanie recorded a hit single in Japan; at age 92, Paul Spangler completed his 14th marathon and Hulda Crooks, 91, climbed Mount Whitney, the highest mountain in the continental United States (Wallechinsky & Wallace, 1993). At 77, John Glenn completed rigorous physical preparation to become the oldest space traveler in history.

At age 61, a California woman named Arceli Keh lied about her age (she said she was 51) in order to become eligible for a fertility program where she was implanted with an embryo from an anonymous donor. In 1996, at age 63, she became the oldest woman on record to have a baby. Another 63-year-old climbed one of the Himalayan peaks in 1998, a peak that only the most elite alpinists can ascend (Kinoshita et al., 2000).

While I marvel at these examples of unusual achievement by aging adults, I do not use them as inspiration for older, or even younger, persons. These models are astonishing, but they do little to enhance the confidence of aging adults who do not believe they can—and oftentimes do not want to—come close to similar achievement.

As Betty Friedan (1993) noted in her book *The Fountain of Age*, older adults "attempt to hold on to, or judge oneself by, youthful parameters of love, work and power. For this is what blinds us to the new strengths and possibilities emerging in ourselves."

Perhaps health professionals should be more cautious about defining good health for older adults. This is the message delivered by Faith Fitzgerald, MD, in an editorial in *The New England Journal of Medicine* (Fitzgerald, 1994). "We must beware of developing a zealotry about health, in which we take ourselves too seriously and believe that we know enough to dictate human behavior, penalize people for disagreeing with us, and even deny people charity, empathy, and understanding because they act in a way of which we disapprove. Perhaps (we need to) debate more openly the definition of health" (pp. 197–198).

## PREVENTION

Prevention is often categorized as primary, secondary, or tertiary (Figure 1.1). Primary prevention focuses on an asymptomatic individual in whom potential risk factors have been identified and targeted. Primary preventive measures, such as regular exercise, good nutrition, smoking cessation, or immunizations, are recommended to decrease the probability of the onset of specific diseases or dysfunction. Primary prevention is different than the term *health promotion* in that it is less wide-ranging in scope and tends to be used by clinicians in a medical setting.

Secondary prevention is practiced when an individual is asymptomatic but actual (rather than potential) risk factors have been identified at a time when the underlying disease is not clinically apparent. A medical screening as an example of secondary prevention is only cost-effective when there is hope of lessening the severity or shortening the duration of a pathological process. Blood pressure screenings, cholesterol screenings, and peripheral bone densitometry at community health fairs have become the most widely implemented forms of secondary prevention.

Tertiary prevention, which takes place after a disease or disability becomes symptomatic, focuses on the rehabilitation or maintenance of

| | | |
|---|---|---|
| No Disease | Preclinical or Asymptomatic Disease | Symptomatic Disease |
| \| | \| | \| |
| Primary Prevention | Secondary Prevention | Tertiary Prevention |

FIGURE 1.1   Three levels of prevention.

function. Health professionals attempt to restore or maintain the maximum level of functioning possible, within the constraints of a medical problem, to prevent further disability and dependency on others.

Tertiary prevention corresponds to phase 2 (rehabilitation of outpatients) and phase 3 (long-term maintenance) of the cardiac rehabilitation of a cardiac patient (phase 1 is the care of a hospitalized cardiac patient). A study of 10 randomized clinical trials involving more than 4,000 patients who had myocardial infarctions revealed that patients who completed a program of tertiary prevention reduced their likelihood of cardiovascular mortality by 25% (Oldridge et al., 1988).

A focus on prevention may be more appealing to some older adults than an emphasis on health promotion. Older adults are likely to be coping with chronic conditions, and the prevention, delay, or reduction of disability and dependency is a much more salient issue for them than it is for most younger adults.

Moreover, among medical professionals the relevancy of the term *prevention* is enhanced, because several prevention activities, like mammograms, are reimbursable through Medicare. Prevention has gotten its foot in the door, so to speak, in the system of health care reimbursement, whereas the activities of health promotion have not.

One advantage of the use of the term *health promotion,* however, is that it encompasses mental and spiritual health concerns. Instead of clients and health professionals becoming fixated on risk factors and the prevention of disease or disability, health promotion or wellness can be viewed as an affirming, even joyful, process. As health professionals who promote health, for instance, we can encourage the joy of bird-watching to an older client and not concern ourselves with its ability to prevent disease or illness.

*Health promotion* is also a more proactive term than *primary prevention,* which tends to imply a reaction to the prospect of disease. Directing a client's anger or frustration into political advocacy work, for example, is a proactive, health promoting enterprise that benefits both the individual and society.

In one (admittedly dated) health study, however, in-depth interviews with older adults who declined to participate in a health promotion study, reported that they were less familiar and comfortable with the phrase *health promotion* than were those who eventually participated (Wagner et al., 1991). The research topic of assessing older adults' attitudes toward different health terms remains largely unexamined, and this ignorance can reduce our effectiveness as health educators.

## WELLNESS

Although the term *wellness* has had many supporters in the health professions over the past 25 years (Jonas, 2000), particularly among persons who conduct health programs at large U.S. corporations (Jacob, 2002), it tends to be embraced less than the terms *health promotion* and *disease prevention*. Nonetheless, wellness conveys an important message—that good health is more than physical well-being. In fact, seven dimensions are usually touted among wellness advocates, as shown in Table 1.3.

Wellness is a welcome and important reminder about the breadth of health promotion that is missing from most other terms. The only limitation to the term *wellness* is that it tends to be identified with the more alternative activities—acupuncture, homeopathy, spiritual healing, aroma therapy—to the exclusion of more mainstream activities like exercise and nutrition. Thus, it conveys flakiness to some.

## ANTI-OLD, ANTI-AGING

Who is healthier: An old person or an older person? Is this a preposterous question? Maybe not. Do the terms *old* and *older* reflect our prejudices? One of the leaders in the field of gerontological language, Erdman Palmore, thinks so. Palmore suggests that most of the synonyms for *old* are unhealthy in some way, words like debilitated, infirm, and frail. An *older person*, on the other hand, is a more neutral term; and perhaps the term *elder* connotes an even healthier role for older persons in society (Palmore, 2000).

And yet I am reminded of a conversation I once had with Maggie Kuhn, the founder of the advocacy organization, the Gray Panthers. She reported on an exchange that she had with a senator when giving testimony in Washington, DC. When she completed her testimony, the senator thanked the *young lady* for her contribution. Maggie replied that she was an *old* woman and proud to have earned that label.

## TABLE 1.3 Seven Dimensions of Wellness

Physical—Exercise, eat a well balanced diet, get enough sleep, protect yourself.

Emotional—Express a wide range of feelings, acknowledge stress, channel positive energy.

Intellectual—Embrace lifelong learning, discover new skills and interests.

Vocational—Do something you love, balance work with leisure time.

Social—Laugh often, spend time with friends/family, join a club, respect cultural differences.

Environmental—Recycle daily, use energy-efficient products, walk or bike, grow a garden.

Spiritual—Seek meaning and purpose, take time to reflect, connect with the universe.

A related concern is the anti-aging movement that has greeted the new millennium. Proponents of anti-aging are referring to the goal of combating the signs of aging. Anti-agers deliver a strong message that aging itself is an unhealthy process that needs to be contested.

I think, however, that we need a "pro-aging movement," one that emphasizes the healthy aspects of aging. No longer needing to impress employers, in-laws, or peers, older adults are free to be themselves. The old not only have an opportunity to be freer, but wiser, more conscious of the present, and more willing to be an advocate for a healthy future. Maggie Kuhn certainly lived a pro-aging lifestyle.

### COMPRESSION OF MORBIDITY

"Although there is little hope for cure of chronic diseases through the traditional medical model, the onset of these diseases may be postponed through modification of risk factors, many of which are possible to control, either personally or socially. As the onset is delayed to older ages and approaches the limit of the human life span, we can envision a society where everyone can expect to live in vigorous health to close to the average life span and then die after a brief period of illness" (Fries & Crapo, 1986).

The prospect of living almost two more decades after reaching one's 65th birthday is bittersweet. Though Americans are living longer today than ever before, we have greater fear of a prolonged period of disability and dependency in late life.

One definition of healthy aging, then, is to be able to live life fully until death. According to one national study, however, only 14% of those who have died after age 64 were fully functional in the last year of their life (Lentzner et al., 1992). Unfortunately, the study did not identify the number of older adults who, despite the fact that they were not fully functional in the last year of life, lived vital and fulfilling lives during that year.

Most of us are greatly concerned with the probability of being severely restricted for a long period in late life. The evidence is not encouraging in this regard, in that the longer we live, the more likely we are to endure a prolonged period of disability prior to our death. Death after age 85 is almost 4 times more likely to follow a period of profound physical impairment than is death between the ages of 65 and 74 (Lentzner et al., 1992).

Examining the length of the dependency period prior to death, at age 65 we have about 17 years left to live, with 6.5 of those years in a dependent state (38% of our remaining years). Also, less than 6% are receiving help in the basic activities of daily living between the ages of 65 and 74. In contrast, at age 85 we have an average of 7 years left to live, with 4.4 years in a dependent state (63% of our remaining years). At age 85, more than one in four are receiving help in the basic activities of daily living (Guralnik, 1991).

Pessimists argue that the period of morbidity preceding death will increase in the future due to: a) limited biomedical research funds available to improve the physical and mental capacity of the very old; b) the fact that some major diseases, such as Alzheimer's, do not have recognized lifestyle risk factors that we can modify; and c) medical advances, such as dialysis and bypass surgery, that will increase the life expectancy of individuals with disease rather than prevent the occurrence of disease.

Optimists, on the other hand, argue that there will be a *compression of morbidity* (see Figure 1.2) in the future due to: a) probable advances in biomedical research that will prevent or delay the occurrence of disease, and b) the continued potential for reducing risk factors such as smoking, blood pressure level, poor nutritional habits, and sedentary lifestyles that will result in better health.

At the same time that the general population will be able to delay the onset of chronic disease due to these factors, the life *span* (the maximum number of years of the species) is fixed. Thus, argue the compressionists, we will not only delay morbidity, but we will also shorten it.

Studies by Manton and colleagues (C. Connolly, 2001; Kolata, 1996; Manton et al., 1998; 1993) analyzed data from the 1982 to 1999 National

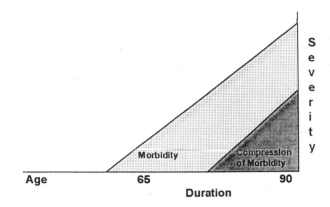

FIGURE 1.2   Compression of morbidity (CoM).

Long Term Care Surveys, a Federal study that regularly surveys almost 20,000 people aged 65 and older. The researchers arrived at the unexpected conclusion that the percentage of chronically disabled older persons—impairments for 3 months or longer that impede daily activities—has been slowly falling. Whereas 25% of people over age 65 reported chronic disability in 1982, only 21% reported this to be the case in 1994 (Manton et al., 1997). Also surprising was the increasing percentage during this time period of those over age 65 reporting no disabilities.

These unexpected findings still need further examination, especially as to whether they are linked more to initiatives in health promotion and disease prevention, such as improvements in diet, exercise, nonsmoking, and other lifestyle factors; or to medical access and advances, such as treatment for arthritis and cataracts; or to increased use of devices, such as canes, walkers, walk-in showers, support rails, and handicapped accessible facilities; or to societal improvements, such as the increase in educational and income levels.

## HEALTH PERSPECTIVES AND AGING

### HEALTH EXPECTANCY VERSUS LIFE EXPECTANCY

Those who live to the age of 65 are likely to live into their 80s. Of the remaining average of 17 years to live after age 65, 12 are likely to be healthy and 5 will be years in which there is some functional impairment (NCHS, 1990a).

Place yourself in the shoes of the person who has just reached age 65. Are you primarily interested in extending your life for more than the 17 years you are likely to live, or are you most interested in how many of your remaining years will be healthy and independent ones?

Your health expectancy, or the number of healthy years you can expect to have left, depends to a great extent on your physical activity, nutritional intake, social support network, access to good medical care, health education, and health services. Health expectancy is more important to older adults than life expectancy (see Table 1.4).

## PHYSICAL VERSUS EMOTIONAL ASPECTS OF AGING

There is a strong reciprocal relationship between the physical and emotional aspects of health. When our physical health is threatened, so typically is our emotional health. The converse is equally true.

As we age, however, it may be the case that good health is less dependent on physical status than on emotional status. One study reported on shifting perspectives of health over time, with older participants expecting physical health problems because of their age and discounting them somewhat because of this expectation (Keller et al., 1989). A study of 85-year-olds living in the Netherlands reported that physical function was not the most important component of successful aging. These older adults were able to adapt successfully to physical limitations. The researchers reported social contacts as the most important factor in well-being, and the quality of the contacts was more important than the number (Von Faber et al., 2001).

Another study of 32 elderly Catholic nuns generated, through open-ended interviews, more than 100 characteristics of health that were important to older adults besides physical health, including the ability to enjoy life and good personal relationships (Huck & Armer, 1995). An examination of multiple studies on declining physical health with age, reported that many older adults who are frail and sometimes disabled did *not* evaluate their health or life negatively (Pinquart, 2001).

Most health professionals subscribe to the notion that health is more than the absence of illness. Were this not the case, they would have to label the vast majority of older adults, 90% of whom are coping with a chronic condition, unhealthy. The chronic diseases that older persons contend with do not necessarily relate to their ability to perform daily activities. Disease, in fact, may not be evident even to the person who has it.

The presence or absence of disease, therefore, may not be a source of great concern to older adults. The ability to perform activities of daily living, however, is of great concern to older adults who desire as much

**TABLE 1.4   Healthy People 2000 Goal**

| |
| --- |
| Healthy People 2000 Goal to increase years of healthy life remaining at age 65 to 14 was not met |
| 1990    11.8 years of healthy life remaining at age 65 |
| 2000    12.2 years of healthy life remaining at age 65 |

independence as possible (M. Duffy & MacDonald, 1990). The definition of health, especially among older adults, should not be linked with disease or its absence, as the medical model suggests, but with independence, the ability to accomplish one's goals, and the existence of satisfying relationships.

A health perspective that emphasizes the psychological status of older adults does not view health as a continuum ranging from physical disability and illness at one end, with a neutral point in the middle where there is no discernible illness or wellness, to a high level of wellness at the other (Kemper et al., 1987; Sarafino, 1990). Critics of this type of health continuum argue that even a person who is functionally impaired or disabled and residing at one end of the alleged continuum can focus considerable attention on a high level of wellness, devoting energy to health awareness, health education, and psychological growth.

Finally, health professionals need to walk a fine line with older clients. On the one hand, they have been accused of ignoring some of the physical needs of older adults and discounting the viability of subsequent medical interventions due to the age of their clients (Ebrahim, 2002). On the other hand, they can fixate on the reimbursable medical needs of older clients and ignore the opportunity to alleviate the emotional deterioration that often accompanies chronic illness.

# HEALTH CARE COSTS

## MEDICARE

Medicare was enacted in 1965 to help persons aged 65 or older pay for medical care. In 2002, Medicare covered 35 million older adults and 5 million younger persons who were disabled. Medicare is a major payer in the United States health care system, spending 238 billion dollars in 2001 and accounting for 38% of public spending on health care.

Medicare Part A is referred to as hospital insurance and most people do not have to pay a monthly premium because they are eligible through the Medicare taxes they paid while they were working. Part A includes

remainder) (McGinnis et al., 2002). Paradoxically, however, the behavioral, social, and environmental components of health care have not constituted a high priority for the health care dollar. In fact, only about 3% of the nation's health care costs were spent on health-promoting and disease-preventing activities.

Most of that 3% goes either to the physician's office or other clinical settings for preventive measures, such as medical screenings and vaccinations (about 35%), or to health protection in the physical environment, such as toxic agent and radiation control (about 30%) (*American Medical News*, 1992a). And only a portion of the remainder is spent on changing unhealthy behaviors.

Although there has been undeniable financial neglect at the federal level for decreasing unhealthy lifestyles among the American people, increasing public attention has been focused on this problem area ever since the publication of the landmark document, *Healthy People: The Surgeon General's Report on Health Promotion and Disease Prevention* (USDHHS, 1979). This report provided considerable credence for the idea that major gains in health and independence in the future are likely to come from personal lifestyle changes.

Dr. John Rowe, director of the MacArthur Foundation's Consortium on Successful Aging, also concluded that our vigor and health in old age is mostly a matter of managing how we live (Brody, 1996). Supporting this contention is a widely cited article in the *Journal of the American Medical Association* (McGinnis & Foege, 1993) that suggested we no longer should view death as being due to heart disease, cancer, stroke, and COPD, but rather due to tobacco, inactivity, diet, alcohol, microbial and toxic agents, sexual behavior, motor vehicles, and illicit or inappropriate use of drugs.

## A HEALTH PROMOTION AND AGING MODEL

Practitioners in the community or clinic who want to promote the health of older clients are limited by time, resources, reimbursement, and training. Although these issues are addressed elsewhere in this book, a succinct conceptual framework for promoting the health of older adults is not. The main components of a model of health promotion and aging might be useful for the training of health professionals (Haber, 2001b, 1996, 1993a, 1992c; Haber et al., 2000, 1997; Haber & Lacy, 1993), and are presented next.

## THE AGING COMPONENT

I criticized the Healthy People 2010 leading health indicators because they were not age-specific. And yet I must confess that the content of this book, *Health Promotion and Aging*, frequently lacks specificity when it comes to aging. Younger and older age segments of the second half of life have little in common. Yet each end of this age continuum is becoming increasingly important to practitioners, educators, and policymakers in the coming years.

The young-old are in their 50s and 60s, people who in all likelihood are not enthusiastic about an oxymoronic label that includes the dreaded term *old*. Nonetheless, the cutting edge of the baby boomers turned 55 years of age on January 1, 2001, with another boomer being added to the ranks every 8 seconds until about the year 2010. And just as the boomers were hard to ignore as babies, and later as Vietnam War protesters, they will be hard to ignore as adults who are eligible for AARP.

People in their 50s and 60s are not old in the sense of physical vitality, mental acuity, or occupational productivity. But none have escaped diminished hearing and vision; few have overlooked the fact that more of their life is behind them than ahead; and most have given considerable thought to their retirement years.

It is during these years that the incidence of major chronic conditions such as arthritis, hypertension, and obesity rises significantly. At the same time, more than 4 million Americans between the ages of 50 and 64 are without health insurance. These persons are too young for Medicare, not poor enough for Medicaid, and not very well protected by the Age Discrimination in Employment Act.

Given the substantial number of years remaining to persons in this age group, and the potential to defer or prevent chronic impairments, it is imperative that a health promotion and aging model follow the lead of AARP and begin to target the aging baby boomers.

The *old-old* are persons age 85 and above (for an interesting essay on the "dwindling years," see Sandock, 2000). Probably half of them are physically frail, mentally diminished, or societally disengaged. These older adults have a challenging and diverse set of problems to solve in order to remain independent. At the same time, their problems are likely to be costly to resolve and bedeviling to solve for future cohorts of politicians. In this era of cutting government budgets, how do you provide home care support that is preferred by most frail old-old, programs to strengthen muscles that are in danger of becoming too weak to maintain independence, and prescription medications that are costly but vital for maximizing functional ability?

On the bright side, some of the nonagenarians are pumping iron for the first time. And the potential to strengthen the old-old, to keep them independent in a home setting, to engage them in society, has never been more promising. This potential for improvement continues through the dying process, when the ability to die in comfort with family and friends visiting in a home environment is also, thanks to the hospice movement, more probable as well.

## COMMUNICATION AND COLLABORATION

Two fundamental assertions within this health promotion and aging model is that it is better for older adults to collaborate with health professionals than to take a passive, compliant (or, equally likely, noncompliant) role; and it is also better to collaborate than to engage in health-promoting activities on one's own.

These assertions are based on two facts: a) that most older adults have medical conditions that require professional supervision, and health-promoting activities can affect these medical conditions, and b) that health professionals who keep up with the health promotion field can make vital contributions to the health-promoting efforts of older adults.

Effective communication between clients and health professionals is an essential component of collaboration, and can lead to better results and more satisfied clients and health professionals.

## HEALTH BEHAVIOR CHANGE

Health assessments help determine where best to focus limited time, energy, and resources. Crucial to this process is selecting the area that the individual (or the collective—ranging from group to state) is most ready to change. It is the rare or mythical person who is attentive to every periodic medical screening and who strives constantly to improve every aspect of a healthy lifestyle. It is more realistic to set a health priority or a set of priorities and devote energy and time to it or them.

Assessments lead to interventions, and interventions should focus on goals that are modest and measurable in order to increase the likelihood of success. Attention must also be paid to the important components of the intervention, such as building and maintaining motivation, establishing the new behavior as a habit, garnering social support, setting the health goal for a short period of time on the way to more ambitious longer-term goals, and problem-solving around the barriers that have prevented success in the past and might be anticipated to arise in the future.

Social cognitive theory underlies assessments and interventions, and suggest social, behavioral, and psychological management techniques for health behavior change. Regarding social support, the most likely sources come from family members, friends, neighbors, and peers. Peer support can be found in community health education programs, intervention programs, and mutual help groups. The medical profession is also a potential source of social support, but because it tends to slight behavioral, psychological, and social interventions, it is underutilized. Regarding behavioral techniques, common strategies include health contracting, self-monitoring, stimulus control, and response substitution. Widespread psychological techniques include stress management and cognitive restructuring.

It is important to learn multiple social, behavioral, and psychological techniques in order to address the unique and multifaceted needs of older adults.

## HEALTH EDUCATION

Health education has advanced considerably beyond the idea that knowledge inspires change. First, given the plethora of information that pours out of the media, bookstores, libraries, and the mouths of experts, it is difficult for individuals to sort out accurate, up-to-date information that is pertinent to their particular health needs.

Second, older adults learn best in andragogical (adult-oriented learning) situations in which new ideas are presented through collaborative relationships, and in small participative groups where they have control over the learning and maintenance process.

Third, education by itself is often insufficient to inspire behavior change. It is far more effective to add behavior and psychological management techniques to the transmission of knowledge, as well as to infuse the educational process with social support.

## DIVERSITY

Unique problems emerge from diversity: a) Asian American elders who become the first generation of their ethnicity to be placed in American nursing homes by their baby-boomer children; b) older women who have inadequate retirement incomes because they spent many years in unpaid caregiving roles; c) rural elders who do not have access to nearby hospitals or health professionals. What do we gain by focusing on the diversity of aging within America, as well as from the study of global aging? At minimum, more sensitivity to the disparate ways we age. At best, innovative strategies for improving the quality of life as we age.

## COMMUNITY HEALTH

Health professionals have limited time, knowledge, and skills with which to help their older clients. It is vital, therefore, that older adults and health professionals be as informed as possible about the community health options that are available to them. These options are proliferating at a variety of community sites, such as religious institutions, medical clinics, businesses, hospitals, educational institutions, community centers, shopping malls, government agencies, professional associations, and non-profit agencies.

Health professionals need to visit these sites, as well as get feedback from clients who visit them, in order to make more effective referrals in the future.

## ADVOCACY

Community health programs cannot meet all the health needs that are not met by the health care system. In recent years, in fact, health care inflation has started to soar again, forcing medical administrators to make tough decisions about limiting the availability of health professionals and other resources. Until utopia comes to America, the health care system will never work for meeting the health needs of all the people, all of the time.

The health care system can be improved, however, and oftentimes through advocacy. By dramatizing their particular plight to community leaders, media representatives, and state and federal legislators, older adults can be effective change agents in ways that health professionals cannot. When health professionals mobilize their clients to political or community action, they may not only help to bring about a more responsive health care system for their clients, but also for themselves. Health professionals can also advocate for change by joining professional organizations and advocacy groups, reaching out to Congress, writing articles, and appearing on the media.

# QUESTIONS FOR DISCUSSION

1. Is it necessary to support the claim that health promotion and disease prevention *save medical dollars* in order to obtain financial

support for such activities from our federal and state governments and through insurance reimbursement? Present a brief argument supporting a positive response, and then a negative response.

2. Are you optimistic or pessimistic about the occurrence of a compression of morbidity? Explain your reasoning.
3. In two or three paragraphs, what is *your* definition of health?
4. Why do we call medical care "health care"?
5. What are two or three of the most important changes that are needed to convert our medical care system into a health care system? How do we make these changes?
6. What do you think is the most important health objective that should be set for older adults for the Healthy People 2010 initiative, and what should federal and state governments do to help?
7. What can both health professionals and laypersons in your community do to help achieve the objective you set in the previous question?
8. If you were writing a book on aging and health promotion, which age range would you cover: 50-plus, 65-plus, 80-plus, all ages, or something else? Justify your answer.

# 2

# Health Professionals and Older Clients

*The art of medicine consists of amusing the patient while nature cures the disease.*

*—Voltaire, French physician and author*

Voltaire knew that most medical conditions are self-limiting, and that benignly amusing the patient is oftentimes all that is needed. Other than for, perhaps, a unique problem with stress management, benign amusement is not enough help to provide older clients who want to collaborate with health professionals on health promotion or disease prevention goals.

## COLLABORATION

"Suffering" is an appropriate adjective for many patients. In fact, the term *patient* is derived from a Latin word meaning "to suffer." Patients, however, are also associated with another adjective—passive. And passivity is no longer appropriate for patients.

Passive patients comply with the decisions of health professionals. When it comes to managing chronic conditions or engaging in health promotion or prevention, aging persons are better off participating in the decision-making process and becoming collaborative clients rather than compliant patients. For this reason, I prefer to use the term *client* in this book, though on occasion I use the term *patient* when it is more relevant for the context.

In order to collaborate, clients must understand the choices available to them. These choices may be profound, such as deciding whether to combine chemotherapy with visualization techniques; or mundane, such as helping to decide on the timing of a treatment plan. Research has shown that client participation, even in mundane choices such as the timing of chemotherapy treatment, can result in fewer side effects (Spiegel & Bloom, 1983).

Similarly, nursing home residents receive health benefits when encouraged to make choices about their environment. Residents who make decisions become more sociable, show improvement in their mental health, and even live longer than do residents who adopt a passive lifestyle in an institutional setting (Rodin & Langer, 1977).

Another example of the benefits of participating in decision-making is demonstrated by clients who improve compliance with their drug regimen after participating in the choice of medication. Clients may make this choice knowing that they are able to live more easily with the side effects of one medication in comparison to another (Lorig, 1992). Or, clients who take multiple medicines may choose a less challenging medication schedule because they know that compliance will improve in a lifestyle that is already characterized by a busy calendar and a faulty memory.

In contrast, many medical decisions are made as a consequence of physician priority rather than client preference. For example, the selection of the best treatment for prostate cancer—surgery or radiation—is controversial. The choice, however, usually depends on whether a patient visits a urologic surgeon or a radiation oncologist. Surgery is also less likely for benign prostate enlargement if physicians involve patients in the decision-making process by educating them about the options ("Controversial Cases," 2002).

## WILLINGNESS TO COLLABORATE

In a 1992 national survey by the Gallup organization, 63% of the 1,514 randomly selected adults reported that doctors did not involve patients enough in treatment decisions (*American Medical News*, June 1, 1992, p. 16). A survey sponsored by the American Board of Family Practice (1987) reported that earlier cohorts of older persons have been less likely to take an active role in the professional-client relationship, but present and future cohorts of older adults have significantly higher educational levels than do their predecessors. Educational levels correlate with client willingness to collaborate with a health professional.

Even older adults with less formal education, however, are more likely than previous cohorts of older adults to encounter health information from television, radio, newspapers, and magazines. This type of informal health education, which prevails today, also correlates with client willingness to collaborate with a health professional.

Nonetheless, clients differ significantly in the degree to which they want to collaborate in an active way in a health care encounter. Some clients want to give up responsibility to the practitioner; others want an active part in the decision-making process (Haug & Lavin, 1981). These two perspectives, however, may not be as contradictory as they appear. A focus group study of coronary artery disease patients, for instance, reported that older patients were likely to prefer that doctors make *certain* decisions for them (Kennelly, 2001). This deference may not mean they preferred to be passive about making *all* decisions, but either the patient or the physician was trying to simplify a particularly complicated or uncertain decision-making process (Braddock et al., 1999; Kennelly, 2001).

Practitioners also vary in their willingness to collaborate with patients. Sometimes the same practitioner will relate to different patients in different ways. One study of patients at primary care clinics, for example, reported that physicians were less willing than they were with younger patients to ask patients aged 65 and older to change their health behavior habits or to provide them with health education or counseling (Callahan et al., 2000).

Philosophical orientations among practitioners vary as well. Some health practitioners want a professional-centered relationship with patients. They want to be in total control of the interaction and prefer brief responses to their questions. This approach is guided by highly structured questions to patients. Others are more client-centered. They ask open-ended questions, value information on the psychosocial aspects of the health problem, restrict the use of jargon, elicit the client's perception of the health problem, and encourage clients to participate in the decision-making process (Sarafino, 1990).

The theoretical middle position is for the health professional to assess each client's willingness to be active in his or her health promotion and medical care decision-making, and then match their strategy with the level of participation desired by the client. Although this approach can theoretically reduce client stress levels and enhance communication, it is based on an untested assumption—that the health professional can accurately assess the client's willingness or potential to be active in their health decisions.

Another option is to encourage clients to be more involved in their health care, regardless of their initial enthusiasm toward this prospect. This stance can be justified on the basis that in this age of managing chronic health problems and promoting health over long periods of time, it is in the best interests of clients that we encourage them to be informed and involved.

## CLIENT EMPOWERMENT VERSUS THE PASSIVE PATIENT

From the client's perspective, empowerment means having the opportunity to learn, discuss, decide, and act on decisions. From the perspective of the health professional, empowerment of clients means not only to provide service to them, but also to collaborate with them, to encourage their decision-making ability.

The role of the *passive patient* evolved from the belief that health care is too complex to be understood or controlled by the layperson, that the doctor knows best. In the past, when acute care medicine reigned supreme, the patient only came to the physician when seeking a cure, and this attitude merited validity.

Today, however, acute care diagnosis and treatment are but two of many important health care activities. Other high-priority health activities include health maintenance, rehabilitation, disease prevention, health promotion, and health advocacy. The one element common to these areas is persistence; one cannot maintain, rehabilitate, prevent, promote, or advocate successfully except on a long-term basis. The *passive patient role*, extended over time, can be dangerous to one's health.

Health professionals frequently encounter older clients who could benefit were they more assertive about improving their health and the health care system in which they participate. Following are some typical examples:

- An older client with unhealthy lifestyle habits expresses the desire to eat less and get more exercise, but no health professional has helped galvanize this client to action.
- A chronically impaired older client, or a member of this client's family, is disgruntled by the lack of some service, such as home care or respite, that could enhance the client's independence or the family caregiver's mental health; however, this service is not covered by Medicare or a medigap insurance policy, and the family cannot afford it.
- A client who is recovering from a stroke (or heart attack, cancer surgery, etc.) appears to be isolated and discouraged. This client could benefit from interacting with people who are coping with similar challenges.

- An older client who takes multiple medications on an ongoing basis is having trouble complying with the medication regimen and needs help in managing the medication schedule and monitoring possible interactive effects.

The passive client or family member has little hope of rectifying any of the aforementioned situations, and health professionals cannot solve all problems for all clients. Health professionals can, however, motivate, educate, refer, and follow up. These interventions can empower the older client or family member.

## How to Collaborate

The U. S. Preventive Services Task Force (USPSTF, 1996) recommendations for patient education and counseling are applicable to how to collaborate with a client. These recommendations are liberally paraphrased as follows:

1. Consider yourself a consultant and help clients remain in control of their own health choices.
2. Counsel all clients, and especially reach out to those who differ from you in age, educational level, gender, and ethnicity.
3. Make sure your clients understand the relationship between behavior and health. Understand, though, that knowledge is necessary, but not sufficient to change client's behaviors.
4. Assess clients' barriers to change, including their lack of skills, motivation, resources, and social support.
5. Encourage clients to commit themselves to change, involving them in the selection of risk factors to eliminate.
6. Use a combination of strategies, including behavioral and cognitive techniques, the identification and encouragement of social support, and appropriate referrals.
7. Monitor progress through follow-up telephone calls and appointments, and activate your health care team, including the receptionist and other office staff.
8. Be a role model.

## Changing a Medical Encounter Into a Health Encounter

Although some persons may enthusiastically discuss health issues with their nurse, physician, or other health professional, many do not. People may simply wish to resolve the immediate medical problem with a health professional. They may not view health promotion as a personal priority, much less an issue to be discussed during an illness-related visit. Moreover, persons who *are* interested in health-promoting practices may not think of their health professional as an authority in this area.

If health professionals are interested in health promotion, what should they do to solicit a collaborative relationship? First, they can inform clients at their first visit that health issues are part of their job. Second, it helps to have an ample supply of health-related materials readily available: health articles posted on bulletin boards, a stock of updated health education materials in the waiting area, and relevant health materials given directly to clients. Third, office personnel such as receptionists need to be trained to distribute and explain health information and health assessment forms to waiting clients.

The likelihood is not great that a nurse, physician, or other health professional will turn an office waiting room into an environment that is conducive to health education. A survey of 150 South Carolina physicians, for instance, found that most thought the office waiting area a potential place for health education, but few had purchased any health education materials. In contrast, most spent over $100 a year on commercial magazine subscriptions (R. Taylor et al., 1982).

## AN OFFICE SYSTEM FOR IMPLEMENTING A HEALTH PRACTICE

A report by the American Cancer Society Advisory Group summarizes the elements of an office system that organizes preventive services (Leininger et al., 1996). The report includes such ideas as writing a practice policy for preventive care and setting performance goals, auditing charts for baseline performance, implementing a plan with office staff for efficient delivery of preventive care, choosing a staff member to be the coordinator of the plan, and monitoring progress.

Every medical intervention can include a brief health assessment of the client, conducted either by a clinician, a health educator, or a trained front office person. The assessment may begin with an evaluation of progress on a health contract or another type of intervention plan and end with a notation on the client's progress in the medical record along with a reminder system to ensure timely follow-ups and reinforcement.

There are a variety of effective tracking systems, including chart inserts, flow sheets, and office computer systems, that facilitate systematic follow-up of clients' attempts to change or maintain health habits. The most effective strategy is to include health issues at each client visit, to keep up-to-date health data, and to make telephone calls to the client (by clinician or office designee) as follow-ups, which are preferable to impersonal written reminders (McDowell et al., 1986). The more intense a client's behavior change goal (e.g., stopping smoking as opposed to including more fruit and vegetables in a diet), the more frequent the follow-up contact needs to be (Sennott-Miller & Kligman, 1992).

## HEALTH EDUCATION MATERIALS

A 1996 Kaiser Permanente survey found that many of their patients were dissatisfied with the current state of patient education. As one physician noted, "Who can blame them? In most cases, patient education consists of an out-of-date brochure, pulled from the back of a drawer, dusted off and handed to the patient following diagnosis" (Hutchinson, 1998).

Even good patient education materials tend to be limited in effectiveness in that they are written for those who need them the least, "well-educated, middle-class, middle-aged, non-minority populations who are highly motivated" (Baker & Wilson, 1996). Moreover, patient education materials tend to be disseminated without explanation (Cherry et al., 1995); if they are distributed directly by health professionals with an accompanying explanation on the importance of the materials and how to use them, they are more likely to be helpful to recipients (Barlow et al., 1996).

Another study reported that patients do not usually help themselves to educational pamphlets but prefer to receive them directly from a health professional. At some of the 18 family medicine practices observed in one study, hundreds of different educational handouts were available. The researchers concluded, however, that the best way to distribute patient education materials was for health professionals to choose a small number of documents that are well suited to their educational style, their patient profile, and the perceived informational needs of patients (McVea et al., 2000).

## PUT PREVENTION INTO PRACTICE

Put Prevention Into Practice (PPIP) was developed by the U.S. Public Health Service's Office of Disease Prevention and Health Promotion in order to improve the delivery of clinical preventive services on a national level. PPIP clinical sites in the community are designated to provide annual health risk assessments to patients and to target risk reduction and health promotion through screening, examination, immunization, counseling, and education (Melnikow et al., 2000). In Texas, primary care sites throughout the state are offered support for implementing prevention services through consultation, protocols, and grants provided by the state health department (Haber, 2002a).

If a health professional is interested in assessing readiness for incorporating prevention into an office, developing a protocol, and evaluating its impact, PPIP offers a manual: *A Step-by-Step Guide to Delivering Clinical Preventive Services: A Systems Approach.* It can be downloaded from the Agency for Healthcare Research and Quality Web site (www.ahrq.gov) or obtained through AHRQ Publications Clearinghouse (800-358-9295) or requested through e-mail (ahrqpubs@ahrq.gov). For more information about PPIP in general, e-mail PPIP@ahrq.gov.

## REFERRALS TO COMMUNITY HEALTH EDUCATION PROGRAMS

Assisting older clients with promoting health and preventing disease is an important component of the health professional-client relationship, but the amount of time available for this endeavor is typically severely limited. It is important, therefore, for the health professional to learn more about the health resources and programs available in the community and to make appropriate referrals.

The past decade has witnessed a proliferation of low-cost or free educational opportunities for older adults within the community. Except in isolated rural areas, a considerable number of health education opportunities for older persons are available.

These opportunities may include programs sponsored by the local senior center, YMCA/YWCA, hospital, religious institution, AARP (formerly American Association of Retired Persons), health professional association, health advocacy group, mutual help group, university or community college, Elderhostel program, shopping center mall-walker program, or corporate retiree wellness program—to name a few possibilities (see chapter 12 on Community Programs).

Once having identified a substantial number of community health organizations or resources, additional considerations come into play. Cost, transportation access, and instructor competency with older persons are obviously important factors in referring clients to community health education programs. Besides being knowledgeable about community health services and programs and referring clients to them, it is important to get feedback on the effectiveness of community health programs. Do clients recommend the program to others? Feedback from clients can be systematically elicited and made available to other clients by computer access or through a card catalog.

Community health programs are likely to be more successful if based on andragogical principles. Andragogy is the art and science of teaching adults based on a set of assumptions about learning that are different from traditional pedagogy. These assumptions, which have received only limited empirical examination (Brookfield, 1990), are twofold:

1. *Active involvement.* Active involvement on the part of older persons is preferable to the more traditional, passive student role. Older adults learn best when actively participating in an experience, such as setting goals, planning instruction, and assessing progress.
2. *Peer interaction.* The participation of older adults is fostered when age peers provide support, information, and assistance to one another. Community health education programs that allow for peer interaction may be more effective than those that rely primarily on didactic educational techniques.

## PERSONALITY CHARACTERISTICS OF A HEALTH PROFESSIONAL "COLLABORATOR"

Certain personality characteristics, such as patience, tolerance, and a positive attitude, enhance the health professional's chances for collaborating successfully on a health goal (Sarafino, 1990). Encouraging health change requires *patience;* client progress tends to be slow, incremental, and characterized by lapses or reversals. Health professionals are unrealistic if they expect to achieve health goals with their clients in the same time period required for the reversal of most acute care problems.

*Tolerant* health professionals are nonjudgmental about the poor health habits of clients. These habits no more should be viewed as character weaknesses than a physical illness would be. If a client senses self-righteous judgment on the part of a health professional, even though it may not be verbally expressed, any mutual health endeavor is doomed to fail.

Health professionals with a *positive attitude* begin any health endeavor by identifying the personal assets of clients that *will* facilitate a change in health behavior. If, for instance, a client has a receptive attitude toward health, the professional should acknowledge it. It is also important to acknowledge past successes in a health area; positive personality traits, such as persistence or a sense of humor; the support of a spouse or friend; or the educational and financial resources that will help the client access community health education programs.

# COMMUNICATION

Effective collaboration between health professionals and clients is dependent upon good communication. Open-ended inquiries and empathic listening skills are important aids to the health professional, increasing the likelihood of good communication with clients. Taking the time to explore the values and beliefs of clients can help the professional overcome communication barriers erected by differences in educational attainment, cultural beliefs, socioeconomic status, religion, gender, and age.

Given the limited amount of time within which most physicians and patients operate, however, it is not surprising that physicians who are similar to their patients are viewed as better communicators and more participatory. Specifically, physicians get rated highest on participatory decision-making style when they and their patients are of the same gender and race (Cooper-Patrick et al., 1999).

One small study in Albuquerque, New Mexico, brought family medicine residents and older patients together to examine provider-client discrepancies in medical encounters (Glassheim, 1992). The elders said they wanted health providers to listen to us more. The providers, in contrast, said they wanted their older patients to focus, tell us what you want.

Communication takes time. The client may need to focus more precisely to help busy health professionals be more effective. But busy health professionals need to be part of a team effort, and some member of the team (e.g., office staff, peer support group members, or trained paraprofessionals) needs to allow the client adequate time to communicate.

Time and caring work together: "the quality of the relationship also may be enhanced through the use of appropriate touch and the acceptance of patient reminiscences during the medical exchange" (McCormick & Inui, 1992). Health professionals who are unable to communicate warmth and unwilling to spend time with older clients put themselves at a severe disadvantage for motivating and encouraging behavior change.

To help an older patient communicate more effectively with a physician, the National Institute on Aging disseminates a 30-page soft-covered book entitled *Talking With Your Doctor: A Guide for Older People.* The book provides many tips for good communication and focuses on getting ready for your appointment, how to share information with your doctor, and how to get information from your doctor and other health professionals. To get free copies for a medical office, or for an older patient, call the NIA Information Center (800-222-2225) or order via e-mail (niaic@jbs1.com), and ask for NIH Publication No. 94-3452

## COMMUNICATION SKILLS

A health professional's message can be viewed as a therapeutic agent, comparable to a prescription of medicine or a surgical intervention. The positive expectations and good communication skills of a person considered to be trustworthy, expert, and powerful should not be underestimated as a therapeutic tool.

Conversely, poor communication skills by health providers are significantly more likely to be associated with patient lawsuits. In one astonishing study, 40 seconds of speaking could distinguish between surgeons with and without prior malpractice claims (Ambady et al., 2002). Surgeons with histories of malpractice claims were significantly more likely to demonstrate dominant and hostile voice tones, while those without such histories were more likely to demonstrate warmth, interest, concern, and sincerity.

The following questions are designed to help assess communication skills. About half were stimulated by a presentation made by Kate Lorig, RN, health educator at Stanford, or borrowed from an article by McCormick and Inui (1992). The rest are based on my personal experience with health education in the community.

## INTERPERSONAL EFFECTIVENESS

1. Do you make eye-to-eye contact?
2. Do you have a caring but not condescending tone of voice?
3. Are you and your clients comfortable with touching? If so, will this enhance rapport?
4. Do you engage in reciprocity of information by self-disclosing when useful?
5. Do you let your clients talk enough, or provide someone who will listen, or refer them to a support group that will listen?
6. Are you well informed about clients' religious or cultural restrictions regarding privacy, touching, speaking to a woman alone, or engagement in other types of intimate interactions?
7. Cross-cultural issues are not just racial, religious, or ethnic issues. We all interpret our health and diseases uniquely (i.e., we try to make sense of things within our belief system). Do you try to be sensitive to your client's unique "cultural interpretation"?
8. Are you able to resist countering clients beliefs that are not harmful and instead just add to them? "Yes, astrology [or, acknowledge to yourself, superstition] may contribute to your pain, but pain is

also caused by other factors." Do you give clients' power by adding to their data bank, rather than contradicting it?

9. Is it possible to gain insight into your client's lifestyle by making a home visit or getting feedback from someone who has?

## INFORMATIONAL PROCESSING

1. Do you know if your clients understand what you said; can they paraphrase it back to you?
2. Do you know what your clients mean; can you paraphrase it back to them?
3. Do you supplement your verbal instructions with clear, unambiguous written instructions?
4. Do you ask your clients to write down their questions between visits and bring the questions with them on their next visit?
5. Do you encourage your clients to bring along a helpful family member or friend to help with communication? Do you talk directly to your client and not primarily to their support person?
6. If appropriate, have you screened for cognitive impairment?
7. Are you aware of the impact that medication side effects may have on your client? Do these side effects interfere with their ability to communicate?
8. Do your clients have interest in the science (e.g., the anatomy and physiology) of their medical problem, or are they just interested in practical skills and knowledge? Do you provide data in a manner that is preferred and easily understood?

## SOCIAL AND BEHAVIORAL SUPPORT

1. Do you motivate through positive incentives, rather than rely exclusively on fear tactics like warning your clients about morbidity or mortality risks?
2. Do you rely exclusively on talk to change client behaviors, or do you combine talk with other strategies like behavioral management techniques?
3. Do you involve the client's social support system, such as family and friends, in the plan to change or maintain a health behavior?
4. Do you have an adequate reminder system to support the healthful behaviors of your clients or to help them avoid health risks?
5. Do you make appropriate referrals to community health programs or services when necessary and, equally important, do you seek

feedback for the benefit of other clients and to help decide about future referrals?

6. When making referrals, do you consider programs and resources that are offered at culturally relevant and supportive sites, such as neighborhood churches?

7. Do you ascertain client goals, see the underlying importance even if seemingly grandiose or trivial, and help your client redefine goals until they are achievable?

8. If you refer clients to support groups with lay leaders, do you know if they are receiving appropriate information? Do the groups invite professional expertise, and are you interested in contributing health education to these groups?

## CRUISING THE NET

Face-to-face communication with health professionals has become increasingly limited in our health care system. Consumers, therefore, rely on other sources of health information. A 1998 Roper survey (Kleyman, 1998) of Americans found that television is their primary source of health information (40%), followed closely by physicians (36%) and magazines and journals (35%).

The fastest growing source of health information, however, is the Internet. A survey of patients in one primary care practice in Providence, Rhode Island, reported that 54% of respondents were already seeking health and medical information on the Internet. The topics most often accessed are nutrition and diet (68%), medical therapy and medications (58%), and alternative medicine (41%) ("Study Looks," 2002).

The fastest growing segment using the Internet is the age 50-plus category. Merely 7% of online users were aged 50-plus in 1996, but that increased to 25% in 1997 (Kleyman, 1998).

As stated by former vice president Al Gore, the wealth of online consumer health information is "a mixed blessing because finding high-quality information that is accurate, timely, relevant and unbiased is a daunting challenge to even the most experienced Web surfer" (Schwartz, 1997). It is important to know the credentials of contributors to Web sites, whether the contributor has a financial stake in the products or information discussed, and if there are other sources of information with competing points of view.

A survey of 160 randomly selected health information sites found that more than half might have contained biased information (Laurence,

1997). Bias was not defined as accuracy but as whether the site's owner stood to gain financially from the products or services mentioned.

Other cautions with using the Internet are lack of privacy, inefficiency (a search using the key word "senior" brings up 57,600 sites, and senior centers turned up 275,992 sites), and high traffic causing delays ("A World of Information," 1998).

A review of the privacy policies of the 21 most trafficked health sites on the Internet concluded that few sites followed their own privacy policies. Most sites shared the personal health information that they collected from visitors, without their knowledge or permission ("Personal Data on Web Sites," 2000).

## A CASE STUDY IN WEB DECEPTION: drkoop.com

During his 8 years as U.S. surgeon general (1981–1989), Dr. C. Everett Koop became one of the most trusted and recognizable public figures on the topic of public health. He was best known for leading campaigns to deter cigarette smoking and to raise AIDS awareness.

In June of 1999, a decade after leaving office, Dr. Koop cashed in on his fame and reputation and launched an online health information Web site. The initial public offering of drkoop.com sold 9 million shares and raised close to $90 million. A bull market for e-health stocks at the time resulted in a start-up value of more than $500 million dollars for this Web site. By August, 1999 it was the most-visited health Web site, with about 3.5 million users.

It was downhill from there, unfortunately, due to a series of ethical lapses. Millions of dollars were made by Dr. Koop and his investment partners when they sold shares of their stock soon after the initial public offering, and in direct violation of securities law (Biesada, 2000). Nor did visitors to the site know that 14 hospitals that were described on the site as "the most innovative and advanced health care institutions in the country" had actually paid a $40,000 fee to be included on this list (Noble, 1999). Repeated examples of the site's inability to distinguish between advertising and health education continued to surface.

By the time I accessed the site in May, 2002, questionable dietary supplement formulas were being peddled by "The Doctor you KNOW you can trust," and free psychic readings were being promoted. A few months later drkoop.com filed for bankruptcy ("DrKoop to Cease Operation," 2002) and in July 2002, its assets were sold for a paltry $186,000 to a company that sells discount vitamins. At one time drkoop.com had been valued at $1 billion.

Drkoop.com was not alone. Medscape Inc., worth $3 billion in February 2000, was sold to WebMD Corp. for $10 million in December 2001. WebMD Corp., in turn, worth $20 billion in May 1999, was down in value to $1.4 billion in August 2002. Most online consumer health information companies have either vanished or have become mere shadows of their former selves (Chin, 2002a).

The problem for companies, and the appeal to consumers, is that most online health information is available free. Internet users seeking health information went from 52 million in 2000 to 73 million in 2001 (Chin, 2002a). The growth rate is even more impressive when you consider that the number of people going online for health information in 1994 was close to zero. The growth rate is explained not only by the increase in computer usage, but also by the fact that 82% find what they are looking for most of the time or always (Chin, 2002a).

## WEB SITES

Potential problems aside, more and more health consumers are finding the Internet to be an incredibly useful tool. Free online health information is available in all forms, including continuing education, consumer education, journal articles, discussion groups, magazine and newspaper articles, book reviews, chat rooms, Web reviews, databases, and so forth. There may be as many as 50,000 Web sites devoted to health (Gearon, 2000).

I have attempted to categorize below a few of the more interesting Web addresses that I have accessed. Generally speaking, government sites (.gov), nonprofit groups (.org), and educational institutions (.edu), are more trustworthy than commercial sites (.com). Two other cautions: a) these sites are very interesting and you might find yourself lost in cyberspace for hours; and b) on one site I read about a condition labeled *cyberchondria,* referring to people who *increase* their anxiety about their health by going online.

To access the Web sites listed below, it is necessary to first type http://www.

### Government

- healthfinder.gov (considered by many to be the premiere site for health information, including publications, clearinghouses, databases, Web sites, self-help or support groups, etc.)
- nih.gov (National Institutes of Health with links to more than 100 government databases, and consumer health publications)

- medlineplus.gov (a database with references to 4,000 medical journals, a medical encyclopedia and dictionary, a drug reference guide, and hundreds of links to reputable health organizations)
- fda.org (U.S. Food and Drug Administration provides latest information on new drugs and recently identified risks)
- odphp.osophs.dhhs.gov (Office of Disease Prevention and Health Promotion provides fact sheets, links to publications)
- aoa.dhhs.gov (Administration on Aging and the aging network)
- ahcpr.gov (Agency for Health Care Research and Quality provides information on best treatments for specific health problems)
- clinicaltrials.gov (details on 5,200 mostly government-funded clinical trials)

## Wellness

- drweil.com (Dr. Weil is director of Integrative Medicine at University of Arizona, this site is broad in scope but focuses on dietary supplements)
- wholehealthmd.com; healthy.net; and healthtouch.com (all three sites focus on complementary and alternative medicine)
- welcoa.org (Wellness Councils of America focuses on worksite wellness programs and products)
- nationalwellness.org (the National Wellness Institute offers conferences, programs, and wellness assessment tools)
- nccam.nih.gov/nccam (National Center for Complementary and Alternative Medicine)
- quackwatch.com (identifying dubious alternative health care claims)

## Professional Associations

- cancer.org (American Cancer Society)
- americanheart.org (American Heart Association)
- diabetes.org (American Diabetes Association)
- lungusa.org (American Lung Association)
- nof.org (National Osteoporosis Foundation)
- geron.org (Gerontological Society of America, focus on research)
- aghe.org (Association for Gerontology in Higher Education, focus on education)
- ncoa.org and asa.org (National Council on the Aging and the American Society on Aging sponsor many community services and educational programs, including a joint conference)
- hospiceinfo.org (National Hospice Foundation will help you find a hospice near you, draft a living will)

## Specific Health Content Areas

- aahperd.org (American Alliance for Health, Physical Education, Recreation, and Dance)
- acefitness.org (American Council on Exercise)
- active.com (event locator for individual and team sports)
- navigator.tufts.edu (Tufts nutrition navigator provides a rating guide to nutrition Web sites)
- eatright.org (American Dietetic Association offers daily nutrition tips and reliable answers to nutrition questions, including where to find a dietitian),
- wheatfoods.org (everything you want to know about grains)
- cspinet.org/nah (Center for Science in the Public Interest, and publisher of Nutrition Action Health Letter)
- healthletter.tufts.edu (Tufts University Health & Nutrition Letter)
- quitnet.org (a quit-smoking site in association with Boston University and a private company)
- niaaa.nih.gov (National Institute on Alcohol Abuse and Alcoholism)
- nida.nih.gov (National Institute on Drug Abuse)
- samhsa.gov (Substance Abuse and Mental Health Services Administration)

## Older Consumers

- aarp.org (AARP provides health news, information on a wide range of activities, and links to other sites)
- seniornet.org (Seniornet teaches adults aged 50 and older to use computers, links to 600 discussion groups)
- thirdage.com (tips on a wide variety of topics, from retirement savings to clothing colors that flatter gray hair)
- seniorjournal.com (daily news stories on topics of interest to older adults)
- assistedlivingstore.com (devices for assisted living)
- seniors-site.com/funstuff (jokes—some off-color, some just off, and some are actually funny)
- webmd.com (click health site—access wide range of health and medical topics)
- elderhostel.org (educational programs for those aged 55 and older throughout the United States and abroad)
- geezer.com (seniors selling handcrafted goods)
- Berkeleywellness.com (University of California, Berkeley Wellness Letter)

- healthandage.com (Novartis Foundation for Gerontology provides interesting articles and information on a wide range of health and medical topics)
- mayohealth.org (Mayo Clinic covers a wide range of health topics)

*Postscript:* It was a tough call, but I decided to include Web site addresses again for this edition of the book. Web site addresses come and go, and sometimes they transform into topics you do not expect or want. For example, as the second edition of this book was going to press, a student of mine took the initiative to review my Web site addresses one last time. One address, which included the word sweat, reported on exercise topics. Or, at least it did at one time. When the student checked it out again, however, it had transformed into a particularly malicious pornography site.

I, needless to say, was quite grateful for that student's initiative and managed (without too much difficulty) to get the editor to make a last-minute change in the second edition. I should note, though, that the student was unavailable for a last-minute review of this edition.

# MISCELLANEOUS COMMUNICATION ISSUES

## CROSS-CULTURAL COMMUNICATION

Some managed care organizations are recognizing the importance of helping health professionals communicate more effectively with minority patients. In Southern California, for instance, Kaiser Permanente has a medical anthropologist on staff to help health professionals work more successfully with minority patients and to develop special programs for minority members.

Cross-cultural communication, however, is not simply an issue of race or nationality. Many cultural differences that emerge between health professionals and clients are based on differences in age, gender, religion, ethnicity, socioeconomic class, and education. Every health professional must deal with these types of cross-cultural issues. Open-ended questions can help the health professional understand the client's point of view: How would you describe your health problem? Why do you think this problem occurred? Do you have sources of relief that I don't know about? Apart from me, who do you think can help you get better? Has anyone made recommendations to you? Did you try any of them?

The following organizations sell videotapes designed to improve communication skills between health professionals and clients: American

Academy of Family Physicians (800-274-2237) on racial and cultural biases; Boston Area Health Education Center (617-534-5258) on geriatric bilingual medical interviews; and the National Alliance for Hispanic Health (202-387-5000) on preventive health care for Hispanic patients.

## END-OF-LIFE COMMUNICATION

Effective communication is important up to the end of life. Some health care professionals believe that discussing end-of-life care issues upsets their clients. One study reported that few older adults are upset by such a discussion (Finucane, 1988). It is important that client's views be clearly recorded before an unexpected crisis develops. Clear thinking is more likely when a patient is relatively healthy and not suffering from anxiety.

Unfortunately, this type of communication is the exception rather than the rule. More than 90% of older adults in one study, for instance, did not clearly understand cardiopulmonary resuscitation (CPR) (Shmerling et al., 1988). Eighty-seven percent of older respondents thought CPR should be discussed routinely with health professionals, but only 3% had engaged in such discussions with them.

Another common example of a serious failure to communicate is the fact that most older adults understand the idea of a living will, but the vast majority have neither signed one nor discussed the issue with a health professional (Gamble et al., 1991). Geriatrician Joanne Lynne, director of George Washington University's Center to Improve Care of the Dying, reported on the importance of clear communication between health professionals and clients. She examined 569 advance directives, but only 22 of them were specific and clear enough to help physicians and family members decide what to do (Lynne, 1997).

Almost 1,200 seriously ill Medicare beneficiaries were interviewed at five U.S. teaching hospitals. Forty percent of the study patients requested a preference for treatment to focus on extending life, whereas 60% expressed a preference for comfort care. Eighty-six percent of the patients who wanted aggressive treatment reported that their care was consistent with their preferences; however, only 41% of those who preferred comfort care reported that their care was consistent with their preferences (Teno et al., 2002).

In October 1997, Oregon legalized physician-assisted suicide through the Death with Dignity Act. As a consequence, patients who requested assistance with suicide spent more time communicating about the issue through discussions with nurses, social workers, and physicians. According to participating nurses and social workers, the primary reason a patient makes such a request is to be able to control the circumstances of death if they so choose, not to end their life because they are depressed, lack social support, or fear being a financial drain on family members (Ganzini et al., 2002). Even among the terminally ill persons who requested a prescription for lethal medication, less than half actually end up taking their lives (Hedberg et al., 2002).

## COMMUNICATING TO CLIENT COMPANIONS

One study of more than 1,000 patients visiting an academic general internal medicine practice over a 3-month period reported that one third brought a companion with them to the doctor's office, and 16% had the companion come into the exam room (Schilling et al., 2002). A majority of physicians, and an even higher percentage of patients, found the arrangement to be helpful. The two major drawbacks were patient confidentiality and whether patients will reveal all they need to when someone close to them is in the room.

Older men are less likely than women to bring a companion when visiting a doctor, but more likely to bring a companion into the examining room to help them communicate with the doctor. Older women tend to bring companions primarily for transportation or companionship, visiting with the doctor alone (Beisecker, 1990).

A client's companion can provide a vital service to both the health professional and the client, serving as an independent monitor of a person's condition and providing helpful feedback on client collaboration with treatment regimens. A companion can make sure that questions are asked, and answers understood. On the other hand, health professionals can be seduced into communicating with companions and ignoring their clients. Problems that may stem from coalition formation (between two of the three participants) have not been examined as yet.

## COMMUNICATION BARRIERS BETWEEN HEALTH PROFESSIONALS AND OLDER CLIENTS

The satisfaction of older clients is positively associated with the length of their visits with physicians, and with physicians' support of topics initiated by the clients (Greene, 1991). Using audiotapes and other tools, however, researchers have found that doctors seem reluctant to discuss psychosocial and prevention issues with older clients and are less receptive to these issues when raised by older clients than when raised by younger ones (Callahan et al., 2000; Greene, 1991; Greene et al., 1987; Kennelly, 2001).

Another study reported that older clients are less likely than younger clients to agree with their physicians on the main goals of their visit (e.g., to discuss medication side effects, physical symptoms, etc.), and the topics that ought to be discussed (Adelman et al., 1989). An exception was with personal habits (e.g., diet, exercise, smoking, drinking). These topics, however, were infrequently discussed with physicians, regardless of a client's age (Greene et al., 1989).

A study of older diabetic clients reported that 42% were unable to discuss with their physicians the symptoms that concerned them (Rost, 1990). Physicians were much less responsive to topics raised by their older clients than to those raised by themselves (Adelman et al., 1989; Greene, 1991). Many of the recognized verbal and nonverbal approaches to good communication are not being practiced between primary care physicians and their patients (Beck et al., 2002).

Physicians give older clients considerably less cardiac risk reduction advice (regarding diet, exercise, weight control, smoking, stress management, and work) than they give younger clients (Young & Kahana, 1989). Thus, older clients are systematically denied the opportunity to lessen their risk of future heart problems by adopting the behavioral advice of their physician.

How well do nurses communicate with older patients? A meta-analysis of 34 studies reported that more patients were satisfied with care from a nurse practitioner than they were with care from a physician. Some of the studies reported that the nurse practitioner gave more time, information, and advice on self-care and management of disease (Horrocks et al., 2002). The key difference between nurse practitioners and physicians—the amount of time spent with patients—may be diminished in the future if nurse practitioners find themselves with less time to spend with patients.

A survey of 552 pharmacists in Indiana reported that 88% were willing to participate in continuing education courses to learn more about health education and promotion. Despite this willingness to learn, however, the pharmacists reported barriers to communication, including lack of time, reimbursement, privacy, training, and management support, when it comes to integrating health education and promotion into daily pharmacy practice (Kotecki et al., 2000).

## JARGON

A study conducted more than a quarter of a century ago on lower-class clients' comprehension of 13 terms used by their physicians found, not surprisingly, that each term was understood by only about one third of the clients (McKinlay, 1975). What *was* surprising is that physicians expected these clients to have even *less* comprehension than was reported.

A scholarly effort a few years later reported that the problem persisted. The reasons physicians continued to use incomprehensible language may have been habit; the belief that accurate comprehension of a medical problem might increase the client's stress level; the fact that hard-to-understand terms are likely to be conversation stoppers, making more time available for seeing other clients; the belief that the use of big words elevates the status and the authority of the practitioner; and the belief that lack of comprehension may make errors harder to detect, thus litigation less likely (Sarafino, 1990).

Clients, however, prefer health professionals who are willing to listen, communicate clearly, and show warmth and concern. When these expectations are met, clients offer more significant diagnostic details, keep more appointments, and litigate less (Sarafino, 1990).

### FOUR COMMON REASONS FOR NOT COMMUNICATING ABOUT HEALTH WITH OLDER CLIENTS

1. *I do not think most of my clients want to communicate about health.* This may be true, given the dry way in which health education is often presented. But many clients become more enthusiastic about health when they are encouraged to identify benefits that are meaningful to them; benefits like more energy, less arthritic pain, better sleep, or more strength. Clients also appreciate help with identifying the best pathway for accomplishing the health goal of their choice.
2. *I am not skilled in doing it.* With a few exceptions in nursing (e.g., Wold & Williams, 1996), medicine (e.g., Haber & Looney, 2000) and allied health (e.g., Haber et al., 1997), health science students do not receive adequate knowledge, skills, and especially practice in providing health promotion and education to older clients during the course of their student training. Given the wealth of continuing health education opportunities for health professionals that are available online and in the community, however, the major barrier to becoming more skilled at practicing health promotion and education with clients is insufficient motivation.
3. *I do not have the time for it.* This is a major concern that permeates the managed care environment. On the other hand, many ideas and

techniques can be presented effectively to clients in a brief period of time, office staff and health educators can assist with providing health education, and informed referrals can be made to appropriate and effective community health programs.

4. *I am not paid to do it.* Health professionals rarely benefit monetarily from offering health promotion and education to clients. But they do receive the gratitude of clients who stop smoking, start exercising, lose weight, or reduce stress. And this, in turn, provides most health professionals with tremendous mental health benefits, not to mention more client referrals from the family and friendship networks of satisfied clients.

## QUESTIONS FOR DISCUSSION

1. Think about an occupation that you wish was more health-oriented (like a nursing home administrator, a physician, a minister, etc.). How could you transform that job to generate more health-promoting activities with older adults?

2. Cruise the Web sites and find a particular health source that you like. Why do you like it, and how can you determine the accuracy and integrity of this source of information?

3. Three important personality characteristics of a *health* provider are mentioned in this chapter. Add a fourth. Why do you think this additional characteristic is important?

4. Describe an example of ageism that you witnessed in a health professional-client or teacher-student encounter. Why was it ageist?

5. The term *empowerment* can easily be viewed as a buzzword (thrown around a lot, signifying much but meaning little). Do you feel that way? Can you give an example of how you or someone you know became a more empowered student, teacher, or practitioner?

6. Suppose you encounter a 70-year-old client who prefers an authoritarian health provider. As a clinician, would you accept this person's attitude or would you encourage more patient initiative? If you encourage more initiative, how would you go about it?

7. How familiar are you with the health-promoting resources in your community? Find one that you are unfamiliar with but believe may be important for older persons. Summarize it sufficiently to answer most questions that older adults might have about it.

8. Which communication skill listed in this chapter are you most in need of improving, and how might you go about improving it?

# 3

# Clinical Preventive Services

## MEDICAL SCREENINGS AND PROPHYLAXIS: CONSIDERABLE CONTROVERSY

For the second edition of this book I wrote the chapter on medical screenings with a lot more certainty about the utility of its content. I began by stating a few of the obvious successes achieved by medical screenings and subsequent interventions. For example, I noted that because of the Pap smear test, cervical cancer mortality dropped substantially during the 1970s and 1980s. I also noted that partly due to the increased screening for, and treatment of, hypertension, the incidence of stroke and heart attack was significantly reduced.

I was not Pollyannaish about the topic, however. I reported that despite considerable support—and in some specific screening instances, universal acclaim—medical screenings were neither systematically nor uniformly implemented by clinicians. I noted that this behavior was due in part to clinicians and researchers failing to agree on the effectiveness of screenings and interventions, that is, the relative benefits versus the risks (medical, psychological, and financial) to individual patients.

I also noted that people with low-income levels were at a disadvantage when it came to medical screenings because of greater time constraints with physicians (Dawson et al., 1987), and persons with low-education levels (including Medicare recipients) were less likely to discuss screening options and other health education matters with their physicians (Gemson et al., 1988).

Obviously, none of this examination in 1998 and 1999 could capture the controversy over medical screenings that emerged in 2001 and 2002.

During this time, there was an explosion of research findings and popular articles on the utility of medical screenings and interventions. Much of the attention was on whether women should get mammograms or hormone replacement therapy. But there were also interesting questions raised about such topics as bone density, blood pressure, cholesterol, prostate cancer, the age at which screenings should begin and end, and whether we should be taking statins as an intervention for just about everything.

Underlying many of the issues raised about medical screenings and subsequent medical interventions were fundamental questions about the validity of the research that had been conducted. Before we tackle these questions, screening by screening, we need to lay some groundwork on what guides clinician decision-making when it comes to medical screenings.

## GUIDE TO CLINICAL PREVENTIVE SERVICES

Almost a quarter of a century ago, routine annual medical screenings were being replaced by periodic reviews, based on the unique health risk factors of individual clients. There is some evidence to suggest, however, that even today the public still believes in the undifferentiated approach of an annual physical examination and testing (Oboler et al., 2002). Health professionals, though, are expected to be better informed about the ongoing research findings that are being published and to educate themselves about the current recommendations for periodic screenings.

In order to simplify and standardize this effort, the Canadian Task Force on the Periodic Health Examination initiated in 1976 the first comprehensive effort to assess the effectiveness of a wide array of preventive services. They began by developing explicit criteria for assessing the quality of the evidence from published clinical research. Decision rules were then developed to guide clinicians.

In a similar effort that began in 1984, the U. S. Preventive Services Task Force (USPSTF, 1989) developed recommendations for clinicians on the basis of a comprehensive review of the evidence of clinical effectiveness. The conclusions were published in the *Guide to Clinical Preventive Services,* which catalogued 60 preventable diseases and conditions and provided guidelines to help health professionals select the primary, secondary, and tertiary preventive interventions that were most appropriate for their clients.

In 1996, the second edition of the *Guide* was published, and the number of topics expanded to 70. More than 6,000 citations to the literature were provided to substantiate the prevention recommendations that were made in this edition. Beginning in 2001, in lieu of a one-volume third edition, the Preventive Services Task Force began to issue new and updated guidelines on a piecemeal basis. Topics included a wide variety of screening and counseling recommendations, such as breast cancer screening, colorectal cancer screening, and counseling to promote physical activity.

These updates are to take place about twice each year and compiled in a 2-volume loose-leaf notebook that can be purchased in installments. All recommendations and supporting materials released over a 5-year period are available at a $60 subscription rate. You can order the subscription by calling the AHRQ Publications Clearinghouse (800)358-9295, or by sending an e-mail to ahrqpubs@ahrq.gov.

The recommendations in the *Guide* are based on a rating system that gives the most weight to research based on randomized controlled trials, followed by well-designed trials without randomization. The least weight is given to the opinions of respected authorities or expert committees, descriptive studies, and case reports.

"A" and "B" recommendations are based on good evidence to support the recommendation that a condition be specifically considered in a periodic health examination; "C" recommendations indicate insufficient evidence for making a recommendation for or against inclusion; and "D" and "E" recommendations are based on good evidence for exclusion.

"A" and "B" medical recommendations include such screenings as mammography, Pap smear, blood pressure, dental care, fecal occult blood tests, sigmoidoscopy, influenza and pneumococcal immunizations, vision, hearing, and postmenopausal hormone prophylaxis. On October 15, 2002, however, the Task Force updated its recommendation toward postmenopausal hormone prophylaxis. It recommended against the use of combined estrogen and progestin therapy for postmenopausal women, and reported insufficient evidence for or against the recommendation of estrogen therapy for women who have had hysterectomies.

In the previous edition of this book I had included a table from the *Guide to Clinical Preventive Services* that listed medical screenings and their recommended frequencies for persons aged 65 and over. You will notice that the table does not appear in this edition of the book. This is due in part to the controversies that I alluded to earlier, which will be examined in more detail later. But it is also due to the fact that the screening tables are outdated, and new guidelines are being released in installments by the U. S. Preventive Services Task Force.

In contrast to the evidence-based *Guide to Clinical Preventive Services* is the *Clinician's Handbook of Preventive Services,* published by the Put Prevention Into Practice initiative of the federal government (USDHHS,

1998). The handbook is divided between children/adolescents and adults/older adults, and within each of these two sections are subsections on screenings, immunizations and prophylaxis, and counseling. This handbook is oriented more toward clinicians than researchers, and includes expert opinion in each prevention area, even when it is not evidence-based.

As a consequence, the handbook includes the recommendations of not only the evidence-based Preventive Services Task Force, but also many authorities like the Center for Disease Control and Prevention, the National Institutes of Health, the American Association of Family Practice, the American Cancer Society, the American Heart Association, and about 30 other health associations. These associations represent a wide range of recommendations. It is up to the clinician to choose the authority or evidence to guide his or her decision-making.

In addition, the clinician handbook differs from the research-oriented *Guide* in that it provides assessment tools, technical information on how to perform each preventive service, a resource list for health providers, and a resource list for patients.

## ACCURACY, RELIABILITY, AND EFFECTIVENESS OF SCREENING TESTS

*Accuracy* refers to the sensitivity and specificity of screening tests. The *sensitivity* of a screening test is defined as the percentage of persons who actually had the disease and tested positive when screened. A test with poor sensitivity will miss persons with the condition and produce a large proportion of false-negative results. Persons who receive false-negative results will experience delays in treatment. *Specificity* refers to the percentage of persons without the condition and who correctly test negative when screened. A test with poor specificity will result in healthy persons being told that they have the disease and will produce a large proportion of false-positive results. Persons who receive false-positive results may experience expensive follow-up tests or unnecessary treatment that might not be completely safe.

Even if the test is sensitive and specific, it needs to be reliable and effective. *Reliability* refers to the ability of a test to obtain the same result when repeated. The reliability of some screenings, such as mammograms and Pap smears, has been increased due to the initiation of federal certification and annual state inspections of facilities. *Effectiveness* refers to whether the test is worth the cost, time, and bother, that is, whether there is a subsequent clinical intervention for a positive finding that can prevent or delay the disease.

# BREAST CANCER

Breast cancer is the leading cause of death from cancer among women, accounting for 46,000 deaths in 1997. In 1995, an estimated 182,000 new cases of breast cancer were diagnosed in women, with 48% of new breast cancer cases and 56% of breast cancer deaths occurring in women age 65 and over (USPSTF, 1996).

The three screening tests for breast cancer are breast self-examination, clinical examination, and X-ray mammography. Breast self-exams have never been proven to reduce breast cancer deaths, but the American Cancer Society—along with many physicians—encourage their use on a regular basis. The encouragement is based on the belief that the procedure may be effective, and it is simple, safe, and free.

A study of 266,000 women in Shanghai factories, however, were randomly assigned to breast self-examination or no intervention. (Mammography is not widely available in China, so self-examination is the best option available). The breast self-examinations were supervised, and were done correctly and regularly. After 5 years there was no difference in mortality between the two groups (D. Thomas et al., 2002). One meta-analysis reported that although larger tumors were more likely to be discovered through self-examination (Hill et al., 1988), the sensitivity of self-examination was quite low and specificity remained uncertain (USPSTF, 1996).

An annual clinical breast examination for women older than 40 is recommended by the U.S. Preventive Services Task Force. A thorough clinical breast examination may be as effective as mammography, but the research evidence is thin in support of this possibility. It is also unclear whether clinical breast examinations provide added benefit when conducted in conjunction with mammography.

Regarding mammography, a consensus on its utility had grown tremendously over the past two decades. A national survey in 1985 reported that the majority of primary care physicians never recommended mammography screening to their female patients, but by 1988, 96% reported having done so (Report on Medical Guidelines, 1991). A national study of primary care physicians by the American Cancer Society in 1988 found that 80% of physicians performed more screenings than 5 years earlier.

The importance of physician recommendations for subsequent mammogram screenings was confirmed in a study of mostly older white women, two thirds of whom had mammograms within the prior year (Brimer et al., 1991). Education and affordability might also have been factors in this study, but such was not the case for two samples of lower-income older Black women, of whom 60% complied with physicians when a mammogram was specifically recommended (Burack & Liang, 1989, 1987).

Compliance with a recommendation for a mammogram was also enhanced in 1992, when Medicare began offering partial coverage for *routine* mammographies conducted every 2 years. In 1998, this benefit was increased to annually for Medicare-covered women. Another factor that contributed to adherence was the improved accuracy and reliability of mammogram screenings. In 1992, Congress approved the Mammography Quality Standards Act, which regulated equipment and personnel, including technologists and physicians, and required federal certification and annual state inspections of facilities.

The specificity of mammograms, however, still left much to be desired. Fifty percent of women who have had 10 mammograms over the past decade or two, will have had one false positive result that required further testing and unnecessary stress and expense. As many as 20% of these false alarms will lead to a breast biopsy in which tissue is removed from the suspected tumor (Elmore et al., 1998).

The effectiveness of subsequent intervention for early detection was also a concern with some cancers, though this issue was not being addressed by many health professionals nor was it generally known by the public over the past two decades. About 20% of the breast cancers being found, for example, were ductal carcinoma in situ (DCIS). There was evidence to suggest that 80% of DCIS will not become invasive if left untreated; nonetheless, DCIS has been routinely treated with surgery, radiation, and chemotherapy (Napoli, 2001).

The *relatively* minor controversies that the public was aware of—such as when breast cancer screenings should begin and how often they should be conducted—did not serve as deterrents to screening compliance. This was especially true because of the substantial federal government publicity in favor of mammograms, the expanded Medicare coverage, and the widespread endorsement of the procedure by physicians. Not surprisingly, the percentage of women aged 50 and older who reported having had a mammogram in the previous 2 years went from 27% in 1987, to 61% in 1994, and 69% in 1998 (Kolata & Moss, 2002).

## THE 2001–2002 MAMMOGRAM CONTROVERSY

Widespread use of mammography as a screening tool began in the United States in the mid 1980s, after seven large studies involving 500,000 women seemingly demonstrated the effectiveness of this screening tool.

The controversies surrounding mammography over the next decade and a half were the relatively minor ones of whether they should start at age 40 or 50, and whether they should be annual or biannual.

On one side of the debate were the National Cancer Institute and the American Cancer Society, which recommended regular mammograms beginning at age 40. On the other side was the National Institutes of Health's consensus panel, which recommended that decisions about starting mammograms before age 50 be left up to each woman and her physician. Taking a middle position, the American Medical Association's Council on Scientific Affairs recommended mammograms every 2 years between the ages of 40 and 49 and annually beginning at age 50.

In the same 2002 issue of *The Annals of Internal Medicine*, two opposing points of view continued to be expressed. The Canadian National Breast Screening Study reported that after 11 to 16 years of follow-up, a randomized screening trial of mammography in women age 40 to 49 did *not* produce a reduction in breast cancer mortality (Miller et al., 2002). The U.S. Preventive Services Task Force, however, reviewed eight randomized controlled trials and still advised women to begin breast cancer screening at age 40 (Humphrey et al., 2002).

The age at which mammography screenings should be terminated also generated a little controversy, but was not generally known by the public. The U.S. Preventive Services Task Force (1996) recommended the discontinuation of mammogram screenings at age 69 in asymptomatic women who had consistently normal results on previous examinations. Other authorities and researchers recommended no discontinuation of mammographies after age 69 (Kerlikowske et al., 1999; McCarthy et al., 2000; McPherson et al., 2002; USDHHS, 1996).

The disagreements in the field continued to generate little public notice in 2000, even when two Danish researchers published a report questioning the effectiveness of mammography at any age (Gotzsche & Olsen, 2000). Perhaps public awareness was muted because the majority of researchers criticized the methodology and conclusions of the Danish researchers. When the report was reissued in October 2001, however, and substantiated with additional statistical analysis (Olsen & Gotzsche, 2001), considerable attention was paid to it by both researchers and the general public. The report challenged the long-prevailing orthodoxy on whether mammography was helpful at any age, and not just the decade between age 40 and 50.

The conventional wisdom up to this point was that the seven previously mentioned studies were convincing and that mammography helped save women's lives by detecting tumors early enough to be treated. The

Danish researchers, however, concluded differently. They reported that five of the seven studies were too flawed to be credible and that the remaining two studies showed that mammography did not save, or even prolong, lives. Their conclusions were endorsed by *The Lancet* and by an expert group sponsored by the National Cancer Institute.

Other researchers, though, took exception to their findings (S. Duffy et al., 2002a; Tabar et al., 2001), and an analysis in Sweden reported that mammograms may reduce deaths from breast cancer by as much as 45% (S. Duffy et al., 2002b).

The surrounding publicity following Olsen and Gotzsche's report in 2001 was nothing short of astonishing. Major professional organizations and experts expressed uncertainty, or they argued either for or against mammograms. In February 2002, Tommy Thompson, secretary of Health and Human Services, declared almost by fiat that if you are a woman age 40 or older, you need to get screened for breast cancer with mammography every year. A not unrelated aside was that Secretary Thompson's wife was a breast cancer survivor whose tumor was detected by mammography.

Scientific controversies, however, are not resolved by fiat. Proponents of mammography noted that breast cancer death rates have declined by a little more than 1% a year since 1990 and mammograms were responsible for this decline. Doubters of mammography suggested that perhaps the decline in breast cancer death rates was not due to early detection but to the increasing effectiveness of treatments like the drug tamoxifen. Despite the secretary's proclamation, the following scientific, economic, and political issues remained:

1. Early detection may prevent a tumor from becoming more deadly. Larger tumors that are discovered later may be more likely to have spread beyond the site in which they arose. And survival chances of a woman with a larger tumor are not as good as those of a woman with a smaller tumor. Or, maybe not. Some tumors may be discovered early by mammograms and despite intervention still spread and become deadly; some may never become deadly, and early treatment (surgery, radiation, and chemotherapy) may be more harmful than doing nothing; and some may be detected later without harmful consequences.

2. There are also economic considerations. The breast cancer screening industry generates $3 billion a year (Kolata & Moss, 2002), and the medical industry has lobbyists who will not be easily dissuaded about the benefits of mammograms. About 30 million women are having mammograms each year as well as additional tests, and the

federal government has compelled insurance companies to cover the screenings.

3. There are other economic influences on mammograms as well. Medicare paid only $81.81 for an initial mammography in 2002 (and many commercial insurers reimbursed even less) for a procedure that most argue costs at least $15 more than that. Given the inadequate reimbursement and the risk of legal liability, postgraduate fellowships in mammography were not easily being filled. On a related note, there were 5% fewer accredited mammography centers in 2002 than in 2001, and the waiting time for routine screenings was rising (Freudenheim, 2002).

4. It is commonly accepted that all radiologists will miss some breast cancer tumors. But it is not generally known that between 15% and 40% of cancers are not detected by mammography clinics (Moss, 2002). Many physicians read too few mammograms to achieve an acceptable skill level, skill tests are not required, and physicians do not receive feedback on what percentage of cancers are detected.

5. Routine breast self-examinations by older women have never been proved to reduce breast cancer deaths, despite the encouragement by physicians and the American Cancer Society. And the idea that this procedure is simple and safe is disputed by researchers who argue that the practice leads to unnecessary biopsies that can be harmful (Baxter, 2001; Hill et al., 1988; USDHHS, 1996).

So what is a woman to do? There may be no enduring answers, but the U.S. Preventive Services Task Force decided to weigh in on the controversy in 2002 through one of their updated guidelines. Their tentative conclusion: the original mammography studies did have flaws, but they were probably not drastic enough to change the recommendations. They encouraged women, particularly between the ages of 50 and 69, and perhaps between the ages of 40 and 74 (Humphrey et al., 2002), to get a mammogram every year or two. For clinical breast examination and breast self-examination, the Task Force reports that the evidence from randomized trials is inconclusive.

## MENOPAUSE

There is no definitive medical screening for menopause. The average age at menopause in the United States is 51, and its existence is primarily documented by the onset and eventual termination of a variety of symptoms. These symptoms typically include irregular menstrual cycles, hot flashes, changes in mood and cognition, insomnia, headache, and fatigue.

Some women do not view their menopausal symptoms as a medical problem and do not seek a consultation with a physician. At the other end of the spectrum, menopause may be viewed as an estrogen-deficiency disease. There is considerable cultural variation in attitudes toward, and the definition of, menopause.

At the start of the new millennium, however, the debate over the use of hormone replacement therapy (HRT) to relieve the symptoms of menopause and prevent disease may have even surpassed the controversy over the use of mammography. And, once again, there were serious questions about the validity of the research that had been conducted over the past couple of decades.

The early studies that provided optimism about HRT were based on observational studies in which large groups of women were tracked for years. In these studies, the patients themselves decided whether to take HRT. We later found out that the sample populations for these studies were more affluent, better educated, younger, thinner, more likely to exercise, and with greater access to health care than women in general. In other words, the sample populations were healthier and had better health habits than other women, and the outcomes they had may have been due more to this sampling bias than to the intervention of HRT.

Under the leadership of Bernadine Healy, the first woman to head the National Institutes of Health (NIH), the Women's Health Initiative was launched in the 1990s and it included the Heart and Estrogen/Progestin Replacement Study (HERS) and its follow-up (HERS II). Using a more rigorous methodology, HERS and HERS II produced surprising results by correcting the previous sampling bias through a placebo-controlled clinical trial with random assignment. This type of randomized study is considered the gold standard in medical research but it is much more expensive to conduct, and ethical questions are raised when some persons have to be randomly assigned to a placebo control group.

To the surprise of many people, the randomized clinical trials did not agree with the earlier observational studies. Even more surprising, the HERS studies reported that there was an increase in heart attacks, strokes, blood clots, and gallbladder disease among healthy women taking HRT, compared with those on the placebo (Grady, 2002b; Spake, 2002). In 2001, the American Heart Association reversed its support of HRT, and for women with cardiovascular illness a recommendation was made to avoid the therapy. In 2002, NIH became sufficiently convinced about the problems associated with HRT to send letters to the 16,000 women participating in the HERS II study and recommend that they terminate the therapy.

Other studies were also raising questions about the effectiveness and safety of HRT. A meta-analysis of 22 HRT trials questioned whether the therapy was effective for reducing bone fracture risk (Grady & Cummings, 2001). There was also evidence of increased breast and ovarian cancer risk among HRT users (Chen et al., 2002; Rodriguez et al., 2001). Finally, a randomized federal study found that HRT did not produce meaningful clinical improvement in quality of life: vitality, mental health, sexual pleasure, memory, or restful sleep (Hays et al., 2003).

Even prior to the publication of these studies, most women who opted for HRT were not staying on it for long. Within 1 year, 53% of 900 HRT users between 1993 and 1995 in one study had discontinued the therapy, and two thirds by the following year (R. Reynolds et al., 2001). Those who discontinued HRT cited the fear of cancer and side effects. Physicians were also becoming more cautious with HRT, using lower doses (Lindsay et al., 2002), focusing on menopausal symptoms, and reassessing its effectiveness after a few years (Grady, 2002a; Spake, 2002). For disease prevention, there appeared to be better options than HRT for heart disease (e.g., statins or aspirin) and osteoporosis (e.g., Fosamax or Actonel).

To offset emerging HRT risks, drug companies have been working on selective estrogen-receptor modulators (SERMs) that appear to reduce the risk of breast cancer and cardiovascular events and have a positive impact (though considerably less than estrogen) on the slowing of bone loss (Barrett-Connor et al., 2002; Mestel, 1997a; Walsh et al., 1998). SERMs, however, do not relieve hot flashes and the other common side effects experienced by about 85% of menopausal women.

Options for alleviating menopausal symptoms have not been as promising as HRT. Over-the-counter herbal supplements like black cohosh were becoming more popular for alleviating symptoms, even though the supporting research on its effectiveness remained inconclusive. Black cohosh and a variety of soy products (i.e., weak plant-based estrogens) work to some degree in the alleviation of symptoms in up to 40% of menopausal women, but this is about the same percentage improvement that placebos elicit.

In October 2002, the North American Menopause Society recommended that HRT not be prescribed for the prevention of heart disease and that alternatives should be considered for the treatment of osteoporosis. For women who want to treat menopausal symptoms, HRT should be limited to the shortest possible duration, and lower doses should be considered. Apparently, women already had gotten the message. On June 21, 2002, 379,581 prescriptions were filled for Prempro, a popular HRT; on September 20, 2002, only 211,249 prescriptions were filled (Elliott, 2002), a decline of 44% in 3 months.

# BLOOD PRESSURE

High blood pressure is defined as a systolic blood pressure of 140 mm Hg or higher, or a diastolic blood pressure of 90 mm Hg or higher, regardless of age. Systolic and diastolic blood pressures tend to increase until age 60; after that, systolic pressure may continue to increase with diastolic pressure stabilizing or even decreasing (Beers & Berkow, 2000). A few years ago, clinicians distinguished between hypertension, or readings over 160/95, and high blood pressure, or readings over 140/90. Now the terms are used interchangeably and the lower threshold applies.

Moreover, researchers are making the case that the threshold should be lowered. High-normal blood pressure (130/85) is associated with elevated risk for heart disease and stroke (3 times more in women, 2 times in men), particularly among older persons (Vasan et al., 2001). In 2001, the National Kidney Foundation lowered the blood pressure target recommended for people with diabetes to 130/80 or below. And, in 2003, new federal guidelines urged that readings between 120–139 and 80–89 be considered pre-hypertensive.

More than 50% of Americans aged 65 and over have high blood pressure (Beers & Berkow, 2000), though the precise percentage is subject to disagreement and may be higher. Researchers associated with the Framingham Heart Study of the National Heart, Lung, and Blood Institute, for instance, report that Americans aged 55 or over face a 90%(!) chance of developing hypertension (Vasan et al., 2002). Complicating the problem of a greater incidence and prevalence of high blood pressure than previously thought is the undertreatment of the problem by physicians, especially among older patients and perhaps up to 75% of them (Hyman & Pavlik, 2001; Oliveria et al., 2002).

Measurement error should be a factor in assessing high blood pressure. Errors can result from the manometer itself; patient physical factors such as anxiety, the timing of the last meal eaten, and recent exertion; and white-coat hypertension, an overestimation of the blood pressure of certain patients in the physician's office (Little et al., 2002; Pickering, 1988). White-coat hypertension may not just be a harmless case of nerves in the doctor's office, but a signal of early heart damage (Grandi et al.,

2001). To offset white coat hypertension, the average of multiple measurements of blood pressure over closely spaced visits may more accurately approximate a person's true blood pressure (Applegate, 1992).

The good news about blood pressure is that there is widespread awareness. It is estimated that three out of four adults and perhaps 90% of older adults have had their blood pressure measured within the preceding year. (See Figure 3.1). Among those with high blood pressure, though, only one quarter remain in treatment and consistently take their medication in sufficient amounts to achieve adequate blood pressure control (National Heart, Lung, and Blood Institute [NHLBI], 1997).

Nonpharmacologic therapies, such as exercise, sodium restriction, weight reduction, decreased alcohol intake, smoking cessation, and stress management, are promising in lowering mildly elevated blood pressure (Appel et al., 2003; Chobanian, 2001; Linden et al., 2001; NHLBI, 1997), but these lifestyle changes can be complicated by biological factors (e.g., hypertensives who are not salt-sensitive) and behavioral factors (e.g., ability to maintain weight loss or sustain an exercise program).

Medicare does not provide specific coverage for blood pressure screening (though it is considered part of the overall care covered by Medicare), despite the fact that uncontrolled high blood pressure among older adults is widespread, with costly consequences (Rigaud & Forette, 2001). If Medicare coverage of blood pressure screenings was instituted, it would provide more attention to the problem, encourage more reliable screenings than the ones currently available in clinics and at community sites, and allow for appropriate follow-up counseling in a timely manner (Haber, 2001).

Finally, although blood pressure screenings have been recommended over the entire adult life cycle for many years, there has been disagreement over whether screenings and counsel might be discontinued at age 80 due to uncertain impact on morbidity or mortality (Amery et al., 1986; Gueyffier et al., 1999; Rigaud & Forette, 2001; Staessen et al., 1998).

# OSTEOPOROSIS

Osteoporosis is a condition in which the bones are thin, brittle, and susceptible to fracture. It is technically defined as a bone density that is 2.5 or more standard deviations below the young adult peak bone density. Osteopenia is a weakening of the bones and can be considered a warning on the way to osteoporosis. It is technically defined as 1 to 2.5 standard deviations below the young-adult peak bone density.

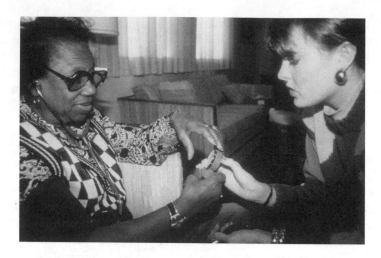

FIGURE 3.1  Nursing student teaching older adult to take a blood pressure reading in one of the author's health education classes.

Without intervention, about 5% to 10% of trabecular bone is lost during the first 2 years after menopause, up to 20% in the 5 to 7 years following menopause, followed by a more gradual loss after that.

A study of more than 200,000 allegedly healthy women aged 50 and older, found osteoporosis in 7% of the women and osteopenia in another 40% (Siris, et al., 2001). The fracture rate of women with osteoporosis in the following year was 4 times higher than the women with normal bones, and 2 times higher in women with osteopenia. The study used a noninvasive, imaging technique (with very low levels of radiation) called single-energy X-ray densitometry on peripheral bone sites, rather than the more accurate double-energy X-ray densitometry that is done on the spine and hip. The authors noted, however, that the fracture prediction rates were not compromised much by the use of the quicker, less expensive, single-energy X-ray readings.

These study results were surprising not only in detecting the widespread prevalence of osteopenia, but also in the researchers' ability to detect within a year a significant increase in fracture rate.

Osteoporosis affects more than 28 million Americans, 80% of whom are women, and causes 1.5 million fractures each year. Almost half the fractures are vertebral (700,000), followed by hip and wrist (300,000 each). Half of women over age 50 will have an osteoporosis-related fracture in their lifetime.

Close to 90% of women with osteoporosis were not being diagnosed with the condition, and only about one third with the diagnosis were offered treatment for the disease during the 1990s (Gehlbach et al., 2002). Diagnosis and treatment are expected to increase markedly due to the growing popularity of screenings for bone density, and coverage by Medicare that started in 1998 for women at risk for osteoporosis. Unfortunately, the definition of risk for osteoporosis was not made clear by Medicare, and physicians are unclear about reimbursement for their older patients.

If almost half the women aged 50 and older have osteoporosis or osteopenia, one can argue that a significant majority of women aged 65 and older are at risk and that all women aged 65 and over on Medicare should be screened. The U.S. Preventive Services Task Force came to the same conclusion in an updated guideline, and recommended that routine screening begin at age 65 for all women (H. Nelson et al., 2002). It is not known, though, how often women should undergo screenings (though some panel members recommended every 2 or 3 years), or when or if they should be discontinued at a certain age.

Others may take a more conservative approach and add up the number of risk factors for osteoporosis for a specific woman before recommending screening. The risk factors in addition to age and female gender are being of Caucasian or Asian race, slender build, bilateral oophorectomy prior to natural menopause, early onset menstruation, smoking, alcohol abuse, physical inactivity, the use of steroid hormones to treat a variety of medical conditions, and getting too little calcium or too much caffeine, protein, and salt from the diet.

Interventions for reducing or reversing bone loss include dietary calcium, calcium and vitamin D supplementation, weight-bearing exercise, hormone replacement therapy, and bisphosphonates (drugs such as Fosamax and Actonel).

Fosamax (alendronate sodium) is a medication approved by the Food and Drug Administration in 1995 that can actually reverse osteoporotic bone loss. It increased bone density 3% to 9% in one sample of postmenopausal women, while a placebo group lost bone (Liberman et al., 1995). That study also reported that women with osteoporosis who took Fosamax were only half as likely to break a hip as women who did not take it. Actonel is a newer drug but it too shows evidence of substantially reducing the incidence of new vertebral fractures (Heaney et al., 2002).

The major drawback to Fosamax is that it is a tablet that must be swallowed without chewing, and it can linger in the esophagus and cause serious ulcers if not taken exactly as directed: on an empty stomach, with a full glass of water, half an hour before the first meal of the day, and standing or sitting upright for at least 30 minutes. Many patients have problems complying with these recommendations (DeGroen et al., 1996).

On a positive note, a once-a-week Fosamax pill was approved in 2001, and a once-a-year intravenous infusion of a bisphosphonate drug has demonstrated positive preliminary results (Reid et al., 2002). A nasal spray called Miacalcin (calcitonin) is an alternative that is easier to use, but only half as effective.

Calcium and vitamin D supplementation is also an effective intervention for osteoporosis and will be examined under dietary supplements in chapter 8 on Complementary and Alternative Medicine.

## CHOLESTEROL

The new cholesterol guidelines have become more confusing since the second edition of this book was published, and it is probably no accident that I waited this long in the chapter to examine them. (Cholesterol was the first medical screening reviewed in the second edition). A few years ago I was able to report that a total blood cholesterol level of 240 mg/dl or higher was considered abnormal (for abnormal cholesterol *ratios,* see Chapter 6 on Nutrition) because it had a substantial association with coronary heart disease (USPSTF, 1996), and about 27% of U.S. adults had this high a level. I was also able to report on an increasing awareness of cholesterol levels with the percentage of adults who had their cholesterol level checked increasing from 35% to 59% of the population between 1983 and 1988 (AARP, 1991).

I also reported that the recommendation for cholesterol screenings after the age of 70 remained an unresolved issue. It had not been determined yet whether the association between higher cholesterol concentrations and atherosclerotic coronary artery disease, for instance, may weaken or strengthen with age (W. Ettinger et al., 1992). Should the association remain the same or strengthen with age, it is an important and modifiable risk factor among older persons. Should it weaken with age, cholesterol testing with older adults would not be effective.

An informal survey of several hundred physicians revealed that the majority considered age 70 the approximate threshold for effective treatment of an elevated cholesterol level. Most expressed some concern about initiating treatment through drugs or diet with patients over age 70. The concerns regarding the use of hypolipidemic drugs related to their cost, side effects, and their potential interaction with other medications (Hazzard, 1992).

Finally, dietary therapy and follow-up by physicians, dietitians, or nutritionists appeared to be effective in reducing dietary fat intake and serum cholesterol in adults of all ages (Insull et al., 1990). However, dietary recommendations—which typically consisted of reducing fat intake to less than 30% of total calories, saturated fat (fat that is solid at room temperature, e.g., butter, cheese, fat in red meat) to less than 10% of total calories, and cholesterol intake to less than 300 mg/day (Report of the National Cholesterol Education Program, 1988)—may foster malnutrition in highly compliant older clients (see Figure 3.2). Malnutrition is not an uncommon issue when it comes to older adults, and cholesterol or fat avoidance that triggers malnutrition is a legitimate concern.

There have been significant changes over the past few years regarding cholesterol screening and—from my perspective as a health educator—not completely for the better. The National Cholesterol Education Program (NCEP) III guidelines were published in 2001 and they are complicated to review (Expert Panel on Detection, Evaluation, and Treatment of High Blood Cholesterol in Adults, 2001). To determine whether you are at risk involves assessing many measurements, such as total cholesterol, HDL cholesterol, systolic blood pressure, the 5-year age category that you are in, gender, smoking status, abdominal obesity, diabetes, a family history of heart disease, and the like.

From a health educator's perspective, the new guidelines make the consumer more dependent on the health professional to calculate risk level. For example, the new guidelines create three new low-density lipoprotein (LDL) categories instead of one, all of which are more aggressive than the previous guideline. An LDL below 100 is optimal, 130–159 is borderline, and 160 and above is high. It is recommended that a physician be consulted for expert advice on the number of risk factors that you have before determining which LDL category is acceptable for you.

In addition, this aggressive approach increases the number of persons who are being recommended to take the new cholesterol-lowering medications—from 13 million under the 1993 guidelines, to 36 million under the 2001 guidelines. This may be reassuring from a medical perspective but raises some nonmedical issues. How many older adults can afford the $1,200 a year for medication costs? If society cannot afford the estimated $300 billion annually that may be needed for statins (Ansell, 2002), what criteria do we use to determine who should receive them (Gambert, 2002)? What are the long-term effects of treating younger persons more aggressively and having them on cholesterol-lowering medications for 40 years or more?

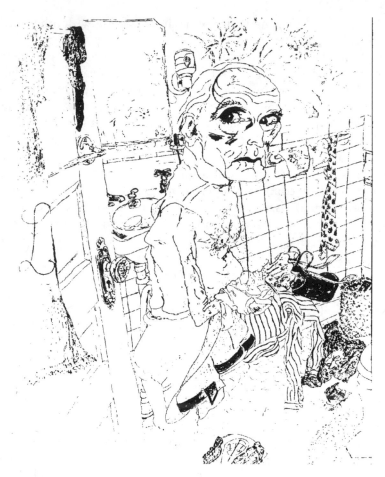

FIGURE 3.2 Elizabeth "Grandma" Layton, popular artist from Wellsville, Kansas, focused her late-blooming artistic skills on her own aging process and that of her husband Glenn, who is pictured on a bathroom scale, concerned about his recent loss of weight. Reprinted with permission.

Paralleling the aggressive new NCEP guidelines, the U.S. Preventive Services Task Force released its new guidelines for cholesterol screening, and eliminated the upper age limit of 65 for cholesterol screening. However, clinical evidence is still more supportive for treating hyperlipidemia in older adults than it is for primary prevention (Hall & Luepker, 2000; Oberman & Kreisberg, 2002).

My last concern with the new NCEP panel guidelines is that while the experts mention diet and lifestyle recommendations, they come close to proclaiming medication as the *only* way to achieve major cholesterol reduction

(Fedder, 2002). The new recommendations also reduce the daily limit on dietary cholesterol to less than the amount in the yolk of a single large egg. This means avoiding, for the most part, eggs, meats, poultry, and cheese. Overly compliant older adults may run the risk of malnutrition.

On the bright side, cholesterol-lowering drugs called statins may not only reduce blood cholesterol by as much as 60%, they also may have benefits for a wide range of conditions like osteoporosis and colon cancer (Ansell, 2002; "Statin Drugs," 2001), heart disease and strokes (Altman, 2001; Heart Protection Study Collaborative Group, 2002; Landers, 2001), breast cancer (Ricks, 2001), and dementia or Alzheimer's disease (Jick et al., 2000; Simons et al., 2001; Yaffe et al., 2002).

These preliminary studies, however, were not randomized clinical trials, and statins may be more efficacious (i.e., likely to succeed in studies) than effective (i.e., likely to succeed in practice) because noncompliance rates increase over time in routine care settings (Benner et al., 2002; Elliott, 2001; Jackevicius et al., 2002). There is also a clinical advisory on the safety of statins, particularly on the risk for myopathy (Pasternak et al., 2002).

# CERVICAL CANCER

Until the 1940s, more American women died of cervical cancer than any other type of malignancy. However, the Pap test, named for its creator, George Papanicolaou, reduced the death rate from cervical cancer by 70%. Pap testing is recommended for women beginning at the age at which they first engage in sexual intercourse, and it should be repeated every 3 years after they have had at least two normal annual screenings. For women age 65 and over who have had regular normal Pap smears, the U.S. Preventive Services Task Force 2003 update concluded that the harms of continued routine screening, such as false positive tests and invasive procedures, may outweigh the benefits.

Many older women, however, have not had adequate screening; nearly half have never received a Pap test, and 75% have not received regular screening. Older women are least likely to have had Pap smears, in part because they no longer visit gynecologists, the specialists most likely to recommend the test (L. Jones, 1992).

Pap screening for older women is important. Recognizing this fact, Congress mandated in 1990 that Medicare cover Pap smears triennially. In 1992, federal clinical laboratory regulations were established. In 1998, benefit coverage improved considerably when the full claim for Pap smears became reimbursable.

As of July 1, 2001, Medicare covered cervical cancer screening every 2 years for women not at high risk for uterine or vaginal cancers, while continuing to cover annual tests for women at high risk. In 2002, new guidelines were established for women with abnormal screening tests. Testing for the human papilloma virus can be done from the original Pap test sample, thus saving follow-up Pap tests and colposcopy costs (Mandelblatt et al., 2002).

# COLORECTAL CANCER

There were 140,000 new cases of colorectal cancer and 56,000 deaths in 1999, making it the second leading cancer (after lung cancer) and cause of cancer-related death. Risk for colorectal cancer increases with age, with most new cancers affecting persons aged 75 and older. Although the Preventive Services Task Force does not recommend one screening method over another, in a 2002 update it *strongly* recommended some type of screening for colorectal cancer for persons aged 50 and over. This upgrades its previous position in 1996 when it simply recommended screening.

The Task Force did recommend annual fecal occult blood testing, though it should be noted that fecal occult blood testing produces a high percentage of false positives (5% to 10%). Digital rectal examinations are of limited value since few colorectal cancers (about 10%) can be detected by this procedure.

In the absence of adequate research, expert opinion recommends a sigmoidoscopy every 4 years for average-risk patients older than 50 (USPSTF, 2000). A sigmoidoscopy, however, only examines the first one-third of the colon (about 2 feet), and research supports the need for a colonoscopy (D. Lieberman et al., 2000; Podolosky, 2000), which examines the entire length of the colon (about 5 feet). Expert opinion recommends a colonoscopy every 10 years.

Medicare covers a fecal occult test annually, and a flexible sigmoidoscopy every 4 years. There is no upper age limit to sigmoidoscopy coverage, though a meta-analysis reported that this test may be discontinued at age 80 with minimal loss in life expectancy (Rich & Black, 2000). Because of the cost of a colonoscopy—$1,200 versus $250 for a sigmoidoscopy—the procedure had not been covered by Medicare, except for high-risk persons. As of July 2001, however, Medicare began covering the cost of routine colonoscopies every 10 years for people who were not at high risk for colorectal cancer.

Although Medicare coverage for colorectal cancer screening has expanded, compliance has not improved much. In 1999, only 14% of Americans over age 65 received a colon cancer screening test, even though the tests were fully covered by Medicare ("Medicare Patients," 2000). The tests remain uncomfortable and embarrassing, and both client noncompliance and physician reluctance to perform the procedure on asymptomatic patients has been reported (USPSTF, 1996).

There was an increase in colorectal cancer screenings, however, after *Today* television show host Katie Couric, whose husband died of colorectal cancer, had the procedure done live on television in March 2000. During the following 9 months colon cancer screenings increased more than 20% (specialists in colonoscopies referred to it as the "Couric effect"). The likelihood, though, was that this increase in screenings was a temporary one.

Some of the discomfort of colon cancer screening may be eliminated through a "virtual" colonoscopy, a scanner that takes hundreds of X rays at different angles from the outside, and then uses sophisticated software to combine the data to produce a 3-D image of the colon. At the current level of technology, however, this type of scan misses growths identified by the traditional colonoscopy, and abnormal results still require a follow-up with the traditional colonoscopy (Fenlon et al., 1999). Another approach to colorectal screening involves the swallowing of a small camera to scan from the inside (Costamagna et al., 2002). Yet another test looks for abnormal DNA in stool samples (Ahlquist et al., 2000). These strategies are in the experimental stage, and a high rate of compliance for colon cancer screening is likely to be dependent on the success of one of them.

## PROSTATE CANCER

At least half of all men over age 50 are bothered by benign prostatic hyperplasia, a gradual enlargement of the prostate that occurs with age and a disease that is second to lung cancer in accounting for cancer deaths in men. Despite the increase in the use of the simple and effective prostate-specific antigen screening test (PSA test), the U.S. Preventive Services Task Force 2002 update concluded that there is insufficient evidence to recommend for or against routine screening for American men.

Although autopsy studies indicate that prostate cancer is present in about 70% of men at age 80, only 3% of men die from it. A large proportion of prostate cancers are latent, unlikely to produce clinical symptoms or affect survival (USPSTF, 1996). Moreover, many men may live with slow-growing prostate cancers that never cause any problems, but removing them can cause incontinence and impotence without providing any benefit. Thus, prostate screening is not yet deemed effective, that is, the screening tool does not yet lead to treatment that reduces the mortality rate (Sox, 1997).

A Scandinavian study of 695 men (mean age, 65) with early prostate cancer were randomized to radical prostatectomy or to watchful waiting. A 6-year follow-up reported that death from prostate cancer occurred significantly less often in the surgery group than in the watchful-waiting group; however, all-cause mortality was not significantly different in the two groups (Holmberg et al., 2002).

Few of the tumors in the Scandinavian study were PSA-detected tumors. In that regard, another study reported that 29% of prostate cancers in White men and 44% of prostate cancers in Black men that are detected by PSA may represent overdiagnosis. Overdiagnosis is defined as the detection of a prostate cancer that otherwise would not have been detected within the patient's lifetime (Etzioni et al., 2002).

When Patrick Walsh, chairman of urology at Johns Hopkins, was asked if he would test a man in his 80s for prostate cancer, he replied "not unless he's brought in by both his parents."

Treatment options for prostate cancer vary, and include drug therapy, surgery, heat, freezing, and herbs. The increasing use of saw palmetto, a plant-based remedy for prostate problems, is promising, providing mild to moderate improvement in benign prostatic hyperplasia (BPH) (Wilt et al., 1998). Long-term effectiveness or ability to prevent BPH complications is not yet known.

## HEARING AND VISION

It is estimated that 33% of Americans aged 65 to 75 have some hearing loss, and the percentage climbs to 50% among persons aged 75 and over. Presbycusis is an age-related hearing loss that results in the inability to register higher-frequency sounds. Consonants with higher-frequency sounds blend together, and a hearing aid that merely amplifies will not be effective.

The intervention for hearing loss has improved over the last several years. Newer digital hearing aids have a precision that the older analog hearing aids lacked, and may be able to create a signal that is more finely tuned to the hearing loss of older adults. Digital aids are expensive (more than $3,000) and cost considerably more than the analog models.

Of an estimated 30 million Americans who could benefit from hearing aids, only 20% use them. This is not surprising, given that aids are not covered by insurance and only about half of hearing aid users are satisfied with their aids. Nonetheless, it is important to deal with hearing loss because a 1999 National Council on the Aging study reported that those with hearing loss are more susceptible to depression, worry, anxiety, paranoia, lower social activity, and emotional insecurity than those who get help ("Time to Deal," 2002).

To buy a hearing aid, clients need to have had a physician's evaluation (preferably by an otolaryngologist or otologist in a soundproof room) within the previous 6 months. After this initial screening, consumers need an audiologist or licensed hearing-instrument specialist to evaluate hearing loss and recommend an appropriate device. Unfortunately, people who dispense hearing aids may receive a commission from a hearing-aid maker, thereby affecting their objectivity in choosing the most appropriate aid for a client ("Age, Hearing Loss," 2000).

Because Medicare and most health insurers do not pay for hearing aids, it may be helpful to contact Hear Now (800-648-HEAR), which can provide hearing aids to persons whose income level qualifies them for assistance. The Better Hearing Institute (800-EAR-WELL) may also help persons locate financial aid in their local area.

Although less common than hearing impairment, blindness is one of the most feared disabilities (Gallup, 1988). Presbyopia, a universal age-related change in vision, begins in most persons in their 40s. Despite age-related changes, visual acuity in the absence of disease should be correctable to 20/20 even in very old persons (Beers & Berkow, 2000).

Macular degeneration, the loss of central vision, is the leading cause of blindness among older adults and can be self-detected by looking at a grid with a dot in the middle of it (the Amsler grid is available through www.macular.org). Approximately 25% of persons over 65, and 33% of those over 80 have signs of macular degeneration.

Though damage from macular degeneration cannot be reversed, early detection may help slow the progression of the disease. The National Eye Institute's Age-Related Eye Disease Study reported that antioxidant vitamins with zinc may slow the progress of macular degeneration in certain subsets of people with the disease ("Preserving your sight," 2002). A vitamin E supplement by itself, however, does not appear to slow the progress of macular degeneration (J. Taylor et al., 2002).

A cataract is a clouding of the lens that reduces visual acuity. Most cataracts can be successfully dealt with through changes in corrective lenses, and more advanced cataracts can be successfully removed through surgery. Surgery should be performed when desired activities cannot be performed, rather than on the basis of which stage of maturation the cataract is in (Beers & Berkow, 2000).

About 3 million Americans have glaucoma, a condition that occurs when fluid in the eye does not drain and the increased pressure can damage the optic nerve. Half of the 3 million Americans, however, do not know they have glaucoma because they do not have their eyes tested often enough, preferably every year or two. As of January 1, 2002, Medicare covered an annual dilated eye examination for persons at high risk of glaucoma. High risk is defined as those with diabetes, a family history of glaucoma, and African Americans. Glaucoma is 5 times more likely to occur in African Americans.

## ORAL HEALTH

The surgeon general in 2000 reported that Americans' mouths are in the best shape ever. Regarding older adults, there has been a steady decline in the level of edentulism (loss of all teeth) among successive cohorts of older adults. Nonetheless, about one third of persons aged 70 and older are still afflicted (P. Marcus et al., 1996).

As the American population ages, visits to physicians increase, but visits to dentists decrease (Ettinger, 2001). More than 90% of adults aged 40 and older in the United States have not had an oral cancer examination in the past year (Horowitz & Nourjah, 1996). The lack of reimbursement by a third-party payment system for dental care is no small factor in this neglect.

Professional oral health care may be particularly important in nursing homes. A study of older residents in two nursing homes reported that professional oral health care given by dental hygienists was associated with a reduction in the prevalence of fever and fatal pneumonia (Adachi et al., 2002).

The surgeon general reported that there are widespread oral health problems among low-income older persons (Allukian, 2000). One public policy initiative that could have positive consequences for older adults is the promotion of water fluoridation in the 38% of communities that are not yet treating their public water supplies. A study of more than 3,000 women aged 65 and older reported that fluoridation not only enhanced the prevention of dental caries, but it also appeared to increase bone density in the hip and spine and slightly reduce the risk of fractures at these sites (Phipps et al., 2000).

# DIABETES

Type II diabetes (previously called adult-onset diabetes until it started showing up in teenagers) is the inability of the pancreas to produce sufficient insulin, the hormone that allows glucose to enter and fuel the body's cells. One study of 3,000 individuals aged 70 to 79 revealed that 24% of the older adults had diabetes, one third of whom were undiagnosed (Franse et al., 2001). This prevalence is due to an increase in obesity and to an increase in the number of older minorities (Asians, Hispanics, and African Americans), who have higher incidence rates.

A U.S. Preventive Services Task Force 2003 update concluded that there is insufficient evidence to recommend for or against routine screening for diabetes mellitus in asymptomatic adults. However, at its 1997 national meeting, the American Diabetes Association, with the endorsement of the National Institutes of Health, recommended that Americans over age 45 have their blood sugar screened every 3 years, and that the blood sugar threshold be lowered from 140 to 126 milligrams of glucose per deciliter of blood. This new level can detect many more cases when diet and exercise can prevent or delay the disease.

It is estimated that about 16 million Americans aged 40 to 74 fall within this new level of "pre-diabetes," when diet and exercise can reduce by 60% the number who eventually develop the more serious disease ("New Diabetes Screenings," 2002). One study compared diet, exercise, and weight loss with the drug metformin (Glucophage) for preventing the onset of diabetes. The changes in lifestyle habits were nearly twice as effective as the medication, particularly in people aged 60 and over who were little helped by the drug (Knowler et al., 2002). Another study also concluded that type II diabetes can be prevented by changes in lifestyle among high-risk older subjects (Tuomilehto et al., 2001).

# DEPRESSION

Lifetime prevalence of depressive disorders ranges from 5% to 17% (Williams et al., 2002a) and is projected to become the second leading cause of disability worldwide by the year 2020 (American Psychiatric Association, 1994). Despite its prevalence and economic significance (Murray & Lopez, 1996), studies have shown that usual care by primary care physicians fails to identify 30% to 50% of depressed patients (Simon & VonKorff, 1995).

The U. S. Preventive Services Task Force issued an updated guideline in May 2002, advising that physicians begin screening adults for depression in the clinical setting. This revises the Task Force's 1996 recommendation, which encouraged clinicians to remain alert for signs of depression but did not recommend for or against regular formal screening. The Task Force's update concludes that there is good evidence that screening improves the accurate identification of depressed patients in primary care settings and that treatment of depressed adults identified in these settings decreases clinical morbidity.

There are a number of formal screening tools available, but asking two simple questions may be as useful as administering longer instruments (Whooley et al., 1997). "Over the past 2 weeks have you a) felt down, depressed, or hopeless? b) have you felt little interest or pleasure in doing things?" An affirmative response to these questions may indicate the need for more indepth diagnostic tools.

Screening adults for depression should take place only when adequate diagnosis, treatment, and follow-up are in place. Treatment may include antidepressants, cognitive behavioral therapy, or brief psychosocial counseling, alone or in combination (Pignone et al., 2002).

## OTHER MEDICAL SCREENINGS

For better and for worse, new medical screenings are developed on an ongoing basis. On a positive note, a quick, finger-stick blood test might detect ovarian cancer before it becomes deadly (Petricoin et al., 2002), and C-reactive protein may predict heart attacks and strokes better than cholesterol testing (Ridker et al., 2002). On a negative note, unnecessary full-body CT scans are becoming increasingly popular and carry a hefty price tag. If this type of scan was widely carried out, the number of false alarms triggered by it would overwhelm the health care system ("Whole-body Screening," 2002).

Routine thyroid screenings are still not recommended, despite the availability of a simple, inexpensive blood test (USDHHS, 1996). A large survey revealed that about 4% of the population had subclinical hypothyroidism (Hollowell et al., 2002), but experts disagree about whether this subclinical condition should be treated (Brett, 2002).

## IMMUNIZATIONS

For many years, the estimated annual U.S. deaths attributed to influenza and pneumonia combined ranged from 20,000 to 40,000. In 2003, however, using improved statistical models, the Centers for Disease Control and Prevention's (CDC) new estimate was that 36,000 persons die from flu-related complications alone each year. This dramatically revised estimate is due in part to the aging of the U.S. population and the fact that more than 90% of the deaths from flu and pneumonia occur in people aged 65 and older.

Researchers report that widespread use of the influenza and pneumococcal vaccinations can prevent up to 60% of these deaths among older persons (Nordin et al., 2001). A recent study reviewed data from 286,000 persons over the age of 65 and found that an older person's chance of being hospitalized for heart disease or a stroke is sharply reduced during the flu season that followed a vaccination (Nichol et al., 2003).

The pneumococcal vaccine should be administered to persons aged 65 and older at least once during a lifetime, with possible revaccination for older persons with severe comorbidity after 5 years. Pneumonia is 3 times more prevalent among those 65 and over than among younger persons.

There was a substantial increase in pneumococcal vaccinations between 1989 and 1998. Only 10% of older adults in the community had received the pneumococcal vaccination in 1989, despite the fact that pneumonia at that time accounted for an average of 48 days of restricted activity per 100 people aged 65 and older (NCHS, 1990a). By 1997, due in large measure to the onset of Medicare reimbursement, 46% of Medicare beneficiaries had received the vaccine. And according to a General Accounting Office report, this rate jumped to 55% in 1999.

Nonetheless, almost half of older adults remained unvaccinated, and there was considerable racial disparity. In 1999, 57% of Whites received a pneumonia vaccination, compared with 36% of Blacks and 35% of Hispanics (Mieczkowski & Wilson, 2002).

The influenza vaccine should be administered annually to all persons aged 65 and older, with an advisory panel at the CDC recommending in April 2000 that it be administered beginning at age 50. Health care providers for high-risk patients should also receive influenza vaccine.

Between 1972 and 1982, the death rate during six flu epidemics was 34 to 104 times higher among older adults than younger persons. Yet only 20% of older adults in the community received influenza vaccines in 1989. This percentage, however, increased to 68% by 1999, several years after Medicare began paying for influenza shots for the nation's older and disabled populations.

Among older Blacks, however, the influenza vaccination rate was 21% lower than among whites (Schneider et al, 2001). About 70% of Whites received flu shots, while only 49% of Blacks were immunized ("Medicare Screenings," 2002).

To increase the compliance rate, the federal government in 2002 approved standing orders for annual flu and pneumonia vaccinations in nursing homes, hospitals, and home health agencies that serve Medicare and Medicaid beneficiaries. These standing orders ensure that older adults are reminded to get flu and pneumonia immunizations, and that the shots can be administered by a nurse without the need for a physician to write a new order.

In the 2000–2001 season, flu vaccinations were characterized by delays and shortages. The distribution system was uneven, resulting in some providers receiving plenty of vaccine and others receiving none. Moreover, the price of the flu and pneumonia vaccines had increased, but Medicare reimbursement had not. Consequently, some providers resisted participating in vaccination programs. These and subsequent challenges will need to be resolved before vaccination rates continue to climb, and certainly before the Healthy People 2010 goal—90% of older adults vaccinated—is met.

Tetanus is an immunization recommended for all adults, including older adults. After a primary series of three doses of the tetanus-diphtheria toxoid, a booster shot should be administered at least once every 10 years. Medicare does not cover tetanus immunization as there are only about 50 tetanus cases reported each year in the United States. About half of these cases, however, occur in persons over age 65 (USDHHS, 1998).

## MEDICARE PREVENTION

Nearly 40 million older adults and disabled persons covered by Medicare became eligible for new prevention benefits in 1998. This was a major step towards providing prevention benefits to the older population in America. Yet much of the content of this prevention package appears to have been influenced more by lobbyists advocating for specific segments of the medical industry (e.g., oncology, urology, orthopedics) than by policy derived from evidence-based medicine (Haber, 2001a).

Mammogram screenings, for instance, increased to annually for all Medicare-eligible women ages 40 and older, and the Part B deductible was waived. The U.S. Preventive Services Task Force, however, noted that the more frequent annual mammogram screenings for women after age 65 will be expensive and may not result in reduced mortality. The Task Force also raised the prospect of more false-positive results and additional biopsies.

New bone-mass screening procedures were approved for high-risk individuals as of July 1998 for women aged 65 and older. High risk was vaguely defined as estrogen-deficient women at clinical risk for osteo-porosis, which could include all women in that age category. While the National Osteoporosis Foundation hailed the new benefit, opponents argued that it is an expensive test (particularly the dual-energy X-ray densitometry), and for most women will not lead to a recommendation that could not have already been made prior to the screening: engage in weight-bearing exercise, good nutritional practices, and calcium and vitamin D supplementation. An opposing argument, however, is that a low densitometry reading will motivate older women to engage in risk-reduction behaviors.

New benefits were also provided for colorectal cancer screenings of all individuals aged 50 and over. Aside from the expense, little criticism can be leveled at the new coverage for flexible sigmoidoscopy and colonoscopy. However, the more relevant issue—how to increase the exceptionally low compliance rate for colorectal cancer screening—was not addressed by Medicare.

New coverage for an annual prostate cancer screening was made available to Medicare-eligible men over age 55 on January 1, 2000. This coverage is made available despite the lack of evidence that early detection among older men improves survival. Prostate screening also carries a strong risk of screening results leading to expensive and invasive inter-ventions, while the original condition may have posed no harm during the individual's life expectancy.

There were also new Medicare prevention benefits in 1998 that were not controversial. There was new coverage for 3 million Medicare bene-ficiaries with diabetes: outpatient self-management training services and coverage for blood glucose monitors and testing strips for type II diabet-ics without regard—for the first time—to whether insulin was being used. In mid-2001, the self-management training was expanded to include up to 10 hours annually to help control blood sugar, though only 1 of the 10 hours was targeted toward nutrition education.

On January 1, 2002, an estimated 4.5 million Medicare recipients with diabetes (and 110,000 persons with kidney disease) became eligible to receive additional individualized medical nutrition therapy to help them eat better to control their disease or to lose weight. Medicare recipients are now able to meet with a registered dietitian to discuss food intake and exercise, review lab tests, and set goals for making dietary changes. Health-promotion advocates were hoping this new benefit for diabetes patients would pave the way for routine nutrition counseling for other Medicare recipients.

Other additions to the collection of benefits provided in the 1998 Medicare prevention package were a new coverage of screening pelvic exams, an enhanced coverage of Pap smears with the Part B deductible waived, and the extension of coverage for influenza and pneumococcal vaccinations.

Given that five of the eight Medicare prevention benefits covered are medical screenings, it is not unfair to question whether prevention from a Medicare perspective is too biomedicalized. Analysts have argued that prevention resources are limited, and we should reexamine policy that is so heavily focused on medical screenings (Mason, 2001; Napoli, 2001). Perhaps it would be more cost-effective to counsel for risk reduction programs, particularly in the areas of inactivity, inadequate nutrition, smoking, and alcohol abuse (Haber, 2001a). This topic will be addressed in chapter 4 on Health Behavior and chapter 14 on Public Health.

*A Final Word*

Medical screenings and immunizations are undeniably important tools for disease prevention, but the data collected by the U.S. Preventive Services Task Force (1996) resulted in a surprising conclusion: "among the most effective interventions available to clinicians for reducing the incidence and severity of the leading causes of disease and disability in the United States are those that address the personal health practices of patients" (p. xxii).

Stated another way "conventional clinical activities (e.g., diagnostic testing) may be of less value to clients than activities once considered outside the traditional role of the clinician," namely, counseling and patient education (USPSTF, 1996, p. xxii).

To be fair to clinicians, however, a recent study reported that the average patient in a family practice waiting room needs 25 preventive services (Yarnall et al., 2003). Using a base of 2,500 patients, the researchers conservatively estimate that 7.4 hours a day would be needed to provide the recommended preventive care in a typical practice. The authors recommend a team approach toward prevention, involving health educators and other practitioners in the clinic, and collaboration with health-promoting practitioners in the community.

# QUESTIONS FOR DISCUSSION

1. What would you say to a client who is asking you for advice on whether to get a mammogram or to start hormone replacement therapy? Why did you answer that way?

2. There has been a trend toward lowering the threshold of medical screenings like blood pressure, blood glucose, and cholesterol. This can allow people to take action before the problem gets too serious. It can also lead to more people being on medications and the greater medicalization of health care. What do you think?

3. What do you believe is the best way, at this time, to increase compliance with colorectal cancer screening recommendations? Why?

4. The author rails against the complicated cholesterol guidelines, but perhaps they foster better collaboration between the patient and the physician. What do *you* think?

5. Even if you felt that older men in general should not be routinely screened for prostate cancer, what would *you* do if you were a 65-year-old male? Why?

6. Densitometry can motivate older women to engage in weight-bearing exercise and consume more calcium and vitamin D. Or, we can save the expense of this screening and apply it to advising and assisting all older women to increase exercise and improve diet. What do you think?

7. What do you believe accounts for the racial disparity in immunization rates, and what can be done about it?

# 4

# Health Behavior

In their article, "The Case for More Active Policy Attention to Health Promotion," McGinnis and colleagues (2002) examine the impact of five spheres of influence on early deaths in the United States. Using the best available data, their estimates are as follows:

- Environmental exposures (5%)
- Shortfalls in medical care (10%)
- Social circumstances (education, poverty) (15%)
- Genetic dispositions (30%)
- Behavioral patterns (40%)

McGinnis and colleagues observe that behavioral patterns are not only the most important contributor to early death, but also to quality of life as well. They noted that "what we choose to eat and how we design activity into (or out of) our lives have a great bearing on our health prospects" (McGinnis et al., 2002, p. 82).

And yet more than 95% of the trillion-plus dollars we spend on health care in America each year goes to medical care, and less than 5% is allocated to improve behavioral patterns. This budgetary allocation may seem out of balance to the health-conscious reader, but it is undeniably good for certain businesses and practitioners, such as medical institutions, medical professionals, tobacco growers, alcohol producers, food manufacturers, and advertising companies.

The health education profession, in contrast, is a modest industry with practitioners who toil away in relative obscurity. There are few millionaires, and few lobbyists who seek concessions from congressional leaders. As a consequence, the health care industry in America is primarily a medical care industry dominated by medical practitioners. In this chapter, however, I will focus on the role of health educators in the health care industry—and more important, their potential role in changing health behaviors. The topics that will be examined are health behavior assessments, interventions, and theories.

# HEALTH BEHAVIOR ASSESSMENTS AND INTERVENTIONS
## HEALTH RISK APPRAISALS

In comparison to *specific* medical screenings that tend to be the focus of research studies and clinical interventions, health risk appraisals and other health behavior assessments are typically *comprehensive* in scope and are implemented in nonmedical settings in the community. Health promotion advocates in the community believe that clients get a broad, holistic perspective through a comprehensive health behavior assessment, and a sense of the priority areas that they may want to work on.

This big picture, though, may also discourage persons who discover an array of lifestyle risk factors that need attention. A good health assessment may be broad in scope, but it also has to guide the client who is able and willing to begin with one achievable health behavior change.

The most common example of a comprehensive health assessment is the health risk appraisal (HRA) instrument that began in work settings and is now implemented in a variety of community settings. HRAs became accepted in the workplace in the 1970s and continue to inspire widespread utilization (WELCOA, 1997). During the 1970s and 1980s the HRAs were used primarily by employers in order to give feedback to their employees on their major health risks. Some companies demonstrated cost savings through the utilization of HRAs (Uriri & Thatcher-Winger, 1995). It was estimated that about 30% of workplaces utilized HRAs in the 1990s, and the number of instruments that they had to choose from had grown to several dozen.

By the late 1980s, health assessments were adapted to the characteristics of older adults in the community (Uriri & Thatcher-Winger, 1995). A program like Senior Healthtrac, based in San Francisco, reached out to 300,000 individuals nationwide who were aged 55 and older, through Blue Cross and Blue Shield plans and Medicare supplemental coverage programs. Periodically, the program distributed a Senior Vitality Questionnaire and followed up with a Personal Vitality Report that included an individual's "vitality age," which may be younger or older than an individual's chronological age. The Vitality Report noted an individual's risk for cancer, heart disease, emphysema, cirrhosis, and arthritis compared to that of other persons of the same age and sex, and suggested lifestyle changes to reduce specific risk factors.

The applicability of HRAs to older adults, though, is still unresolved (RAND, 2001). Risk calculations based on younger and middle-aged adults may be inaccurate for older adults, and HRAs tend to focus on premature mortality rather than on lifestyle risk and the progression of illness and disability. The process of evaluating the suitability of HRA instruments for older populations is ongoing.

I reviewed summaries of 20 HRAs, including ones from such well-known organizations as the National Wellness Institute and Johnson & Johnson Health Management. They were being used in work and other community sites, and all claimed to have versions of their instrument that were appropriate for, or adaptable to, specific age groups, ranging from high school to older adults.

Among the instruments that I reviewed I noted the following:

1. They were computerized and available for commercial use. Most offered individual and aggregate reporting, as well as data security.
2. They included, at minimum, medical questions like blood pressure and cholesterol level, and health habits like smoking, exercise, and nutrition.
3. There was no consensus on length. Some instruments were deliberately short, about 15 questions; others included upwards of 150 questions.
4. They were quantifiable, comparing actual age with an earned age. The apparent assumption is that learning whether your days are running out faster or slower than expected, is motivating to clients.
5. They used outdated or debatable scientific evidence. This is not surprising since research results are changing more rapidly than patented HRA instruments.
6. They had a health education component to motivate individuals to change undesirable health behaviors in order to reduce specific risk factors. In most instances, this health education component relied on tailored written resource materials, although some provided follow-up by a health educator. In some cases the specific risk factors identified by the HRA were linked to appropriate health programs in the community.

## A REFLECTIVE HEALTH ASSESSMENT

In contrast to specific responses to a series of narrowly focused risk reduction questions posed by health risk appraisals, Dr. Andrew Weil at the University of Arizona's Integrative Medicine Clinic offers his patients a unique health assessment tool that encourages patient reflection and initiative. ("Broadening your View," 2000). Dr. Weil begins with the questions, What does good health mean to *you?* And how do *you* attain it? Additional questions in this vein include, Does your life have meaning to you? Are you happy?

Dr. Weil also asks clients unique questions about specific content areas. What is your relationship with food? What is your relationship with exercise? Do you have satisfying personal relationships? How do you deal with your stress?

When you complete these questions, it is time for you to reflect on your answers. You may never have examined your health in this way. You will explore your attitudes toward your health, identify your health goals, recognize the obstacles to achieving your goals, and discover the personal resources you can assemble to accomplish them.

At the end of these reflections you may have a better understanding of what is contributing to your health problems. You may be more aware of what kind of support you would like from your family, friends, and health care providers. And you may feel more empowered by defining terms for yourself, assessing your own priorities, and designing self-tailored strategies to achieve your health goals.

## STAGES OF CHANGE

Another type of health assessment, one that is typically *not* comprehensive in scope, is the "stages of change" instrument (also referred to as the transtheoretical model). This popular assessment tool was developed by Prochaska and colleagues (1988; Prochaska & DiClemente, 1992) to help health professionals assess an individual's readiness to change a specific health habit. The specific stages of change are as follows:

1. Precontemplation—no intention to change behavior in the foreseeable future
2. Contemplation—awareness that a problem exists but no commitment to action
3. Preparation—intention to take action in the next month and, typically, unsuccessful action was taken in the past year

4. Action—modification of behavior, experiences, or environment for a period of from 1 day to 6 months in order to overcome a problem
5. Maintenance—an indeterminate period, perhaps a lifetime, in which to prevent relapse

The authors report that relapsing and recycling through the stages of change is the rule rather than the exception, and this process could be viewed as a spiral rather than a linear model. If individuals become more aware of the relapsing phenomenon they might feel less guilt, embarrassment, and discouragement after an unsuccessful attempt. If health professionals become more aware of the relapsing process, they might be more patient with their clients' attempts at change.

Persons who are in the precontemplation stage are, by definition, not ready for action-oriented programs (Prochaska & DiClemente, 1992). A study of 20,000 people found that only 20% of the population is ready to make a specific behavior change (Health Promotion Inter-Change, 1997). So what happens to those who are *not* ready? According to Prochaska and colleagues (1993), they can be helped through the stages by giving them stage-matched messages and support. Precontemplators, for instance, are denied immediate support (justified on the basis of limited personnel resources) and are offered literature in the hope that some day they may be more ready to make a behavior change. Contemplators, however, receive information about the pros and cons involved with changing a behavior, and support to increase confidence and to explore ways to overcome barriers.

Despite the enormous popularity of the stages of change framework, not everyone is a true believer. One analyst reports that the vast majority of studies testing this model are cross-sectional and not longitudinal. As a consequence there have been serious flaws in the assignment of an arbitrary time period to a particular stage, the overlap in the definition of the different stages, and the overpromotion of meager and inconsistent results (Sutton, 2001).

My first reservation with the stages of change framework occurred when I was interviewing several older people in an African American church. They reported to me that they were not interested in exercise and also not interested in joining my soon-to-be-launched church-based exercise program (Looney & Haber, 2001). Had I allowed this initial report of disinterest to result in my labeling them precontemplators, I would have offered them literature and moved on to seek other people who may have been more ready to join my exercise program.

Instead, a few days later I gave a 20-minute demonstration of the exercise program, along with several of my health science students, to a group of older adults who met weekly at that same church. Accompanied by church music, easy banter, humor, and scripture that I read ("to take care of God's temple [the body]" and "above all else, guard your heart for it provides health to a man's whole body)," many people signed up for, and then successfully completed, the 10-week program—including the several alleged precontemplaters!

Another behavioral scientist questioned the ethics of too quickly ignoring the reputed precontemplaters, or postponing interventions with them, when they constitute the sections of the population who have the greatest need. She suggested that this model may lead to discrimination against those who are poor, those less educated, and those who are frail (Whitehead, 1997).

An interesting variation on the stages of change framework is to assess different aspects of a particular behavior change. A team of researchers examined the topic of weight loss, and instead of asking people whether they were ready to make changes leading to weight loss, the researchers asked which changes they were most interested in making. Six aspects of weight loss were targeted: dietary fat, portion control, vegetable intake, fruit intake, increasing physical activity, and planned exercise. The researchers found that respondents may have been precontemplaters in some aspects of weight loss, but they were ready to make a change in others (Logue et al., 2000).

Another strategy is to present older persons with completely different types of potential behavior change goals to choose from. If given sufficiently diverse options, older adults may be more motivated to choose one behavior change that is of high priority to them (Haber, 1996). Here is a partial list of diverse prevention categories that I have presented to older adults, accompanied by a brief and personalized health assessment in each of the categories (Haber, 2001b):

- Complete one of several medical screenings or immunizations
- Increase physical activity level; begin a brisk walking program; join an aerobics, yoga, or tai chi class; start a strength-building program; or begin a flexibility routine
- Decrease dietary fat; implement portion control; increase vegetable or fruit intake; or increase fluid consumption
- Initiate a stress management routine
- Establish a sleep hygiene routine

- Implement a fall prevention or home safety plan
- Join a smoking cessation program
- Enroll in a memory improvement course
- Join one of the peer support groups in the area
- Implement an alcohol-moderation plan.

Among 48 older adults who were presented an array of health promotion options, 44 were willing to select a health goal. Using the technique of a health contract, 75% achieved substantial success with their goal (Haber & Looney, 2000).

## HEALTH CONTRACTS

A health assessment and intervention tool that I use with older adults is a health contract (Figure 4.1)/health calendar (Figure 4.2), which is based on a self-management application of social cognitive theory (Bandura, 1977) that will be examined in more detail later in this chapter.

Self-management refers to clients who, with the help of a health educator, can choose an appropriate behavior change goal and create and implement a plan to accomplish that goal. The statement of the goal and the plan of action can be written into a health contract format. A health contract is alleged to have several advantages over verbal communication alone, especially when the communication tends to be mostly unidirectional, from health professional to client. The alleged advantages of a health contract, which still need additional empirical testing, are that it:

1. is a formal commitment that enhances motivation;
2. clarifies goals and behaviors and makes them explicit;
3. requires the active participation of the client;
4. enhances the therapeutic relationship between provider and client;
5. provides a structured means for involving significant others (family, friends, etc.) in a supportive role;
6. provides a structured means of problem-solving around barriers that previously interfered with the achievement of a goal;
7. provides incentives to reinforce behaviors.

The health contract includes a set of instructions that help older adults state a health goal (see Table 4.1); identify benefits that provide motivation; establish a plan of action that helps the older adult remember to do new behaviors and to elicit social support for them; and identify potential

# Health Contract

My **health goal** is: I will perform an aerobic activity--brisk walking for the most part, but I may substitute dancing by myself at home. I will do it 3 days per week, for at least 20 minutes per day, and on 2 days I will complete a 10 minute strength-building session for the first two weeks of the contract. During the second two weeks I will increase the aerobics to 4 days and 30 minutes, and the strength building to 15-20 minutes.

My motivation for my health goal is:

1. to increase my energy level
2. to help me maintain my weight

## My Plan of Action

For social or emotional **support** I will... Share my health goal with my son and my daughter, and ask each of them to check up on me and ask me about my progress each week. I will also share my goal with my pastor and ask him if he would inquire about my progress on a periodic basis. I will call my friend, Sandy, and share with her each time I successfully do my exercise routine. After two weeks of success, I will also ask Sandy to join me in my exercise routine.

To **remind** me of new behaviors I will... Attach my health calendar to the refrigerator. I will also write my exercise activities into my appointment book. I will attempt to set up a regular routine, such as exercise just before the dinner hour. For the next month, I will keep my walking sneakers by the front door as a reminder.

**Problems** that may interfere with reaching my health goal and **solutions**:

Fatigue is my primary problem. If I find myself too tired before dinner I will consider moving my scheduled exercise time to first thing in the morning. I will also remind myself that a regular exercise routine is invigorating and that over the long run fatigue should become less of a problem.

Motivation is also a problem. My son Stephen should be particularly helpful in this area, especially if I remind him how much help he is to me in this area. I may also have to ask Stephen to write me into his schedule so he does not forget to call with encouragement. I also find gospel music very motivating, and I will put on my headset about the time I plan on exercising.

My husband's health can be a major distraction. I become stressed about his health and then I forget to take care of my own. I will implement a daily routine of deep breathing as a preventive measure for keeping my worrying under control.

Negative thoughts, like dwelling on my past failures to sustain exercise, can be a barrier as well. I will make a conscious effort to correct my negative thinking as soon as I become aware of it, and substitute a positive phrase, like: I can do it.

| | |
|---|---|
| *John Brown* | *Jane Smith*  4/1/03 |
| My support person's **signature** | My signature  and date |

FIGURE 4.1  Health contract.

Fill in activities and make a ✓ on each day you complete them.

**Month:** November, 2003

Backup plan: I will participate in Sunday morning mall walking for back-up exercise session.

| Sunday | Monday | Tuesday | Wednesday | Thursday | Friday | Saturday | *Weekly Success* #days completed/ #days contracted |
|---|---|---|---|---|---|---|---|
| | | | | | | 1 | |
| 2 | 3 Aerobics/S-B  20/10-minutes | 4 | 5 | 6 Aerobics/S-B  20/10-minutes | 7 | 8 Aerobics  20 minutes | 3/2 |
| 9 | 10 Aerobics/S-B  20/10-minutes | 11  call / assess | 12 | 13 Aerobics/S-B  20/10-minutes | 14 | 15 Aerobics  20 minutes | 3/2 |
| 16 | 17 Aerobics  30 minutes | 18 Aerobics/S-B  30/15-minutes | 19 | 20 Aerobics/S-B  30/15-minutes | 21 | 22 Aerobics  30 minutes | 4/2 |
| 23 | 24 Aerobics  30 minutes | 25 Aerobics/S-B  30/20-minutes | 26 | 27 Aerobics/S-B  30/20-minutes | 28 | 29 Aerobics  30 minutes | 4/2 |
| 30 | 1 Assessment | | | | | | |

**FIGURE 4.2  Health calendar.**

## TABLE 4.1 Health Contract Directions for Exercise

**Exercise Motivation:** Review "Motivation" handouts. Help client choose "function" and "disease prevention" motivations, and record up to three of these motivations on the health contract.

Clients may also want to write down one motivation and keep it in their wallet, or post it in a conspicuous place. Or clients may want to state the motivation out loud on a daily basis. (This may be included under problem/solutions, for bolstering motivation).

**Exercise Modality:** Review "Exercise Modality" handouts. Help client choose an exercise modality before working on the health goal. (Community exercise programs, aerobic movement options, walking alternatives, increasing physical activity, strength-building, flexibility and balance).

**Exercise Baseline:** If client is sedentary, set a minimum goal; if client is not sedentary, assess the baseline. Review last week for exercise/physical activity frequency, duration, and intensity. If last week was not typical, substitute a typical week.

Frequency and duration should be assessed by number of days per week and total minutes each day. Intensity should be assessed by asking the client about body warmth and breathing rate during each specific session of exercise/physical activity.

Aim for a goal of slightly above baseline for the first week, gradually increase over the remaining weeks, and reach modest goal that was set for the last week of the month.

**Health goal:** Write a specific statement about what the client will do by the end of the first month, and consider including how often (# days/week); how much (duration/day); how intense (light/medium); where; when.

The goal should be modest and measurable, not more than 5 days a week, half-hour a day, one unit over baseline for the first week, with week-by-week gradations until the health goal is reached during the last week of the first month. Client may choose to exceed these parameters, but not as part of the stated health goal.

Reassess the health goal at the end of the first week. Determine then whether the health educator will contact client during the remaining part of the first month. Set a day and time to meet at the end of the first month and record on health calendar.

**Plan of Action:** *Social Support:* See "Social Support Possibilities" handout. Clients should select socially supportive people from the list of categories, select the ways that they want support to be given, and determine frequency of support.

*(continued)*

**TABLE 4.1   Health Contract Directions for Exercise** *(continued)*

*Reminders:* Attach health contract to the refrigerator. Have friend or family member call with reminder. Associate new behaviors with an established habit, like engaging in brisk walking just before dinner. Keep exercise reading materials visible around the house. Keep workout shoes by the door. Exercise at the same time each day. Hang a picture on the wall that shows the client or others exercising.

**Problems/Solutions:** Consider previous problems that arose when similar goals were set in the past, or anticipate new problems that might arise in the future.

*Positive*—A solution for the negative thinker is to deliberately verbalize positive thoughts about achieving the health goal on a daily basis. The positive thought can also be written on paper and read, e.g., "I am confident of success, though not perfection."

*Reinforcement*—Seek praise: swallow modesty and tell people about successes and solicit additional praise from them. Seek internal motivation: pay attention to the signs of feeling better. Seek external motivation: buy theatre tickets, or another nonedible treat if success is achieved at the end of a week or a month.

*Environmental support*—Alter immediate surroundings. Place walking sneakers by the front door, distribute exercise reading material around the house, place exercise band on the coffee table, have pictures of healthy people exercising on the wall.

*Stress management*—Stress can sidetrack person from their goal. To manage stress, consider some of the following options: deep breathing, muscle relaxation, meditation, prayer, music, playing with a pet, taking a walk, or doing whatever the client usually does to relieve stress. Schedule these things on a regular basis.

*Problem Solve*—Brainstorm about problems that arose from past attempts at behavior change. Brainstorm about problems that might arise in the future. Find solutions. Record under Problems/Solutions.

**Signatures:** The client signs the contract, along with someone who will be offering support to them and is willing to sign the contract as well. If no one comes to mind, the health educator should sign it.

**Health Calendar:** Follow directions for recording activities on the health calendar.

problems to achieving the health goal and encourage solutions to overcome these barriers. The contract is signed by the older adult and a support person. Progress is typically assessed after 1 week, and the success of the contract is reviewed at the end of a month.

The health contract directions refer to exercise handouts. If you are interested in obtaining copies of some of these handouts, please write your request to me at: David Haber, Ball State University, Fisher Institute for Wellness and Gerontology, Muncie, Indiana 47306.

Health contracts have been applied with varying degrees of success to a wide variety of behaviors, such as drug use, smoking, alcohol abuse, nutrition, and exercise (Berry et al., 1989: Jette et al., 1999; Leslie & Schuster, 1991; Lorig et al., 1996; Neale et al., 1990). A cardiac rehabilitation program in Canada reported that participants who signed health contracts adhered to their 6-month program more faithfully (65%) than did members of a control group (42%) or people who were asked to sign an agreement but did not (20%) (Oldridge & Jones, 1983).

Another study of health contracts came to a predictable conclusion: specific goals and ongoing feedback led to higher client performance than did vague goals and inconsistent feedback (Latham & Locke, 1991). Other studies have been less predictable. Clients who selected their own health goals, for instance, were not more successful than those who had health goals set by their health providers (Alexy, 1985).

Research on health contracts, however, is often marred by a lack of random assignment to treatment and control groups, small sample sizes, and lack of replication (Janz et al., 1984). When a study is replicated, the results may be inconsistent, as was the case with studies that compared health contracts that used external versus internal incentives (Strecher et al., 1995).

In addition, there are several uncertainties about the effectiveness of health contracts in terms of ability to identify which components work better than others (e.g., health education, social support, the professional-client relationship, memory enhancement, motivation building, contingency rewards, etc.); whether contracts work better with one type of person than another; and determining the content and amount of training that is required for health educators or clinicians to administer health contracts effectively.

Even without a definitive body of research, health contracts are widely used. They are simple to administer, time-efficient, and even cost-effective when medical personnel assign the completion of health contracts to a health educator or trained office worker.

## PRECEDE

The PRECEDE framework (Green & Kreuter, 1999) offers a conceptual guideline that can also be used for assessing the readiness of adults to change or maintain a health behavior. PRECEDE is an acronym (perhaps the worst one, in terms of being convoluted, in the history of health education) for *pre*disposing, *re*inforcing, and *e*nabling *c*onstructs in *e*ducational/*e*cological *d*iagnosis and *e*valuation.

*Predisposing* factors are the knowledge, attitudes, and beliefs a person holds about a health behavior. For instance, if an older woman believes exercise will aggravate her arthritis or cause her unnecessary fatigue, exhortation to exercise will be difficult. Because older adults, especially minority older adults or those over age 80, frequently have lower formal educational levels than adults in general and may be prone to act on less information or on misinformation, it is necessary that health professionals ascertain the barriers to changing health behaviors.

Oftentimes it is not necessary to change a belief, just to add a new one. If older persons believe, for example, that God will take care of their health, the health professional can agree with this assertion and then simply add Sophocles' declaration, "Heaven never helps the man who will not act" (Lorig, 1992).

Predisposing factors can be determined by finding out what the clients know about the health area of concern, whether they believe they have a problem, whether they have cultural habits that need to be taken into consideration, and whether they believe behavior changes will help. Older adults, for instance, may believe (or espouse) that because of their age, it is too late to change or to do themselves any good. It may be helpful to respond with specific data on how rapidly health improvements can take place after the age of 65. A significant number of older adults may believe they get all the exercise they need when, according to indicators of exercise frequency, intensity, and duration, they actually do not.

*Enabling* factors are those resources necessary for engaging in health-related activities, specifically, access and skill level. Before making recommendations to clients, health professionals need to determine whether there are appropriate programs with experienced leaders who are trained to work with older adults, whether these programs are accessible to those with limited transportation and financial means, whether clients have the necessary skills for modifying their behavior, whether recommended materials needed by older adults are affordable and available, and whether older adults perceive their environment to be safe enough to implement a program.

Practitioners need to be resourceful; it may be necessary to help older adults find accessible programs or gain necessary skills. It is also important that health professionals facilitate ways in which older persons can help themselves, rather than solve problems for clients and thereby foster dependency.

*Reinforcing* factors refer to the peers, significant others, and health professionals who can support the continuation of new health behaviors. Older adults may be widowed, uninvolved in former occupational groups, and relatively isolated from other persons who are interested in maintaining health. Practitioners ought to consider whether their clients have sufficient family, peer and professional support to reinforce health behavior changes.

It is best that clients have more than one source of support rather than overburden a single person. A team approach can be useful. Supportive spouses of clients, for instance, can attend a health program with an older adult. Receptionists in the offices of health professionals can play supportive, follow-up roles for clients attempting to change health behaviors. Many health professionals believe they are too busy to be involved in health education, but there are time-efficient strategies that can allow them to play a role.

Green and Kreuter (1999) added an additional step called PROCEED to their PRECEDE model. PROCEED stands for *p*olicy, *r*egulatory, and *o*rganizational *c*onstructs in *e*ducational and *e*nvironmental *d*evelopment. This follow-up step shifts the focus from assessment (the PRECEDE portion of the model) to implementation and evaluation.

## TEN TIPS FOR CHANGING HEALTH BEHAVIORS

After years of working with health science students to help older adults change health behaviors, it would be outstanding if I could offer the reader a simple formula for increasing the probability of success. Unfortunately, I fall victim to the "kitchen sink" syndrome that I think also afflicts the PRECEDE model just described. There are many factors that can influence the success or failure of an individual's attempt to change a health behavior, and research has not helped us much to understand which factors are more important for which types of people.

Over the years, therefore, I have developed my own framework for helping older adults make a desired health behavior change. "Model" is too sophisticated a word to describe this framework, so I refer to it as the Ten Tips approach. With each older client willing to attempt a behavior change, a review of the Ten Tips is likely to produce strategies that will help the person be successful. From personal experience, rather than research, (I am currently working on a project to assess these ten tips) I believe this approach will be helpful. And if you examine the health contract/calendar technique that was previously summarized, along with the directions for completing it, you will notice that the ten tips are incorporated into this technique.

In order to make these ideas more practical, I will focus on the specific goal of increasing exercise or physical activity. This also happens to be the health goal most likely to be chosen by older adults when given a choice among many (Elder et al., 1995; Haber & Looney, 2000).

If you work with older adults to change a health behavior and want to commit these Ten Tips to memory, it may be helpful to note that the first four start with the letter M, the next five form the acronym PRESS, and the tenth one is a P.S., as in a postscript for a letter you are writing.

1. Motivation
2. Modest
3. Measurable
4. Memory
5. Positive thoughts
6. Reinforcement
7. Environmental support
8. Stress management
9. Social support
10. Problem-solve

1. *Motivation.* It is obvious that a person must be motivated to change a health behavior. I have found, however, that the first motivation identified by an older adult is not necessarily the one that lights up their eyes with authenticity. If someone is contemplating a reason for overcoming their sedentary ways, they may first come up with a politically correct motivation that elicits the approval of others, including the health educator they may be working with, rather than one that is genuinely felt.

For instance, avoiding heart disease may truly be the most motivating reason for someone to take on the challenge of a new exercise routine. Or it may not be. With a little probing on the part of the health educator, it may come to light that the person is more passionate about seeking better sleeping habits, or achieving regularity in bowel habits, or increasing energy in order to play longer with the grandchildren. It is best to spend a sufficient amount of time discussing what motivates the client and to examine their facial expressions for clues to its importance.

To help in this regard, I present the client with a list of possible motivations to choose from. This list includes disease categories that the client may want to avoid or alleviate, such as arthritis, stroke, obesity, hypertension, heart disease, peripheral vascular disease, diabetes, osteoporosis, colon cancer, and depression; and areas of potential function improvement, such as constipation, forgetfulness, low energy, sleeplessness, stress management, imbalance, muscle weakness, stiffness, and fall prevention. Once you feel confident that the primary motivation has been identified, write it down (on the health contract if that is the technique of choice), and encourage clients to remind themselves about their motivation on a regular basis.

Also, discover the mode of exercise that motivates best. Is it brisk walking, joining an exercise class, increasing physical activity, or something else they are likely to persist with? Motivation is enhanced by enjoying the intervention, or at least by avoiding the more burdensome options. Other sources of motivation, like finding social support, are included among the remaining tips.

2. *Modest.* No one is ever disappointed if they exceed the goal they have established. And everyone who does not accomplish a desired goal is disappointed. Nonetheless, it is a rare event when an older adult initially declares a goal that is modest enough to elicit the confidence of the health educator that it can be achieved or exceeded. It is common, for instance, for someone to state a goal of exercising every day. It is important, however, to make that daily goal more modest. If a client sets the goal at four times a week and meets or exceeds that goal, motivation will be sustained. But if the goal is set as an every day event, the client then may view exercising on only 4 days that week as a failure and the motivation to continue may be compromised. As a general rule, I limit stated health goals to a maximum of 5 days a week.

If the person establishes 60 minutes of walking a day as the goal, reduce it by half and give "extra credit" (perhaps in the form of more praise) for exceeding that goal. Moreover, encourage the sedentary client to build up to the 30-minute goal by establishing a target of 10-minute sessions for the first week, 20 minutes for the second week, and 30 minutes for the third and fourth week. Also, allow the client to accumulate 30 minutes a day, rather than limit them to only one option of 30 consecutive minutes.

The opposite problem can also reduce motivation: setting a goal that is too easy and then losing interest in it. This is an unusual occurrence in my experience, especially if the person has identified the appropriate motivation. Once you understand what motivates clients, help them modify their goal during the first month so that it is neither grandiose nor timid.

Finally, a modest goal is short-term. I have had success with the 1-month time period, hence the contract/calendar. One month does not extend too far into the future, and with the use of the monthly calendar, the end is in sight. It is also a long enough period of time to allow for an adjustment of the goal, or the behaviors to achieve the goal, in the first week or two in order to increase the likelihood of achieving success. Even if the 1-month goal turns out to be less motivating than was initially thought, the client may still have a good chance of successfully completing it and carrying over that confidence to another, more motivating health goal the following month.

3. *Measurable.* Measurability has several components to it. How much will the older adult be doing, that is, how many minutes of walking and on how many days of the week? How intensely will the person be doing it, that is, will they establish a brisk walking pace that is twice the pace of their normal walking? Will they monitor their breathing, making sure that they achieve sufficient intensity to produce deep breathing, but not too much intensity that makes talking while walking difficult? Over how long a period of time will they be doing it?

If the client is doing strength building, how many exercises will they be doing, how many repetitions in each set, how many sets, how much poundage or what level of elastic band thickness, and how many days each week?

Measurability also implies record keeping, another reason why the contract/calendar is appealing. People are used to recording on their calendars the activities that they need reminding of. I encourage clients to measure and compare the number of days they actually complete the contracted behavior each week with the number of days they had contracted. Monitoring weekly success can lead to greater confidence, or to the need to revise the health goal.

4. *Memory.* Habits take up a large part of the day. We give little thought to many of the activities that constitute our daily routine, and at the same time we rarely forget them. How do we convert a new behavior, one that is a bit challenging to adopt, and make it a new habit? The answer is by enhancing our memory in as many ways as possible.

What cues can be established to help remind us? Do we need to place our walking shoes by the front door? Should we place the health contract on the refrigerator door? Can we ask a family member or a friend to remind us, or perhaps monitor how well we are remembering to do the new behavior? Can we associate the new behavior with an established one, like walking before dinner every night (perhaps supplementing this associative behavior with a well-placed cue—a note near the dinner table, "Did you walk yet?").

5. *Positive thoughts.* Substitute positive and hopeful thoughts for negative, self-defeating ones. For each negative thought like "I've never been able to maintain exercise routines before," substitute a positive argument: "It may be difficult, but this time I will persist and accomplish my goal." It may be helpful to record affirmations and place them in conspicuous locations. Other avenues of positive support are to find books or magazines that inspire the client, encourage them to associate with persons who model what they are attempting to accomplish, and to seek friends or acquaintances who are willing to be supportive of their goal.

For those who like irony and want to try negative reinforcement to promote positive thinking, keep a rubber band unobtrusively around your wrist, and when a negative thought about the health goal occurs, snap the band and replace the negative thought with a positive one.

6. *Reinforcement.* Most psychologists rely on positive reinforcement rather than negative reinforcement. If successful at the end of the first week, for instance, encourage clients to treat themselves to a movie or purchase a book. If successful at the end of the month, encourage them to buy theater tickets. Reinforcements tend to be more effective when they are in close proximity to the achievement being rewarded.

External reinforcement does not necessarily involve spending money. Praise can be an important reinforcement. Encourage the client to speak highly of themselves when they are doing well with their goal, and ask them to be a bit immodest in their solicitation of praise from others. External incentives are helpful to some people and not to others. If the motivation to achieve a goal is strong, the successful behaviors themselves may be sufficiently rewarding. External incentives may, in fact, distract from identifying internal rewards.

Though most psychologists prefer positive reinforcement to negative reinforcement, I heard of a diabolically clever form of punishment that I will pass along. Identify an issue about which a person feels strongly (e.g., euthanasia) and then have the client make out several small checks to an organization that promotes a belief *contrary* to their own. When punishments are to be administered, the checks are mailed to the offending organization by someone other than the client.

7. *Environmental support.* Another term for environmental support is *stimulus control.* The best example of it applies to weight management. If you want to contribute to weight maintenance or loss, make sure that the client does not keep junk food in their house.

Exercisers, however, also have options in this regard. Placing sneakers by the front door is an example of environmental support. Hanging pictures on the walls of older adults exercising is another example.

Distribute reading materials around the house that can be easily accessed and boost motivational levels. Place the stair-stepper in front of the television set to encourage its use. Keep the elastic exercise band on the coffee table as a visible reminder to use it. These are examples of creating a supportive environment, or controlling stimulus, to elicit a more favorable response.

8. *Stress management.* It is the rare person who does not feel stress these days. Not only do we live in a fast-paced society, we are also likely to contend with an automobile driver who is experiencing road rage, cope with a physical disability that frustrates us, struggle with an interpersonal loss, or encounter countless other hassles and annoyances, big and small. Stress is a common barrier to achieving a health goal. If possible, therefore, build into the plan of action a few stress management techniques that can be practiced on a preventive basis, preferably daily.

My favorite stress management technique is deep breathing. I combine that with an everyday occurrence, and stressor for me, driving—typically done too fast and too aggressively. (It's hereditary, as I was born into a family of fast-driving New Yorkers). Every time I am driving a car, therefore, I prompt myself to take periodic deep breaths. This not only helps me control my stress but has a wonderful side effect—I am much more likely to drive sanely.

9. *Social support.* This tip is next-to-last, but definitely not next-to-least in importance. I suggest some thought be given to social support for every client. For most older adults, social support is desirable; for some it may be essential. It may be a good idea to build social support into the statement of the health goal itself.

Ideally, a person has multiple sources of social support. In addition to a health educator's being supportive, a spouse or friend can help out in some designated way that is specified in a health contract. If possible, have the client inform their physician or another relevant clinician who may then provide advice and perhaps even emotional support. A pastor might be notified by your client that they are attempting to improve their health, and offer periodic encouragement and support. If not objectionable to the client, have them announce their health goal to others in general, such as acquaintances and neighbors, in order to increase the chance that additional people will offer support and approval.

Clients who unexpectedly find the social support of a spouse or friend inconvenient (they do not always want to walk when I want to walk), unreliable (they do not always show up), or overly critical, will need to seek other sources of social support. Clients who have a physician who does not muster enthusiasm for their health goal may at least consider the prospect of finding another more health-oriented health care professional. Clients needing more social support than is currently available to them may need to explore the option of joining a class in the community.

Community classes that have a leader of the same age and perhaps gender may provide a role model for the older client. Fellow classmates who are also peers in age, gender, disability, or other relevant variables may also provide extra social and emotional support for behavior change and maintenance.

And, yes, there are clients who do not want social support. It is not essential to employ any of the Ten Tips, but a consideration of each is likely to be helpful.

10. *Problem-solve.* Finally, chances are good that you have tried to achieve this exercise goal or a similar one before. It typically takes multiple efforts to achieve a goal. What went wrong and what might go wrong in the future? Spend a little time identifying likely barriers, and ways to overcome them. It may turn out that problems are likely to be solved by addressing some of the previous nine tips. Or the client may have to develop their own additional tip.

An example of a problem to be solved is the older adult who likes to walk briskly outside—but not in the rain, and who lives in Seattle. This person, of course, needs a back-up plan if she does not like to get wet. The plan may include walking in a shopping mall, turning on music and substituting dancing by herself in the living room, or dragging out the vacuum cleaner and doing an energetic sweeping of the entire house.

Another problem—quite common among older adults based on a study of mine in progress—involves working around aches, pains, and fatigue. The solution may be to modify the exercise or to alter the time it is to be performed. The challenge is to identify problems from the past, imagine possible problems in the future, brainstorm solutions, and increase the chances of success.

## HEALTH BEHAVIOR THEORIES

Theories can help us understand what influences health behaviors, and based on these ideas, help us plan effective interventions. Theories may focus on different levels (e.g., psychological, social, institutional, or community) and are subject to change based on new evidence. They may also be applied singly or in combination in order to address behavior change challenges.

A few well-known behavior change theories, along with models and concepts, will be presented to the reader after three brief definitions. A *theory* of behavior change attempts to explain the processes underlying learning. A *model* draws on a number of theories to help people understand a problem. A *concept* is the primary element of a theory.

## BEHAVIORAL AND COGNITIVE MANAGEMENT

Operant conditioning, B. F. Skinner's (1953) model of behavior control, is based on the premise that behavior is determined by its consequences, that is, the kinds of rewards and punishments that follow behavior. Behaviors followed by rewards will increase in frequency, whereas behaviors followed by punishments will decline.

Operant conditioning has spawned a number of principles. Immediate rewards and punishments are much more effective than delayed ones. Intermittent reinforcement is more resistant to extinction than constant reinforcement. And careful observation of conditions that promote or discourage behavior can help shape behavior by altering those conditions.

Cognitive conditioning, unlike operant conditioning that focuses on external behaviors, deals with internal changes in thoughts and feelings. Cognitive conditioning advocates assert that behavior and feelings are influenced not by their consequences but by antecedent thoughts.

The first step toward cognitive restructuring, therefore, is the identification of undesirable and unrealistic thoughts. The next step is the substitution and regular repetition of positive thoughts in order to shape future affect and behavior. Having positively restructured our thoughts, we engage in fewer cognitive distortions, experience less emotional distress, and perform fewer maladaptive behaviors (Burns, 1980).

Because behavior and cognitive conditioning are practiced universally, they do not appear to constitute a formal learning model. All of us use praise and punishment to influence the behavior of others as well as ourselves, and we often substitute positive thoughts for negative ones, leading us to question why these techniques are labeled learning models. Unlike informal methods for influencing others or ourselves, however, formal behavioral and cognitive management techniques are applied systematically. This systematic application of management techniques to behavior change includes:

1. *Clear definition of the problem.* A need to exercise is vague. To be able to climb the steps in one's home without having to stop to rest is clear.

2. *Implementation of a systematic and measurable response to the problem.* To exercise as often as possible is also vague. To exercise three times a week, 30 minutes at a time, and periodically assess perceived exertion is both systematic and measurable.
3. *Scheduled evaluations.* To feel we are making progress is vague. To assess the effectiveness of our plan on a weekly or monthly basis and alter our plan of action or our health goal as necessary is explicit.

## HEALTHY PLEASURES

In contrast to the behavior and cognitive management theories that are based on structure and self-discipline, there is the theory of healthy pleasures. Advocates of this theory propose that healthy behaviors will be sustained when these behaviors are based on joy, intuition, and self-trust. Some advocates suggest that a growing reliance on one's own ability to listen to the body's internal cues for feeling good can replace behavior-change decisions based on scientific guidelines (Field & Steinhardt, 1992). For additional ideas, read *Healthy Pleasures* (Ornstein & Sobel, 1989).

My own bias is that awareness and management techniques are not an either/or proposition. Joyful and intuitive activities may be appreciated in their spontaneous form, or they can be converted into healthy routines. Self-disciplined routines can be enjoyable and effective, or they can evolve into stale and counterproductive activity. It is not a question of choosing between awareness and management strategies—both are important.

Self-monitoring can be viewed as a strategy that is a cross between increasing internal awareness and a disciplined and systematic management technique. Self-monitoring is the process of systematically observing one's own pattern of behavior for a specific period of time, without an effort to control this pattern of behavior.

One example of self-monitoring is to keep a written record, or diary, of everything you eat and drink. During a 3-day period (including a weekend day if your weekend eating pattern differs from that of weekdays), record what you eat, how much you eat, the time of day, the location, your companions, and how you feel when you are eating. Make no effort to control this pattern of behavior, and make no effort to *not* control it. Just be aware of what you are doing, how you are feeling, and record it.

When you carefully observe your eating behaviors, you not only increase your awareness of what triggers unhealthy eating patterns but you also often begin to modify them as part of the monitoring process.

You might realize through self-monitoring that you eat automatically, and in greater quantity, in front of the television set or when you socialize in certain settings—even when you are not hungry.

## SOCIAL COGNITIVE THEORY

Several researchers have endorsed a broad learning perspective, referred to as social cognitive theory (Bandura, 1977, 1997; Rodin, 1986; Rotter, 1954), that addresses both the psychosocial dynamics underlying health behavior and the methods of promoting behavior change. This perspective actually encompasses a wide range of learning theories that include operant and cognitive conditioning, modeling, guided mastery of tasks on a step-by-step basis, verbal persuasion, social support, self-efficacy, health locus of control, and personal control.

Role-modeling is an important component of social learning theory. Modeling is most effective when the role model shares many characteristics with the participant (e.g., age, physical impairment, sex, ethnicity, and socioeconomic status). Professional leaders of health education classes who are not role models in this sense should consider sharing teaching with, and deferring problem-solving to, class members who are.

McAuley and Courneya (1993) suggest that role-modeling with older program participants "may be particularly salient. In such cases it is common to look to other people, especially those that bear similar physical characteristics to ourselves, for motivation and information regarding our own prospects of success" (p. 73).

Persuasion is another social cognitive strategy, one that is probably more popular than effective (Lorig, 1992). Persuasion is most effective when health providers and educators ensure that it is accompanied by realistic goals and includes opportunities for guided mastery of tasks on a step-by-step basis. It is also important that messages are positive and direct (You can do it, not try and do it) and delivered by a respected source.

Social cognitive theory is also likely to be more effective when its ideas are applied through several strategies, rather than the application of a single technique (USPSTF, 1996).

## SELF-EFFICACY

Self-efficacy may be the most widely utilized and tested concept in social cognitive theory. It is a belief in one's capabilities to implement a course of action. Self-efficacy is synonymous with having confidence about behavior change or maintenance within a specific behavioral domain (Bandura, 1997). It is fostered by guided mastery, modeling, and persuasion.

*Guided mastery* involves learning and practicing appropriate behaviors through the assignment of small, graded tasks that are accomplished in a short period of time. *Modeling* refers to teaching and leadership responsibilities by persons who are as much as possible like the clients being taught in terms of age, race, gender, and physical limitations. *Persuasion* focuses on identifying the risk, the intervention to reduce the risk, and convincing the client that they can successfully engage in the intervention.

Self-efficacy is often predictive of health behaviors, especially in regard to sustaining behavior change (McAuley, 1993). One researcher concluded that "self-efficacy affects the amount of effort devoted to a task, and the length of persistence when difficulties are encountered" (O'Leary, 1985).

Self-efficacy can be manipulated experimentally with success. In one study, psychological tests were administered to a group of volunteers in a smoking cessation program. Half the subjects were then randomly assigned to a treatment group and told that in their tests they had demonstrated great potential to quit smoking. The other half were told the truth, that they had been *randomly* assigned to a control group. Fourteen months after treatment, smoking frequency had been reduced by 67% among the efficacy-enhanced group, and by 35% among the control group (Blittner et al., 1978).

After reviewing the literature McAuley and Courneya (1993) concluded "If practitioners and clinicians fail to organize, present, and develop their programs in such a way as to cultivate efficacy beliefs, participants are likely to perceive the activity negatively, become disenchanted, discouraged, and discontinue. On the other hand, adequately organizing [programs] in a manner such that a strong sense of personal efficacy is promoted will result in the individual displaying more positive affect, evaluating their self-worth more positively, embracing more challenging activities, putting forth more effort, and persisting longer. In short, they will be in a position to successfully self-regulate their behavior" (p. 72).

An increasing number of researchers believe that the relationship between self-efficacy and behaviors is interactive, not unidirectional (Goldsteen et al., 1991; Lorig et al., 1989; McAuley, 1994). Just as enhancing self-efficacy beliefs may increase the likelihood of sustaining a new health behavior, ongoing adherence to a new health behavior may continue to increase self-efficacy.

Several cautionary notes emerge from research findings. Bandura (1997) reports that behavior change and maintenance are also a function of outcome expectations. Enhancing your belief about your ability to behave in a particular way (self-efficacy) needs to be supplemented by the belief that your performance will lead to a desired outcome (outcome expectancy).

*Extreme* optimism regarding one's self-efficacy may relate *inversely* to successful performance (Rakowski et al., 1991). Also, self-efficacy is limited to an individual's belief in a specific, not a general, ability. For example, people may perceive themselves to possess the self-efficacy to implement a walking program but not to follow through on a diet. Self-efficacy in one area of behavior does not generalize to another.

Also, the perceived ability to change a health habit or adopt a new health behavior does not guarantee that a person has the necessary skill level, role model, peer or professional support, or access that might be required. Self-efficacy may be a necessary but not a sufficient condition for clients attempting to improve a health behavior.

Self-efficacy is an important part of the Arthritis Self-Help (ASH) course (Lorig et al., 1989) developed at Stanford University in 1978 by Kate Lorig, a nurse and health educator, and physicians Halsted Homan and James Fries. More than 100,000 persons with arthritis have completed the ASH course, usually in groups of 15 individuals or less, and typically led by nonprofessionals who have arthritis. During the 12-hour program, students are taught about arthritis and about how to design an exercise program, manage pain through relaxation techniques, improve nutrition, fight depression and fatigue, and communicate more effectively with physicians.

Participants who complete the program report, in general, about a 15% to 20% reduction in pain, are more active, and visit a physician less frequently. Among those who are depressed when starting the program, fewer depressive symptoms are reported by the end of the program.

The researchers were surprised to find that while changes in behavior, such as exercise and stress management, occurred as a consequence of the program, the factor most closely linked to outcomes (improvements in pain control, depression management, and activity level) was an increase in self-efficacy. In one group of successful patients, self-efficacy was still 17% higher 4 years after they completed the course (Lorig et al., 1989).

## HEALTH LOCUS OF CONTROL

Health locus of control (Wallston & Wallston, 1982) refers to the idea that an individual's health can be controlled through that person's ability to control his or her behavior (i.e., internal locus) or by external forces (i.e., powerful others or luck).

One's health locus of control orientation, similar to perceived self-efficacy, is of limited utility when individuals do not place much value on their health (Lau, 1988; Wallston & Wallston, 1982). Also, medical practices and outcomes, unlike health practices, may not be within one's sphere of influence (Sechrist, 1983). Therefore, it is important that health professionals who encourage their clients to take personal responsibility for their health practices discourage them from overestimating their personal control over medical events.

It may be necessary to help clients differentiate between the realistic goals—increasing energy, reducing stress, enhancing feelings of well-being, and increasing knowledge and decision-making ability—and the less realistic goal of staving off a deteriorating medical condition. Research in the future, however, may suggest that even mortality may be influenced by behavioral interventions.

Spiegel and colleagues' (1989) 10-year follow-up study of metastasized breast cancer patients, for instance, reported that patients who participated in supportive therapy groups lived twice as long as those who did not. (A review of subsequent and conflicting studies in this area will be provided in chapter 11 on Mental Health). Also, nursing home residents who were able to exert control over their environment lived twice as long as those who were given assistance without responsibilities (Rodin & Langer, 1977).

As people move from adulthood to old age, their belief in self-efficacy may increase in specific areas (Sarafino, 1990), perhaps because experience has taught them what they can and cannot do. Their belief in health locus of control, on the other hand, may become more external with age (Lachman, 1986). Older patients are more likely than younger ones, for instance, to prefer that health professionals make health-related decisions for them (Haug, 1979; Woodward & Wallston, 1987).

This increased externality among older adults, however, may be due to *cohort factors* such as a) the cultural orientation of specific older cohorts who believe in an authoritarian health professional role, or b) the lower education levels of the oldest cohorts, which lead to their reluctance to engage with health professionals in a dialogue they might not understand.

Increasing externality with age, on the other hand, may be due to *maturational factors.* For example, the increased physical vulnerability that occurs with age may, over time, discourage an individual's sense of personal control. And yet an external health locus of control may correlate with a positive attitude toward the future. A belief in powerful others, like physicians, who can influence the course of an illness, may lead older patients to become more hopeful about the future (Marks et al., 1986).

On the other hand, older adults with an internal health locus of control may be more sanguine about the future. Older adults may not believe they can control the outcome of their disease states, but they may feel hopeful that they can affect other aspects of their future, such as the ability to control their perception of stress or the ability to acquire the information they need to cope as well as possible with health problems (Wallston & Wallston, 1982).

Information seeking does not necessarily lead to better adjustment. Information about an illness can raise, as well as lower, anxiety. When combined with the adoption of a relaxation technique, however, information seeking may lead to a more desirable outcome (S. Taylor et al., 1984).

One interesting study matched subjects by their health locus of control profiles. Internals in self-directed programs and externals in peer support groups were more satisfied and lost more weight than nonmatched subjects (B. Wallston et al., 1976). Unfortunately, another possible, perhaps more powerful, explanation was not examined—that combining *both* internal and external sources of support may lead to better perceptions and results.

The success of Alcoholics Anonymous (AA) may be attributable to its reliance on both internal and external sources of control. On the one hand, AA members must take responsibility for their problem; on the other hand, they are required to acknowledge their inability to control alcoholism without the help of a higher power and the other members of AA (Strecher et al., 1986).

Related to the study of locus of control is the topic of personal control. Two classic studies in personal control reveal that seemingly simple or minor opportunities to control events can affect both physical and mental health. In one study, the residents of two floors of a nursing home were given responsibility for such activities as taking care of a plant, deciding on when to see a movie, and rearranging furniture. The residents of the other two floors were also the beneficiaries of a plant, weekly movie, and furniture, but were given no control over these activities; the staff took care of the plants, decided when the movie would be shown, and rearranged the furniture.

Despite the fact that the residents were similar in physical health, mental health, and prior socioeconomic status, the residents with personal control were physically and mentally healthier, and 18 months later only 15% of those with enhanced control had died, versus 30% of those without (Langer & Rodin, 1976, Rodin & Langer, 1977).

Schulz's (1976) experiment with residents of a retirement home revealed that student visits to residents led to more active, happier lives among the residents. However, unlike the nursing home experiments of

Langer and Rodin (1976) in which personal control opportunities for residents were on a continuing basis, the removal of the students from the retirement home precipitated a significant decline in health.

The rationale underlying perceived control is that control over decisions and actions will more likely produce desirable outcomes. Studies show that perceived control is associated with reduced stress, increased motivation, improved health, and enhanced performance (McAuley, 1994; Peterson & Stunkard, 1989). Perceived control, however, can have negative effects under specified conditions: when perceived control or confidence exists without sufficient information or skill to support a positive outcome; when excessive demands are made on a person's time, effort, and resources; and when individuals erroneously accept responsibility and blame for health problems, regardless of origin (Rodin, 1986).

## HEALTH BELIEF MODEL

One model of health behavior change focuses on perceived threats, benefits, and barriers. The health belief model, developed during the 1950s to explain why people did not participate in free tuberculosis screenings and other prevention programs (Becker, 1974; Rosenstock, 1990), states that individuals choose to take or not to take preventive action depending upon these perceptions.

*Perceived threats* refer to the individual's perception of his or her susceptibility to a particular condition and the degree of severity of the condition that the individual fears. Persons who perceive no threat lack a reason to act.

Perceived susceptibility to, and severity of, a condition together produce fear. Fear is an effective motivator, yet the optimal level of fear for motivating client behavior is unknown (Sutton & Hallett, 1988). Too little fear may not motivate, but too much can lead to denial and inaction. An important consideration in fear-inducing interventions is that fearful individuals, regardless of their motivation, may lack the necessary skills or confidence to change their health behaviors.

*Perceived benefits* refer to the belief that specific actions on the part of an individual will reduce the threat of negative outcomes or increase the chance of positive outcomes. Perceived benefits must outweigh perceived barriers before a person will initiate an action. *Perceived barriers* may include financial considerations, inconvenience, lack of transportation, lack of knowledge, or potential pain or discomfort.

Evaluations of the health belief model conducted exclusively with older persons have been limited. One such study assessed health beliefs related to osteoporosis—specifically, the likelihood that the older adults in the study would adopt exercise behaviors and increase their calcium intake (Kim et al., 1991). The authors concluded that it is important to focus on overcoming perceived barriers, such as the difficulty of changing old habits and the incorporation of new habits into a daily routine.

Each of these belief measures—susceptibility, severity, benefits, and barriers—has a significant but limited relationship to subsequent preventive behaviors, such as participation in flu vaccination, breast self-examination, tuberculosis skin tests, and smoking cessation activities (Kirscht, 1988).

The predictability of the model is limited because of the uncertainty surrounding how rationally a person will act in a given circumstance. In addition, beliefs are not in themselves sufficient conditions for action. "Researchers must seek out that constellation of conditions, including beliefs, which accounts for major variations in behavior" (Rosenstock, 1990). Some of these additional factors are physiological dependency, economic limitations, environmental influences, skill development, and self-efficacy.

## OTHER THEORIES

The theory of reasoned action focuses on attitudes that precede potential behaviors (Fishbein & Ajzen, 1975). One interesting aspect of this theory is its focus on taking into account what relevant others think a person should do. An older person may finally relent and join a smoking cessation program because of his or her perceived belief of what their physician or the spouse wants them to do. The theory of planned behaviors, an extension of the theory of reasoned action, has an additional focus on the perceived ease or difficulty of performing a behavior (Ajzen, 1988). The older smoker may intend to quit but does not believe there is access to a program that will provide the skills to quit.

There are theories that focus more on community than individuals. One example is empowerment theory, a process of collective education and social action that promotes the participation of people, organizations, and communities in gaining control over their lives (Wallerstein & Bernstein, 1988). This theory involves collective attempts to address problems by surmounting cultural, social, and historical barriers.

Community-Oriented Primary Care (COPC) is another community-level theory that encourages clinicians to view their patient populations, not just individual patients, and to involve other community organizations and community leaders to help with population-based behavior change (Nutting, 1987). Examples of applying COPC in the community are provided in chapter 12 on Community Health.

## A FINAL NOTE

The reader may be asking at this point (granted, the likelihood is quite small), Why do you place health behavior theories at the end of this chapter? Should you not start with them, as they help shape the health assessments and interventions to follow? I can only answer this by offering a personal, and perhaps politically incorrect, view. I do not think that the behavior change theories are sufficiently powerful to stimulate the shaping of a health intervention. Instead, I believe that several concepts embedded in different theories may be useful once a health intervention has already entered the development phase.

Theories, moreover, are too rich for my research blood. A theory attempts to relate a set of concepts systematically to explain and predict events and activities. Concepts, however, are the primary elements of theory, and each theory has a concept or two that is particularly well developed and helpful to me in guiding a community intervention and evaluation.

Therefore, I begin my community health education projects based on questions raised from my professional experience: How does the practicum vary among gerontology programs (Haber, 2003)? How is a health promotion directory being utilized by older adults (Haber & Looney, 2003)? How effective is a health contract/calendar for behavior change (Haber & Looney, 2000)? Are African American churches good sites for exercise programs (Looney & Haber, 2001)? How effective are health science students as exercise leaders (Haber et al., 2000, 1997)? How effective is a health promotion intervention with older adults (Haber, 1986; Haber & Lacy, 1993)? At some point after project development has begun, I examine key concepts from different theories and refine my interventions and evaluations accordingly.

## QUESTIONS FOR DISCUSSION

1. Do you think a health risk appraisal by itself has value for the client, or does it require substantial health education followup in a particular risk area? Support your answer.
2. Do you think encouraging a precontemplater to change a health behavior is an inefficient waste of limited personnel resources? Explain your answer.
3. Write a health contract for yourself for a 2-week period of time. What techniques are you going to employ to increase your likelihood of completing it successfully? At the end of the 2 weeks, discuss your success, or lack of such, with others.

4. Which of the Ten Tips is the most important tool for *you* to use in changing a health behavior? Which one is the least relevant for you?

5. If you were forced to describe yourself with one term, are you more of a healthy-pleasure type of person, or a behavior management type of person? What percentage of personal trainers would you guess fall into the healthy-pleasure category? Explain your answer.

6. If you were writing a grant proposal to help older adults exercise more in the community, which health behavior concepts do you find most helpful for guiding your intervention? Explain your answer.

# 5

# Exercise

## 1996 SURGEON GENERAL'S REPORT ON PHYSICAL ACTIVITY AND HEALTH

In her exercise video "Shopping for Fitness," Joan Rivers espouses walking the malls for aerobic conditioning, hefting shopping bags for weight training, and trying on jeans that are one size too small to motivate oneself for weight reduction. According to Rivers, "Everybody's got a tape out, Buns of Steel, Breasts of Iron and Bunions of Teflon. They just don't get it, that it should be fun." Although many of her comments are satirical, much of the *Surgeon General's Report on Physical Activity and Health* supports what she espouses.

The July 11, 1996, *Report* represented a 2-year collaborative effort between the Centers for Disease Control and Prevention and the President's Council on Physical Fitness and Sports. It is the most comprehensive review of the research on the effects of physical activity on people's health. In short, 60% of adults did not achieve the recommended amount of physical activity, and 25% of adults were not physically active at all. Inactivity increased with age; by age 75 about one in three men and one in two women engaged in no physical activity. Inactivity was also more common among women and people with lower income and less education.

Previous reports of the Surgeon General on national health risks, such as the health hazards of tobacco published in 1964, have had a major influence on public awareness and the policies of government and business. It remains to be seen how influential this report on physical activity will be. Acting Surgeon General Audrey F. Manley, MD stated, "This report is nothing less than a national call to action. Physical inactivity is a serious nationwide public health problem, but active and healthful lifestyles are well within the grasp of everyone."

The report agrees with Ms. Rivers in that most sedentary Americans are not going to rigorously pursue buns of steel, and among those who do, all will fall short of the goal. Instead, it is important to make the first step for most Americans achievable and to do so requires a large degree of modesty in setting goals and at least a small degree of enjoyment. Hence, the emphasis on being more active, such as shopping while walking briskly, than adherence to a rigid exercise regimen.

*The basic premise of the Surgeon General's report is that Americans should get at least 30 minutes of physical activity, most days of the week.* This statement provides a major perspective shift from previous recommendations by government and exercise leaders. In summary, this new message recommends that Americans become more concerned about total calories expended through exercise than about intensity level or length of activity session. Regarding intensity level, the report stresses the importance of raising respiratory and heart rate—physiological changes that are apparent to the participant—but not to be too concerned about raising intensity level to a target heart rate, particularly if you are sedentary or have a less than active lifestyle.

Regarding the length of activity session, it is no longer deemed essential to obtain 30 consecutive minutes of exercise. For Americans, the large majority of whom are not too active, accumulating shorter activity spurts throughout the day is effective. Got a spare few minutes? Then briskly walk the shopping malls with Joan or climb a few stairs. A review of the research literature concludes that accumulating several 5 or 10 minute bouts of physical activity over the course of the day provides beneficial health and fitness effects (DeBusk et al., 1990; Jakicic et al., 1995; I. Lee et al., 2000; Murphy et al., 2002; Pate et al., 1995). One study reported that if you time these bouts of activity right you can also use them to gain the added benefit of replacing junk food snack breaks (Jakicic et al., 1995).

Regarding exercise itself, it is difficult for adults to go from inactivity to an exercise routine. Thinking about how to accumulate short bouts of activity is a useful way to get started on better health and fitness. For example, wax your car or wash your floor more briskly than you normally do (even if it means doing it in segments throughout the day), or put more energy into leaf raking or lawn mowing, gardening with enthusiasm, or dancing by yourself to music on the radio.

Finally, the Surgeon General's report urges Americans to be active most days of the week. Aim for the habit of everyday exercise, but do not allow the occasional lapse to discourage you. Making exercise a near-daily routine is more likely to become an enduring habit than the previously recommended three times per week.

In September 2002, I was disappointed to learn that 21 experts at the Food and Nutrition Board of the Institute of Medicine had produced a 1,000 page report (see Dietary Reference Intake report, September 5, 2002, at www.iom.edu) that recommended that Americans exercise at least an hour a day. The exercise recommendation was based on biochemical measurements, rather than on practical considerations. The board inexplicably seems to be recommending that even though few Americans were getting the half hour a day of exercise most days of the week that was recommended by the Surgeon General's report—a recommendation that was based on considerable research to support the substantial health benefits of this routine—why not ignore practicality and raise the bar of expectation even more, to an hour every day?

Despite the Institute of Medicine's report, the evidence is clear. Exercise does not need to be that onerous. It should also be noted that the Institute of Medicine's report was not focused on exercise, but on the new nutritional guidelines called Dietary Reference Intakes, which will be examined in the next chapter on Nutrition (along with, I believe, a few questionable nutrition recommendations that were made by the institute).

## THE MOST POPULAR ACTIVITY OF ALL: WALKING

Older adults need not become triathletes or engage in other high-intensity activities to reap the benefits of exercise. For most older adults, a brisk walking program will provide sufficient intensity for a good aerobics program. An 8-year study of more than 13,000 people indicated that walking briskly for 30 to 60 minutes every day was almost as beneficial in reducing the death rate as jogging up to 40 miles a week (S. Blair et al., 1989). The authors of a study of 1,645 older adults reported that simply walking 4 hours per week decreased the risk of future hospitalization for cardiovascular disease (LaCroix et al., 1996).

The Nurses' Health Study is a long-term research project that began in 1976, involving 122,000 nurses. A prospective study of 72,000 of these nurses over an 8-year period revealed that brisk walking 3 hours a week offered as much health benefit as engaging in vigorous exercise. Brisk walking is defined as about 3 miles per hour (twice the normal pace), and 3 hours a week comes to about 30 minutes per day. Among the brisk walkers, the incidence of coronary events (nonfatal myocardiac infarction or death from coronary disease) was reduced between 30% and 40% (Manson et al., 1999). A subset of this sample containing 5,100 diabetic walkers produced a similar reduction in heart disease risk (Hu et al., 2001).

The National Center for Health Statistics reports that walking has much greater appeal for older adults than high-intensity exercise. A national survey indicated that a smaller percentage of persons aged 65-plus (27%), in comparison to the general adult population (41%), engaged in vigorous activities, whereas people of all age groups were equally likely (41%) to walk for exercise (National Health Interview Survey, 1985).

Brisk walking is the most popular aerobic activity for older adults. As the acting surgeon general emphasized in her report, most Americans can benefit from activities like brisk walking and not concern themselves about target heart rates. Many older adults are concerned about unfavorable weather, though, and may abandon their walking routine as a consequence. Prolonged hot or cold spells may sabotage a good walking program. Rather than discontinue this activity because of the weather, adults may choose to walk indoors at their local shopping malls. Shopping malls—about 2,500 nationwide—open their doors early, usually between 5:30 and 10:00 a.m., for members of walking clubs.

Another option for older adults is to join a noncompetitive walking or hiking club, or participate in a nearby walking or hiking event. Two opportunities in this regard are the American Volkssport Association at 800-830-9255, or at www.ava.org; and the local Sierra Club at www.sierraclub.org.

Traveling to another city can also be an excuse not to exercise. Or it can be an opportunity to gather information from the local newspaper or chamber of commerce about a walking tour for an enjoyable way to get exercise and a unique way to learn about offbeat aspects of a city's history. Most if not all big cities have walking tours (e.g., Los Angeles, 213-623-2489; Atlanta, 404-876-2041) and some sound particularly intriguing (Oak Park, Illinois,' self-guided walking tours of Frank Lloyd Wright homes, 708-848-1976; and the Big Onion tours of New York City's ethnic communities and restaurants, 212-439-1090).

Walking is so popular that it has spawned many magazines, newsletters, and books. It may appear that there is not much to walking—we have been doing it, after all, since we were toddlers—but proper technique improves benefits and reduces injuries. Good walking technique involves proper posture (head erect, chin in, shoulders relaxed, and back straight), a bent-arm swing, and a full natural stride. Good walking shoes should have flexible soles, good arch supports, and roomy toe boxes.

# EXERCISE FOR DISEASE PREVENTION AND FUNCTIONAL IMPROVEMENT

According to the *Surgeon General's Report,* regular exercise and physical activity improves health in a variety of ways, including a reduction in heart disease, diabetes, high blood pressure, colon cancer, depression, anxiety, excess weight, falling, bone thinning, muscle wasting, and joint pain. A few years earlier, in 1992, the American Heart Association (AHA) had added physical inactivity as a new risk factor to its list, joining hypertension, smoking, and high blood cholesterol. It was the first new risk factor the AHA had added in almost 20 years.

The American Heart Association also recommended routine screening of all patients for inactivity. If the physician has time constraints, the AHA recommended that exercise counseling be coordinated through a nurse, allied health professional, or other type of health educator (Fletcher et al., 1992). As a number of gerontologists have noted, if exercise could be encapsulated in a pill, it would be the single most powerful medication a physician could prescribe.

At the time of this writing, I was a member of an expert panel reviewing evidence-based outcomes of exercise in older adults. This CDC-funded project was led by Thomas Prohaska of the University of Illinois at Chicago, and he and his research team were reviewing 2,334 studies published in peer-reviewed journals between 1980 and 2000. While this systematic evaluation is still in progress, I report below—unsystematically—on recent studies that show evidence that exercise demonstrates considerable promise in the areas of disease prevention and improved function.

## CARDIOVASCULAR DISEASE

Inactivity is the most powerful predictor of mortality from cardiovascular disease among healthy persons, surpassing smoking, hypertension, and heart disease (Myers et al., 2002). Studies report, moreover, that interventions as accessible as brisk walking are associated with a reduced risk of coronary heart disease for elderly men (Hakim et al., 1999) and elderly women (Manson et al., 1999). Although walking is sufficient by itself to lower the risk of cardiovascular disease, brisker walking lowers the risk (Manson et al., 2002), and more vigorous exercise lowers the risk further (Tanasescu et al., 2002).

Exercise is also a major prognostic factor in patients with existing cardiovascular disease. Patients who are physically active after a first heart attack had a 60% lower risk of fatal heart attack or a second nonfatal heart attack than those who did not stay active (Steffen-Batey et al., 2000). For a number of years, exercise was contraindicated for patients with chronic heart failure (CHF). Now, exercise is recommended for CHF patients, provided the heart problem is stable (Gielen et al., 2001). Exercise also appears to extend the protective effects of angina—chest pain due to an insufficient supply of blood and oxygen to the heart (Abete et al., 2001).

Though aerobic conditioning has been considered the exercise of choice for improved cardiorespiratory function, other forms of exercise have proved beneficial as well. Tai chi (Lan et al., 1999) and resistance exercise (Tanasescu et al., 2002; Vincent et al., 2002a), for example, provide cardiorespiratory benefits. Resistance exercise, in fact, appears to reduce blood pressure level (Kelley & Kelley, 2000) and cholesterol level (Kraus et al., 2002; Prabhakaran et al, 1999), outcomes primarily obtained previously through aerobic exercise interventions.

A study of peripheral vascular disease (PVD) reports what may seem incongruous to some—that an effective treatment for clogged or narrowed arteries of the legs is aerobic walking (Stewart et al., 2002). Walking increases muscle metabolism and may improve circulation to the legs, allowing more oxygen to get to tissues otherwise starved by blockages. The two caveats to walking interventions for PVD are to avoid extreme pain and to avoid exercise if pain continues when legs are at rest ("Peripheral vascular disease," 2000).

## CANCER

Epidemiological findings have established an association between the risk of cancer and physical activity and exercise. Higher levels of adult physical activity, for example, appear to afford modest protection against breast cancer, perhaps by reducing body fat where carcinogens accumulate (Dirx et al., 2001; Rockhill et al., 1999), or by lowering the level of estrogen in the blood (McTiernan et al, 2002). Also, women with substantial leisure-time physical activity had a 27% lower incidence of ovarian cancer (Cottreau et al., 2000). Men who exercised reduced their risk of prostate cancer by 24% and upper digestive and stomach cancer by 62% (Wannamethee et al., 2001).

High activity level is also associated with a substantial reduction in risk, up to 50%, of colon cancer (Martinez et al., 1999; Slattery et al., 1999; White et al., 1996). Although the mechanisms by which exercise appears to protect against colon cancer are not known, it is speculated that exercise speeds food through the bowel and shortens the time car-cinogens in fecal matter spend in contact with cells that line the colon.

There is not one primary theory being offered for the positive influ-ence of exercise and physical activity on the risk of cancer. Instead, sev-eral have been offered, and they tend to differ with the varying types of cancer. The theories range broadly and include the immune, nervous, and endocrine systems.

## DIABETES

Exercise appears to impact on type II diabetes, in terms of both prevention of the disease and the risk of mortality among those who already have the disease. The onset of diabetes can be delayed or prevented when high-risk people make lifestyle changes that include increased exercise. Finnish researchers investigated 522 people over a 4-year period and the incidence of diabetes was 11% among those who received exercise and other counsel, and 23% among controls—a significant difference (Tuomilehto et al., 2001).

A study of 70,000 female nurses who did not have diabetes at baseline, documented 1,419 incident cases of type II diabetes over an 8-year peri-od. There was a substantially reduced risk in obtaining type II diabetes, however, among those who exercised regularly, even among those who engaged in moderate-intensity physical activity such as brisk walking (Hu et al., 1999).

Being active also increased the chances that a person with diabetes will stay alive. Researchers studied 1,263 men with diabetes over an average of 12 years, and reported that the physically inactive had a 70% greater chance of dying than did men who reported being physically active. The overall risk of death shrank as the level of fitness rose (Wei et al., 2000). Another study of 2803 men with type II diabetes reported that physical activity was associated with reduced risk of cardiovascular death and total mortality (Tanasescu et al., 2003).

High-intensity resistance training also improves glycemic control in older patients with type II diabetes (Dunstan et al., 2002). The study authors were surprised at the magnitude of the effects, as they equaled those typically seen with drugs for diabetes. They noted that muscles are major clearance sites for circulating blood sugar, or glucose.

## DEPRESSION

Exercise may be just as effective as antidepressant medication in treating some cases of depression (Lawlor & Hopker, 2001), though medication may initiate a more rapid therapeutic response than exercise (J. Blumenthal et al., 1999). After 16 weeks of treatment, however, exercise was equally effective in reducing depression among patients with major depressive disorder (Blumenthal, et al., 1999). Another study reported that, conversely, individuals who stop exercising lose the long-term mood-enhancing effects (Kritz-Silverstein et al., 2001).

A study by Singh and colleagues (2001) reported that supervised weight-lifting exercises significantly benefited depressed older adults in comparison to control persons who attended health lectures. (I suppose one could argue that if you had lectured the older weight lifters as well, both groups would have remained depressed). What was interesting about this study was that the antidepressant benefits were sustained even after supervision was terminated and the participants were exercising on their own. After 26 months, one third of the elderly exercisers were still regularly weight lifting.

## COGNITION

A longitudinal study of physical activity among older women over an 8-year period reported that those with higher physical activity levels were less likely to experience cognitive decline. This association was not explained by difference in baseline function or health status (Yaffee et al., 2001). Another study of 349 healthy adults aged 55 and older reported that older adults with higher levels of fitness—as measured by a standard treadmill exercise test, experienced a slower rate of cognitive decline over a 6-year period (Barnes et al., 2003).

Examining the relationship between aerobic fitness and in vivo brain tissue density, high-resolution magnetic resonance imaging scans from 55 older adults revealed that declines in tissue densities as a function of age were substantially reduced as a function of fitness, even when other relevant variables were statistically controlled (Colcombe et al., 2003).

Exercise may not only stem a decline in cognitive functioning, it may improve it as well. Researchers found that older men and women who engaged in aerobic exercise improved the higher mental processes of memory and executive functioning—such as planning and organizational abilities—that are based in the frontal and prefrontal regions of the brain (Khatri et al., 2001; Kramer et al., 1999).

## BONE DENSITY

Both weight-bearing aerobic exercise and resistance training increase bone density in older women (Jakes et al., 2001; Rhodes et al., 2000). Of most relevance to older adults, though, is a study that reports that even low-impact aerobic exercise such as brisk walking can increase bone mass. A review of 24 studies that examined aerobic exercise and bone mineral density in women reported a 2% bone mass gain among exercisers versus nonexercisers, and that walking was the most common form of exercise used in these studies (Kelley, 2001). The Nurses' Health Study of 61,200 postmenopausal women concluded that moderate levels of activity, including walking, are associated with substantially lower risk of hip fractures (Feskanich et al., 2002).

A study of healthy older persons who engaged in 6 months of resistance training showed 2% greater bone density in the hip area, and signs that bone metabolism had shifted toward generating more bone than was being lost (Vincent & Braith, 2002). Another study reported that resistive back-strengthening exercises reduced the incidence of vertebral fractures among postmenopausal women (Sinaki et al., 2002).

## FALL PREVENTION

Home-based exercise programs result in significant fall reduction and other benefits. One individually tailored exercise program in the home improved physical function, reduced falls, and decreased injuries in a sample of women aged 80 years and older. Over a 1-year period, persons in the exercise program reduced falls by 46%, compared with a usual care control group that received an equal number of social visits (Campbell, 1997). Another home-based exercise program with older adults aged 70 to 84 reported significant fall reduction in comparison to groups that received home hazard management and treatment of poor vision (Day et al., 2002).

A meta-analysis of seven FICSIT Trials (Frailty and Injuries: Cooperative Studies of Intervention Techniques) revealed that a variety of exercise interventions—examined by way of randomized, controlled clinical trials—led to a reduction in falls among elderly patients (Province et al., 1995). Subjects in the seven trials were older adults (minimum ages ranged from 60 to 75 years), and were mostly ambulatory and cognitively intact. The exercise interventions were successful even though they varied in duration, frequency, intensity, and content. The content of the interventions included endurance training, resistance training, flexibility training, and tai chi.

## OSTEOARTHRITIS

People with osteoarthritis of the knee often experience progressive deterioration in the cartilage of the knee joint until they reach the point of being disabled. Both aerobic and resistance exercise with patients who have osteoarthritis of the knee reduced the incidence of disability in activities of daily living by about 50% (Penninx et al., 2001). Another sample of older adults with knee osteoarthritis experienced significant improvement in physical function and reduced pain as a consequence of a strength-training program (Baker et al., 2001).

Another simple home-based exercise program significantly reduced knee pain from osteoarthritis (K. Thomas et al., 2002); and an exercise program combined with medication for knee osteoarthritis was more effective than medication alone for improving physical function and reducing activity-related pain in a sample of older persons (Petrella & Bartha, 2000).

## SLEEP

Older adults with sleep complaints improved self-rated sleep quality by completing a moderate-intensity exercise program. Exercising subjects reported significant improvement in subjective sleep quality, reduced sleep latency (average time in minutes needed to fall asleep), and increased sleep duration (average number of hours of actual sleep per night) (King et al., 1997). Even a sample of healthy older adult caregivers who were without initially reported sleep complaints but who engaged in stressful caregiving with family members reported improvements in subjective sleep quality after they completed a moderate-intensity exercise program (King et al., 2002).

## OTHER CONDITIONS

Exercise has proved beneficial for a wide range of other medical and functional conditions. A sampling of these studies include a reduction in stress among older women caregivers (King et al., 2002); a reduction in functional decline among nursing home residents (Morris et al., 1999; Lazowski et al., 1999); enhanced improvement for elderly women following hip surgery (Henderson et al., 1992); a reduction in the symptoms of chronic fatigue syndrome (Powell et al., 2001); increased function in chronic obstructive pulmonary disease patients (Hernandez et al., 2000); improvement in psychological well-being (McAuley & Rudolph, 1995); a reduction in obesity (Andersen et al., 1999); improvement in motor function among stroke survivors (Duncan et al., 1998); and relief from the symptoms of carpal tunnel syndrome (Garfinkel et al., 1998).

## CAUTION

It takes an act of supreme skepticism to deny the overwhelming evidence supporting the benefits of exercise. Nonetheless, I have met such skeptics who disparage the rigor upon which most exercise research studies are based. Though I most happily do not side with these cynics, the evidence on the benefits of exercise does need to be viewed with a degree of caution. Some studies, for instance, are epidemiological in nature and reveal correlation rather than causality. In other words, exercise may be more the product of being in good health than a contributor to it. Many of these observational studies attempt to compensate for this limitation by employing analytical controls on a variety of baseline variables.

Other methodological limitations are also common among exercise studies. Many of these studies utilize unrepresentative samples, oftentimes relying on volunteers; lack randomization between treatment and control groups; do not restrict awareness of who is in the treatment versus control group (unblinded studies); employ inadequate measurement tools, especially a reliance on self-reports; and report high drop-out rates or do not include dropouts in the data analysis (intention-to-treat analysis). Exercise interventions, therefore, may not be as miraculous as some of these studies seem to indicate.

Nonetheless, the breadth and depth of research on exercise interventions with older adults—including more than 200 randomized clinical trials published between 1980 and 2000—can only lead one to conclude that exercise is an astonishing health intervention, and no amount of methodological nitpicking will seriously diminish its overall wondrous effects.

## THE FOUR COMPONENTS OF MY EXERCISE CLASS

The four components of my community exercise class are aerobics, strength-building, flexibility and balance, and health education. In a typical 60-minute class, I begin with 25 minutes of aerobic exercise, warming up for the first 5 minutes and cooling down the last 5 minutes. I begin with aerobics in order to warm up the muscles not only for higher intensity aerobic levels, but for the subsequent periods of strength-building (15 minutes) and flexibility and balance (10 minutes). These three components—aerobics, strength-building, and flexibility and balance—typically last 50 minutes; the final 10 minutes of class is devoted to health education.

With the aid of students in health science classes (see Figure 5.1), I have implemented this exercise class over the past 25 years. It has undergone continual refinement over this time.

This exercise program was selected for the directory, *Best Practices in Health Promotion and Aging,* compiled by the Health Promotion Institute of the National Council on the Aging (NCOA). To obtain the manual with its brief summaries of selected best practices around the country, contact the NCOA at www.ncoa.org, or call 202-479-1200.

## THE AEROBICS COMPONENT

Aerobic means "with oxygen." An aerobic activity moves large volumes of oxygen, employs large muscle groups (like the arms and legs), and is sustained at a certain level of intensity over a period of time. Aerobic exercise is rhythmic, repetitive, and continuous, and includes such popular activities as brisk walking (about twice as fast as one normally walks), swimming, and bicycling.

Aerobic activity can be contrasted to anaerobic ("without oxygen") activity, which depends on short bursts of energy (like a 50-meter sprint or barbell press), quickly depletes energy resources, and has limited cardiovascular benefit. This type of activity is, however, essential for strength-building purposes.

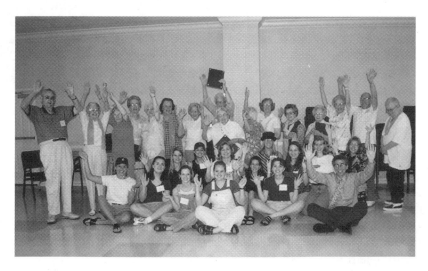

FIGURE 5.1   The end-of-the-semester photograph of one of my exercise classes, taught by occupational therapy students.

Aerobic capacity, or maximum oxygen uptake ($VO_2$ max), is the maximum amount of oxygen that an individual can utilize during strenuous exertion. Aerobic capacity is considered to be the best measure of cardiorespiratory fitness, and although it tends to decrease with age, it can be increased through a regularly practiced aerobic regimen.

Most aerobic exercise programs are designed to stimulate the heart and lungs for a sufficient period of time to produce an increased and sustained heart rate. Traditional programs encourage participants to sustain exercise for a minimum of 20 to 25 minutes and to gradually raise the normal heartbeat, about 60 to 80 beats a minute, to the "target zone" of the individual, the upper and lower limits of which are based on age (see Table 5.1).

The target zone typically refers to between 60% and 75% of the estimated maximum heart rate, which is calculated by subtracting a person's age from 220 and multiplying the remainder first by 60% and then by 75%. The target for the beginning exerciser should be near the 60% level (or less if the person has been sedentary), and gradually increase to the higher level over succeeding months. Individuals can assess the intensity of their aerobic exercise program by counting their pulse beats for a 10-second period and multiplying by 6. Many aerobics instructors ask their students to conduct this assessment at periodic intervals.

The advantage to calculating target heart rates for some older adults (decidedly a minority) is that the older adults believe this is the most scientific approach and prefer this method. The disadvantages are a) a significant minority of older adults have difficulty obtaining a pulse count, b) medications like beta-blockers can limit maximum heart rate intensity, and c) there is controversy in the literature as to whether the commonly used equation to estimate maximal heart rate (220 – age) is valid for older adults (Tanaka et al., 2001). Bailey (1994) reports that the formula for the target heart rate is inappropriate for 30% to 40% of adults. These persons have hearts that beat faster or slower than the age-predicted maximum.

### TABLE 5.1  Target Heart Rate by Decades

| Age | Target Heart Rate* (60% to 75% of Maximum) | Maximum Heart Rate* (220 – age) |
|-----|--------------------------------------------|---------------------------------|
| 50  | 102–128 | 170 |
| 60  | 96–120  | 160 |
| 70  | 90–113  | 150 |
| 80  | 84–105  | 140 |

* Beats Per Minute

My own experience with exercise programs with older adults has led me to appreciate Fries' comment (1989): "We generally find this whole heart rate business a bit of a bother and somewhat artificial. There really are not good medical data to justify particular target heart rates. You may wish to check your pulse rate a few times to get a feel for what is happening, but it doesn't have to be something you watch extremely carefully" (p. 69). Typically, I implement periodic checking of target heart rates during the first or second class, and then encourage those who are receptive to it to periodically check their heart rate on their own.

The technique that I use throughout my exercise class is my version of the Borg (1982) technique, a subjective assessment of how hard one is working. Most older adults prefer the Borg technique. It has the advantage of being easy to gauge, and it serves another purpose: it encourages older adults to become more aware of their bodies and how they feel (see Table 5.2). One study of more than 7,000 men (mean age, 66 years) reported that the individual's perceived level of exertion is a better predictor of risk of coronary heart disease than whether they met current activity recommendations (Lee et al., 2003).

Ideally, the inactive older adult should seek an intensity level of very light, about 1 on the modified Borg scale, or about 50% of maximum heart rate. The active older person should be about 8 on the scale, or approximately 70% of maximum heart rate. Generally speaking, we tell participants that the exercise level should be of sufficient duration and intensity for them to break into a sweat (indicating a rising internal body temperature), but not so intense that they are unable to conduct a brief conversation (if desired) while exercising.

Regardless of whether target heart rates or perceived intensity levels are utilized, exercise is discontinued immediately if shortness of breath, chest pain, dizziness or light-headedness, confusion, or pain occurs.

My exercise classes are led by health science students after they complete a brief period of training. Regarding the aerobics component of the class, we offer the students and the older adults two options, which tend to be equally preferred:

1. A series of arm and leg movements that gradually increase, and then decrease, intensity level. I usually come up with funny names for the movements (my favorite is the Haber Hula—I'll leave that one up to your imagination) and make sure that all parts of the body are moved. If students run out of movement ideas, I encourage them to draw ideas from one of several memory-jarring techniques. For example, a) playing one of a number of imaginary musical instruments (drums, trombone, violin,

**TABLE 5.2  Modified Borg Scale of Perceived Exertion**

| Level | Perceived Exertion | Physical Signs and Equivalency |
|---|---|---|
| 1 | Very light | None |
| 2 | | |
| 3 | Fairly light | Breathing rate increased |
| 4 | | |
| 5 | Somewhat hard | Warmth, slight sweat and |
| 6 | Somewhat hard | breathing rate increased |
| 7 | | |
| 8 | Hard | Sweat, heavy breathing |
| 9 | | |
| 10 | Very hard | Heavy sweat, difficult to talk |

etc.) and pretending to generate the music that is playing in the background, b) mimicking an activity of daily living (drying one's back with a towel, vacuuming the rug, spooning food into one's mouth, weeding the garden, etc.), and c) mimicking a movement in a sport (boxing, baseball, etc.).

2. An imaginary trip is acted out, perhaps a cruise to Spain, or attendance at a local baseball game. The cruise might include climbing up the boat (taking big steps in place with knees raised high), putting away clothes in one's cabin, dancing that evening with an imaginary heart-throb, getting off the boat (more big steps), visiting a bullfight, becoming the matador, and so forth. The baseball game may entail walking to the stadium (walking around the room, sometimes in a haphazard fashion to promote social interaction among fans walking to the game), to being unexpectedly called upon by the manager to pinch hit (swinging an imaginary bat in both directions) or to do some relief pitching (using right and left arms).

The class is not targeted to older adults at a particular fitness level. The class participants may range from wheelchair-bound or walker-dependent, to the very fit. One student typically leads the frail or less fit participants, often from a seated position; another student leads the more fit participants; and the remaining students are free to roam and to individualize movements for older persons with special needs or to promote safety among participants.

If the older adult has a specific health problem like Parkinson's disease, stroke, an orthopedic condition, or mild confusion, the roaming students pay particular attention to helping them keep movements simple, avoid quick action, and provide caution with twisting movements. Before the first class, students will meet one-to-one with older adults to find out if additional cautions need to be observed and, if relevant, to discuss the importance of timing medications for maximal effect during classes.

Deconditioned older adults in the class are encouraged to perform at 1 or 2 on the modified Borg scale, or at 50% of the maximum heart rate for their age. Fit older adults may perform at 8 on the Borg scale, or at 70% of the maximum heart rate. The majority of older adults are at the 5 or 6 level, which is equivalent to the moderate effort required for brisk walking. People tend to be reliable self-raters using the Borg scale.

The emphasis in the class, however, is on having fun, and only secondarily on moving up the scale to higher intensity levels. Several earlier studies have supported the surgeon general's findings that even activities of low to moderate intensity level not only improve the aerobic capacity of older adults, but are less likely than more vigorous activities to result in injury, and are more likely to be maintained as a routine over time (Buchner & Wagner, 1992).

And though low to moderate intensity activity does not provide the fitness benefits of higher intensity exercise (Duncan, 1996), it can be sustained over a longer exercise period because it depletes only fat, the body's richest store of energy. Higher intensity exercise depletes carbohydrates and cannot be sustained for as long a duration (Keim, 1995). This is relevant to older adults in classes like ours that meet only two or three times a week. The older adults in our classes are encouraged to comply with the surgeon general's advice and engage in aerobic exercise at least a half hour in duration on most of the other days of the week.

On days when there is no class, therefore, older adults are encouraged to engage in longer sessions of walking, swimming, cycling, dancing, gardening, yard work, or other activities that can be performed at low or moderate intensity level for a half hour or longer.

Finally, aerobic movement in our classes is always accompanied by music. One small study reported that music can promote adherence to a regular exercise routine (Bauldof et al., 2002). About two thirds of the musical selections in our exercise class, like big band music, are targeted toward the preferences of older adults. The students choose the remaining music, however, with an eye toward eclecticism (rock, rap, theatre music, international music, etc.). Musical variety not only promotes greater interest in the class, but also generates humorous discussions about the quality of the musical selection.

We start and end the class with slow tempo music, and pick up the pace in between. When the musical cadence is faster, the slower-moving older adults are encouraged to time their physical movements to every other beat of the music. Occasionally students will choose soft background music for the strength-building and flexibility and balance components of the class.

## THE MUSCULAR STRENGTH OR ENDURANCE COMPONENT

Experts did not always believe that strengthening exercises were as important for older adults as other components of exercise (Fries, 1989, p. 66), and many geriatric exercise manuals ignored strengthening exercises altogether. Now, experts and community health leaders realize the importance of strength-building for maintaining an independent lifestyle with age. Preserving leg strength allows an older adult to get up from a chair in a restaurant or help regain balance before falling. Preserving arm strength allows an older adult to carry groceries, pick up household items, twist off jar lids, and make minor repairs.

Experts, therefore, are beginning to develop resistance training guideline recommendations for older adults (Porter, 2000). And though strength-building exercise programs are still the exception rather than the norm, the popularity of including a strength-building component into an aerobics exercise class has been growing quickly the past several years.

Muscular strength or endurance is the ability of the muscle to exert force (strength) or to repeat action over time without fatigue (endurance). As people age, lean muscle tissue tends to decrease and the percentage of body fat increases. Thus, muscle strength and endurance tend to decline with age, and bones tend to weaken. Strength training, however, will increase muscle mass, functioning ability, and bone density. When the skeletal frame is strengthened, the likelihood of bone fractures resulting from osteoporosis is reduced (Gorman & Posner, 1988; Jakes et al., 2001; Rhodes et al., 2000; Vincent & Braith, 2002).

In the spring of 1990, attitudes toward strength-building for older adults began to change. A strength exercise program captured the health headlines—which previously had been dominated by popular aerobic activities or unusual aerobic accomplishments (such as the exploits of Johnny Kelley, who completed the Boston Marathon race 58 times and ran his last one as an octogenarian).

This highly publicized strength exercise program involved 10 (including 1 dropout) frail, very old nursing home residents who, after completing an 8-week training program, almost tripled their leg strength, expanded their thigh muscles by more than 10%, and were able to walk 50% faster (Fiatarone et al., 1990). The participants ranged in age from 87 to

96 years! One 93-year-old participant reported "I feel as though I were 50 again. Now, I get up in the middle of the night and I can get around without using my walker or turning on the light. The program gave me strength I didn't have before. Every day I feel better, more optimistic. Pills won't do for you what exercise does!" (Evans et al., 1991). Another resident who at first could not rise from a chair without using his arms was able to do so after the training, and two others no longer needed canes for walking (Fiatarone et al., 1990).

Most community exercise classes do not have the luxury of providing weights or exercise machines to older participants. That is the case with my exercise class as well. I have found the most affordable and safest option for strength-building to be elastic bands (such as the Thera-Bands or Dyna-Bands sold by Fitness Wholesale, go to www.fwonline.com, or call toll free 888-396-7337), and gravity-resisting exercises like modified push-ups, raising arms to shoulder level and making circles, half-squats, toe raises, and others.

Elastic bands are a good alternative to free weights that are more likely to lead to injury, and to resistance machines, which are less accessible. In addition to being safe and portable they are inexpensive. By buying elastic bands in large rolls and cutting off 4-foot strips, I can provide bands to older students for about $1.60 apiece.

I typically include four or five different upper-extremity exercises to strengthen the biceps, triceps (see Figure 5.2), deltoids, trapezius, pectoralis, and latissimus. I then follow up with three or four lower extremity exercises to strengthen the quadriceps, hamstrings, and gastrocnemius. The elastic band manufacturers provide the buyer with a range of illustrated exercises to follow. The booklets also include tips like warming up, practicing smooth and slow movements in eccentric and concentric directions, breathing while exercising, and emphasizing technically correct movements over squeezing out additional repetitions.

Elastic bands come in increasing resistance levels. Typically, I start most older adults using Dyna-Bands at the pink level, and increase repetitions and sets before I consider moving up to the green level. Although the bands can be utilized at increasing levels of intensity, they are less precise than free weights or weight machines for measuring improvement.

I choose the resistance level that allows the participants to perform about 12 repetitions of an exercise. A larger number of repetitions places greater emphasis on endurance, a smaller number of repetitions emphasizes strength. When it comes to repetitions, older persons should err on the side of endurance over strength.

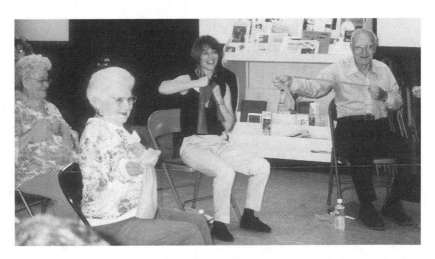

FIGURE 5.2  Horizontal tricep press performed in one of the author's exercise classes.

In my class, the number of different strength-building exercises and number of sets per exercise (usually one or two sets) are chosen to fit within a 15-minute exercise period. I do not try to fit all the strength-building exercises into one 15-minute component of the class, but instead offer a few basic exercises each time, plus a few new exercises.

The elastic band fits easily into a pocket and is convenient to take to class, or anywhere else for that matter. A potential disadvantage to the band is that it can be hard to grip with arthritic fingers. This limitation can be overcome by buying handles, or tying the band into a circle and exerting power through wrists or forearms. Another disadvantage to the band is that eventually it will break (which can startle, to say the least, when it occurs mid-exercise) and it needs to be replaced in a timely fashion.

The preferred schedule of activity for improving or sustaining strength or endurance for older adults is 2 or 3 days a week, with at least 1 day of rest between workouts. One study reported that muscle strength gains achieved during a 12-week progressive resistance training program can be maintained by resistance training *only once per week thereafter* (Trappe et al., 2002). Another study reported that even *light* resistance can help older adults get stronger, while at the same time reducing the possibility for injury (Vincent et al., 2002b).

A good alternative exercise for increasing strength in older adults with painful arthritic joints is isometrics, the contraction of a muscle without movement at the joint. The typical way to engage in isometrics is to pull or push against a stationary object, usually against a wall or against another body part. Each contraction should be held for about 5 seconds, and repeated 3 times. Many exercise physiologists are reluctant to recommend isometric exercise for heart patients because of the increased likelihood of performing the Valsalva maneuver (i.e., holding one's breath). It is possible, however, to avoid this maneuver when doing isometrics.

Because there is no movement, you can do isometrics any place, any time, and at no cost. The muscle that you select tightens but does not change length, thus there is no movement of the joint or the bone to which the muscle is attached. Isometrics, therefore, has the advantage of allowing you to build muscle at a fixed angle, avoiding those joint positions that may be affected by arthritic pain. On the other hand, unless you systematically alter the angle (at least 20 degrees) you do not develop strength over the range of motion.

There are several problems to avoid with all strength-building techniques, but they can be especially problematic with isometrics. To avoid the unhealthy Valsalva maneuver, for instance, count slowly out loud to trigger continuous breathing. To improve range of motion, it is not only important to vary the isometric angle, but to develop opposing muscle groups. Finally, the Borg scale for estimating appropriate intensity level should be used frequently with isometric exercise.

My favorite isometric exercise for older adults in my class takes place in a seated position. The adult places the palms of both hands about 4 or 5 inches above one knee, pushing down with the hands and up with the knee. The angle of the knee is altered by raising it slightly off the ground, and then raising it slightly higher two more times (see Figure 5.3). Repeat with the other leg. This exercise targets the important quadriceps muscle, the largest muscle in the body. It is also a good alternative to leg squats, which can exacerbate knee pain.

In addition to building strength and endurance, my resistance-training component includes safety tips on how to lift objects and how to move one's body to avoid muscle strain, backaches, hernias, and the like. Injuries from weight lifting are not uncommon, and they increased by 300% from 1978 to 1998 for middle-aged women and men ("More people lifting weights," 2000). In weight rooms around the country you can observe frequent examples of incorrect techniques that lead to injury. Men typically are hoisting too-heavy weights, arching their backs, holding their breath, swinging the weights or otherwise using momentum, and dropping the weights (either free weights or machine weights) when done.

Instead, manageable weights and proper technique should be used. Lift slowly and smoothly and return the weights under full control,

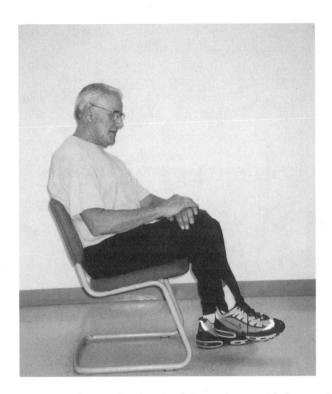

FIGURE 5.3   Isometric exercise for quadriceps that avoids knee pain.

maintain the natural curve of your back, exhale on exertion and inhale as you relax. If you break form, the weights are too heavy. Weight lifters who use correct form actually reduce injuries by strengthening joints and ligaments (Marcus, 1997). Machine weights are safer than free weights because they help foster proper technique and prevent the weight from falling on you (Hesson, 1995).

Sixty percent of weight lifters are males, but women are joining them at a very quick pace. Women strength-builders more than doubled between 1987 and 1996, from 7 million to 17 million, to join the 26 million men (M. Marcus, 1997). Women have learned that they need not fear building bulging muscles because they have less testosterone and fewer cells that make up muscle fiber. In addition to working toward a better appearance, women weight lifters enjoy the benefits of improving strength and balance, and preventing osteoporosis.

Two research leaders who extol the benefits of resistance exercise (free weights, machines, isometrics, and rubber tubing), exercise physiologist

William Evans and physician Maria Fiatarone, believe that strength-building may be even more important for older adults than aerobic exercise. Although many physicians recommend walking because they think it is the safest activity, people who are weak have poor balance and are more subject to fall. Prescribing resistance exercise can give older adults the strength and confidence they need to begin aerobic activity in the first place.

## THE FLEXIBILITY AND BALANCE COMPONENT

Different types of exercise activities for older adults result in different types of benefits. A study by King and associates (1997) reported that although programs emphasizing aerobics and strength-building provide an array of benefits for older adults, flexibility exercises may be particularly well-suited for improving the range of motion and reducing arthritic and other types of pain among older adults.

Ballistic stretching, using quick and bouncy movements, works against the protective reflex contraction and can result in muscle tears, soreness, and injury. Static stretching is the type of stretching that I use in my exercise class and involves the slow and smooth advancement through a muscle's full range of movement until resistance or the beginning of discomfort is felt. The maximum position is then held 10 to 30 seconds, which allows for the reduction of the protective reflex contraction and additional range of movement.

Stretching should always be preceded by a brief aerobic warm-up in order to increase heart rate, blood flow, and the temperature of the muscles, ligaments, and tendons. Conversely, stretching while muscles are cold may sprain or tear them. In my class, therefore, aerobics always precedes stretching.

A good way to develop different flexibility routines for older adults is to complete the arthritis Foundation's 2-day PACE (People with Arthritis Can Exercise) training program to teach stretching to older adults. In addition, you receive the PACE manual, which includes a brief description of the purpose of each of the 72 movements, an illustration that demonstrates how to do each stretching movement, an explanation of the functional benefits of each movement, and the identification of special precautions—particularly for persons with arthritis or osteoporosis. There is also a separate section on teaching tips. To find out more information about the training program or the manual (the manual can be obtained separately), contact the local chapter of the Arthritis Foundation, or call the national office in Atlanta at 404-872-7100.

In each of my 10-week to 15-week classes I attempt to bring in a yoga or tai chi instructor (preferably both) as an alternative activity in one or more of the stretching components of the class. The graceful movements and inner awareness of these techniques affect one's mind as well as body, and are popular with people of all ages, especially older adults. In several Chinese cities that I visited over the summer of 1978, I observed several outdoor groups of tai chi practitioners during my early morning jogging, and noticed that a substantial number of the participants were older adults (Haber, 1979).

To demonstrate the popularity of yoga among older adults in the United States I like to share the story of Sadie Delaney with the older students in my class. Sadie Delaney reported in her book that she began her yoga practice in her 60s and continued it for 40 years, the last several of which she followed a yoga program on television (Delaney et al., 1993). Sadie died in 1999 at the age of 109. She noted in her book that when her sister Bessie turned 80 she decided that Sadie looked better than she did and Bessie then began doing yoga too. Bessie, however, probably started too late to reap the same longevity benefits as did Sadie. Her life ended prematurely in 1995, at the tender age of 104.

The most popular yoga activity is hatha yoga, a sequence of stretching, bending, and twisting movements that causes each joint to move slowly through its maximum range of motion, then is held for several seconds and repeated (see Figure 5.4). These practices improve body awareness, reduce stress, improve balance and coordination, and increase the maximum range of motion by expanding joint mobility (Christensen & Rankin, 1979).

Hatha yoga and other types of stretching, twisting, and bending exercise programs, possess two characteristics that make them highly desirable for older adults. They are well suited to all adults, even the very frail elderly (Haber, 1979, 1988a), and are exceptionally easy to incorporate into a daily routine. The movements of a stretching program, for instance, can be performed while one is watching television or talking on the telephone. Also, for people who engage in regular aerobic or strength-building activity, a brief flexibility routine can be added on at the end.

Performing yoga exercises in a group setting has become very popular with older adults. It is estimated that 18 million Americans are practicing yoga, a number that tripled during the 1990s ("Baby boomers turning to yoga," 2000). For more than a decade, I worked with older adults through the Easy Does It Yoga for Older People program (Christensen & Rankin, 1979), a widely used yoga program for older persons. I implemented yoga and related programs at senior centers (Haber & George,

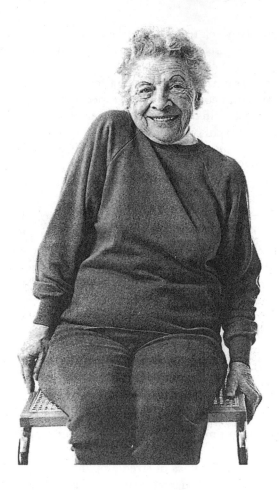

FIGURE 5.4    Shoulder roll from Easy Does It Yoga for Older People.

1981–1982), congregate living facilities (Haber, 1986), nursing homes (Haber, 1988a), churches (Haber & Lacy, 1993), and other sites. Without exception, the programs were enthusiastically received and individual benefits were demonstrable.

For those interested in practicing yoga for therapeutic purposes, the International Association of Yoga Therapists will locate therapeutic yoga instructors in local areas. Call 707-928-9898.

Though not as popular as yoga in the United States, tai chi has increased in popularity as well over the past 15 years. Tai chi consists of slow, graceful movements that are derived from a martial arts form in Oriental cultures. It is gentle in nature and well suited to young and old. Persons of all ages in China can be observed practicing tai chi in groups in urban parks and in front of congregate housing (Haber, 1979). In addition to improving flexibility, tai chi is conducted with a lowered center of gravity (knees and hips held in flexion) and can contribute to lower-extremity strength-building, body awareness, and balance control.

Balance issues emerge slowly and subtly over the life cycle, beginning in the mid 40s and becoming obvious by the mid 60s. Losing one's balance is a major contributor to falling, and each year about a third of persons age 65 and older experience a fall, as do about half of persons over age 80. Even the *fear* of losing one's balance can curtail activity, and this strategy can be particularly counterproductive. Less activity leads to more weakness, and more weakness to more falls.

In terms of balance control, two rigorously controlled studies—part of a 3-year exercise research project sponsored by the National Institutes on Aging and the National Institute for Nursing Research—support the contention that tai chi has favorable effects upon the prevention of falls (Wolf et al., 1996; Wolfson et al., 1996). One tai chi group endured 48% longer than a comparison group before a first fall (Wolf et al., 1996). By practicing the tai chi movements, older participants learn to stabilize their balance and regain it before they begin to fall.

Regarding balance exercises, I include one or more of the following exercises at the tail end of some of my classes. All the exercisers stand next to a wall, chair, or something else that can be grabbed on to when needed.

1. Toe raise: Rise to tiptoes 10 times, reaching for support only if necessary. Repeat with eyes closed.
2. One-legged stand: Stand on one leg, flexing the other knee slightly. Balance on one foot for 10 seconds. Repeat with eyes closed.
3. Tandem walk: Walk across the floor, heel-to-toe, remaining next to a wall for support if necessary.
4. Sitting upside-down (Figure 5.5): No way! I took this photograph of two Chinese acrobats while I was in China on a gerontology study tour.

It is important to remind older adults that loss of balance can be due to a number of conditions in addition to the physical losses that accumulate through a sedentary lifestyle. These conditions include problems with the inner ear, medications, poor posture resulting from arthritis or

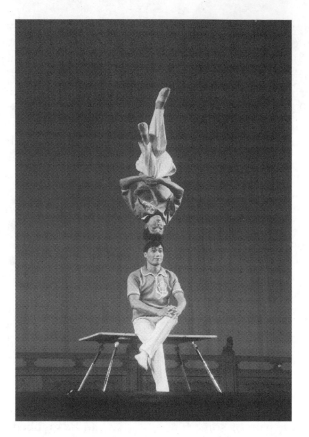

**FIGURE 5.5    A photograph of two fellows with pretty good balance that the author took in China.**

osteoporosis, poor vision, and muscle weakness. To rule out these problems, nothing takes the place of an evaluation by a health professional.

## THE HEALTH EDUCATION COMPONENT

One of the student instructors or one of the participating older adults will facilitate the health education topic (with volunteers obtained at the end of the previous class). The health education topic for the class can be one of an endless number of subjects: describing an experience with a complementary medicine technique, providing a brief description of another health-promoting class in the community, sharing a healthy recipe, discussing fall prevention ideas, sharing a list of sleep hygiene techniques, discussing tips for improving memory, and so forth. The topic may also be presented as a demonstration, rather than pedagogically, such as leading a stress management exercise like deep breathing or progressive muscle relaxation.

## OTHER EXERCISES

*Power yoga* (an Americanized version of *astanga* yoga) is a blend of flexibility and strength building that has become popular mostly in New York and California. It was introduced into America by the aptly named Beryl *Bender* Birch (1995). Power yoga differs from traditional stretching programs that encourage relaxation into a pose while stretching, in that proponents advocate for isometrically tensing specific muscles while relaxing the opposing muscles.

*Vinyasakrama* is another yoga variant that blends flexibility with aerobics, instead of strength-building. Rather than holding postures for a long time, students do a series of yoga movements without pause, synchronized with deep yoga breathing.

*Pilates* (pronounced pi-LA-tees) is a technique that uses specially made exercise equipment with pulleys and springs to stretch and to strengthen your midsection. Trained instructors guide you through breathing exercises and a routine to help you move in a balanced way. To find a Pilates instructor in your city, call 800-474-5283. The Alexander technique also attempts to promote balance and to retrain your body to carry itself properly, with particular attention to head, neck, and spine alignment. The technique combines good posture with simple movements to reduce muscle tension. To see if there is a program near you, call 800-473-0620. The Feldenkrais method is a third alternative to train your body to move with efficiency and ease. A trained practitioner gently manipulates your muscles and joints to find the most comfortable ways to use your body. For more information, call 800-775-2118.

Two programs that emphasize muscle toning and stretching are:

1. The Sit and Be Fit program. Developed by a registered nurse, Mary Ann Wilson, the program has been shown on public television for many years. If a program is not televised in your area, you can purchase a videotape for a general audience of older adults, or for persons with specific health problems—arthritis, stroke, osteoporosis, Parkinson's, multiple sclerosis or COPD. Contact Ms. Wilson at

509-448-9438, or by mail at Sit and Be Fit, P.O. Box 8033, Spokane, WA, 99203-0033.
2. Body Recall. Dorothy Chrisman began her classes for persons aged 50 and older more than 30 years ago. For more information about the program, the location of classes around the country, teacher certification, or the Body Recall manual, contact Ms. Chrisman at Body Recall, Box 412, Berea, Kentucky 40403.

For those readers who have found no variation of exercise to their liking, there is always the work of Dr. Sanders Williams, dean of the Duke University School of Medicine. Dr. Williams is working on chemical pathways that muscle cells use to build strength and endurance. This could lead to the development of a drug that will let people get the health benefits of regular exercise by just taking a pill! If you run out of patience waiting for this pill, try obtaining one of the products that recently received these patent numbers:

- #6,024,678: Vacuum cleaner leg exerciser. This invention consists of shoes with bellows, so that when you walk around your house you create suction that pulls dirt into a cleaning wand and then into a tank strapped on your back.
- #6,042,508: Remote-control dumbbell. This remote is built into a contoured weight that you lift up and down to switch television stations. It also counts your pulse.
- #5,984,841: Shower step master. This device makes you pedal in order to shower, with elastic bands that provide resistance. A side benefit is that you won't even know when you are sweating.

Special thanks to WellnessLetter.com for alerting me to these patented gems.

## DIFFERENT STROKES FOR DIFFERENT FOLKS

As the following chart of five exercise activities indicates, there is considerable variation in the types of benefits that can accrue, suggesting the importance of engaging in a balanced approach to exercise (Table 5.3). It should be noted that each of the exercises below can be performed in such a way as to improve its ranking in each of the three categories (e.g., power yoga increases strength, high repetition weight lifting improves endurance, etc.).

TABLE 5.3   Different Exercises and Benefits

| Exercise | Endurance | Strength | Flexibility |
|---|---|---|---|
| Swimming | High | Low | Medium |
| Brisk walking/jogging | High | Low | Low |
| Yoga | Low | Low | High |
| Tai chi | Medium | Medium | Medium |
| Weight lifting | Low | High | Low |

# THE ACTIVITY PYRAMID

Most people have heard of the USDA's food guide pyramid (see chapter 6 on Nutrition). Now, several organizations have developed an *activity* version of it. Not having seen one that I like without modification, I offer my contribution in Figure 5.6.

Sedentary behaviors—like eating the junk food at the top of the food pyramid—should be done sparingly. It is acceptable to watch television and play computer games, and even to eat junk food while doing it, but doing it to excess is dangerous to your health. On the other hand, slothfulness every now and then is an excellent antidote for wellness self-righteousness.

Two to three "servings" of structured strength-building exercises per week are recommended. Medium or vigorous aerobic intensity, such as jogging and some recreational activities, is recommended three or four times a week for those who have left the ranks of the sedentary far behind. Light to moderate exercise, such as stretching, brisk walking, and finding additional activity bouts in the course of a day, can be done *every* day.

Incorporating additional activity bouts into your everyday routine can be done in a variety of ways. Park your car farther away from the store, use stairs instead of escalators, walk the dog, work in your garden and, the most devious of all, do not use the remote control when watching television. People who are sedentary need to focus their attention on the base of the pyramid.

The everyday activity at the base of the pyramid is different from the exercises above it. Activity can be defined as any body movement produced by skeletal muscles that results in energy expenditure. It is in the lower sector of the pyramid that we can emphasize the healthy pleasures of spontaneity and enjoyment. Activities can be enjoyable when, for

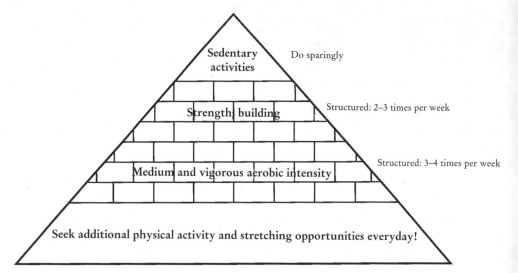

FIGURE 5.6   Activity pyramid.

instance, they are turned into social occasions with family and friends. Or you can take advantage of spontaneity in the lower sector of the pyramid by stepping up the intensity level of, let's say, vacuuming. You not only get your housecleaning done, but you also obtain a free bout of exercise in your home using your vacuum cleaner (or your duster, mop, or other household exercise tool).

Exercise, on the other hand, is planned, structured, and emphasizes repetitive body movement. It is in these upper sectors of the pyramid where maintaining a routine, rather than spontaneity, is desirable. Routine exercise can be enjoyable too, though for me, the highlight is when I am done with it and can savor the way my body feels for several hours afterwards.

# ARTHRITIS:
# A BARRIER TO EXERCISE AND ACTIVITY

This story, entitled "The Joys of Aging," has been circulating anonymously for years. It goes like this: "I have become quite a frivolous old gal. I'm seeing five gentlemen every day. As soon as I awake, Will Power helps me get out of bed. When he leaves I go see John. Then Charley Horse comes along and when he is here, he takes a lot of my attention. When he leaves, Arthur Ritis shows up and stays the rest of the day. He doesn't like to stay in one place very long so he takes me from joint to joint. After such a busy day, I'm really tired and ready to go to bed with Ben Gay. What a day!"

One of the major barriers to performing resistance training, yoga, calisthenics, aerobics, and other types of exercise is arthritic stiffness and pain. In November 2002, the Centers for Disease Control and Prevention announced that 70 million Americans have arthritis or chronic joint pain, up from the previous estimate of 43 million. This public health problem is age-related, with 19% afflicted among persons between the ages of 18 and 44; 42% between 45 and 64; and 59% age 65 and older.

Osteoarthritis (degenerative joint disease), the most common type found among older people, ranges in intensity from occasional stiffness and joint pain to disability. This disease is affected by genetics, obesity, injuries, and overuse of joint movement. Rheumatoid arthritis is less common, but can be more disabling. Although the cause is unknown, scientists believe it may result from a breakdown in the immune system.

Many people with arthritis think that any type of exercise will be uncomfortable, that is, cause joint or muscle pain or swelling of the extremities, or be downright harmful and lead to decreased functional abilities. These indicators of exercise intolerance, however, will typically not take place if exercise is performed properly. In fact, it is more likely that the joints will stiffen, the muscles will weaken, and the ability to function will decline if regular flexibility and exercises are *not* performed. To counteract arthritic stiffness, it may be necessary to briefly engage in flexibility exercises three or four times a day.

It is also helpful to engage in strength-building exercise to strengthen the muscles that surround and support the joints and to force lubricating fluid into the cartilage that helps keep it nourished and healthy. Rall and colleagues (1996) found that even people with severe rheumatoid arthritis could safely increase their strength almost 60% in a 12-week progressive resistance training program. A randomized trial comparing aerobic exercise and resistance exercise on older adults with knee osteoarthritis concluded that both types of programs are effective (P. Ettinger et al., 1997).

The advice of a physical therapist, occupational therapist, or nurse can be especially helpful when developing an individualized exercise program that balances exercise and rest. One way to minimize aches and pains is to relax joints and muscles prior to exercise by applying heat (or soaking in a warm bath) or ice packs, and gently massaging muscles. Weight control can also help keep unnecessary stress from joints.

Another technique for conquering the challenge of aches and pains in order to exercise is to choose a time of day when one is subject to the least amount of discomfort, stiffness, and fatigue. People who are on medication may find that their optimal time coincides with the period during which their medicine is having its maximum effect. Many persons with arthritis depend on anti-inflammatory drugs to alleviate aches and pains and to allow them to exercise.

Many others hold out hope for a miracle medication that will not only alleviate their arthritic pain, but also reverse the disease process. One prospect in this regard, discovered by the public several years ago, coincided with the publication of *The Arthritis Cure* (Theodosakis, 1997). The book touted two supplements, glucosamine and chondroitin sulfate, to stimulate the growth of cartilage and keep it from wearing down. Although many arthritis sufferers are already convinced of the benefit of these supplements, others may want to wait until the research sponsored by the National Institutes of Health is completed.

Another option for avoiding arthritic discomfort is finding a more appropriate exercise routine, such as water exercise. An older adult, for instance, who believes she is aggravating an arthritic knee during her walking program may find an aquatic program more desirable than a land-based exercise program. Water provides buoyancy and can relieve some of the stress and strain of other exercise where gravity and weight are greater influences. Body weight in water is less than 10% of its weight on the ground. Also, if the water is sufficiently warm it will allow greater range of motion since muscles stretch better when they are warm.

A free brochure from the Arthritis Foundation explains how to set safe exercise limits and includes tips for easing into exercises, such as taking a warm shower before engaging in exercise in order to loosen up. To obtain, contact the foundation at 800-283-7800, or its Web site: www@arthritis.org.

## OTHER BARRIERS AND CAUTIONS

There are several barriers to exercise besides the belief that it is painful, unenjoyable, and perhaps even harmful. Some older adults, for instance, engage in a level of exercise that is inadequate or that lacks the proper intensity to meet their needs yet are under the mistaken belief that they are sufficiently active. Others have a problem with overexuberance, tackling an exercise program too strenuously and too quickly, and suffering the consequences of injury (Kannus et al., 1989).

It is necessary to begin and end an exercise routine with an adequate warm-up and cool-down period consisting of gentle aerobics and stretching. It is important that the warm-up period begin with aerobics (walking, or a slow version of the exercise to be engaged in) and not stretching ,as the latter can create damage to the muscles and joints if the body temperature is not warmed up first. The cool-down period prevents blood from pooling in lower muscles, which reduces blood flow to the heart and brain and can cause faintness or worse. Cooling down may also prevent muscle stiffness and soreness by restretching muscles that are shortened during exercise. One meta-analysis of randomized research trials, however, reported no significant effect of stretching on either muscle soreness or injury (Herbert & Gabriel, 2002).

Another inhibitor of activity is the fear of falling. More than one third of community dwelling elderly fall each year (Speechley & Tinetti, 1991). The potential for falling has been used as a justification for physical restraints in the nursing home (Evans & Strumpf, 1989). Fear of falling, imposed by a caregiving spouse, may be a significant barrier to exercising. Some risk, however, may have to be tolerated, but the risk may be reduced by exercising in a seated or lying position or by a change in medication.

Medication usage can contribute to falling. Medications may require that exercise participants modify their exercise routine by decreasing the duration and intensity of an exercise, increasing fluid intake, or foregoing exercise for a period of time (Kligman & Pepin, 1992). One should be alert for dizziness, faintness, and fatigue that may result from a wide variety of medications, especially ones that belong in these categories: antiarthritic, psychotropic, antihypertensive, antiarrhythmic, antiparkinsonism, antihistamine, decongestant, and barbiturates.

To treat injury to a muscle or ligament in the form of a strain, sprain, or tear, and keep it from becoming worse, the most commonly recommended guideline is the acronym RICE, which stands for rest, ice, compression, and elevation. Rest the injured area immediately to cut down on blood circulation to that part of the body. Apply ice immediately, which shrinks blood vessels and reduces swelling. Compress the injured area with an elastic bandage or cloth to also help reduce swelling. Elevate the damaged part to a level higher than the heart.

Other barriers to exercise may include lack of transportation to an exercise facility, limited financial resources for joining a program, medical concerns, lack of access to consultation with a health professional, lethargy, inability to identify a pleasurable exercise that can sustain one's interest over time, and lack of time. Creative problem-solving can overcome most barriers.

Some health professionals erroneously believe that older adults have considerably more discretionary time than younger adults (Haber, 1993a). A perceived lack of time, however, is as likely to be a problem among older adults as among younger adults (Dishman et al., 1985). In fact, a common response among older adults is that they lack the time for exercise because they provide care for a family member who is frail. Other older adults may also have a busy schedule that consists of sedentary hobbies, family events, and volunteer obligations.

In general, exercise is a safe activity. "Indeed, a remarkable aspect of research on exercise in the elderly has been the virtual absence of reports of serious cardiovascular or musculoskeletal complications in any published trials. Thus, exercise should be viewed as safe for most older adults" (Elward & Larson, 1992, p. 45). This is not to suggest that exercise is hazard-free. Walkers and joggers oftentimes share a path with persons on bicycles, and rare collisions do occur. Overexertion in hot weather can lead to heat exhaustion (with symptoms of dizziness and a rapid or weak pulse) or potentially fatal heat strokes. High humidity is dangerous because the air is saturated with moisture, which prevents heat from leaving the body through perspiration.

Occasionally, older persons with unsuspected heart problems embark on exercise programs. To avoid this problem, individuals may consider an exercise stress test prior to beginning an exercise program. This test—consisting of treadmills, cycle ergometers, and steps—is designed to identify individuals without symptoms who may be at high risk of suffering a medical complication during exercise because of undetected heart disease. A review of several studies on stress tests, however, found that they are expensive, of unproven benefit to healthy older persons, and may serve as a deterrent to individuals who delay exercise until they get one (Firestone, 2000; Gill et al., 2000).

Individuals with known or suspected heart disease, however, should consider the test. Abnormal responses to a stress test may consist of a failure of the blood pressure level to increase as work intensity increases, or a slow recovery of ventilation and heart rate, or an excessive shortness of breath, chest pain, or electrocardiogram changes, such as dysrhythmias. There are, however, an unusually high percentage of false positives (abnormal stress-test results for people who can exercise) and false negatives (normal results for persons who should not exercise).

## MISCELLANEOUS

### HOW TO RESPOND TO AN EXCUSE

AARP's (now defunct) Staying Healthy After Fifty Program (SHAF) listed the most common excuses for not exercising: fatigue, fear of heart attack or hypertension, trouble catching breath, need to relax, too old, bad back, and arthritis. Each excuse was examined during the SHAF program and exposed as a myth or a general misunderstanding that can keep an older adult inactive.

Some examples of responses to these excuses are, respectively: improved strength makes daily tasks easier and less tiring; an exercised heart is stronger, works easier, and can lower blood pressure; heart, lungs, and muscles become more efficient through exercise and make breathing easier; exercise can help relaxation; it is never too late to exercise—even nonagenarians benefit; bad backs are commonly caused by inadequate exercise, improper lifting, and poor posture; and exercise can alleviate the pain and stiffness of arthritis.

## BENEFITS

A negative attitude also can be a barrier to exercise. When motivating someone to exercise, it is important to shift the emphasis from the negative—what will happen if you do not exercise—to the positive—how you will benefit if you do. The SHAF program listed benefits of exercise that are likely to motivate old and young alike: having fun, sleeping better, feeling more energetic, controlling body weight, feeling more relaxed, feeling stronger, increased joint flexibility, maintaining an independent lifestyle, improving heart, arteries and lungs, new social contacts, improved morale and confidence, and enhanced agility and mobility.

If these benefits do not appeal, the humorist Erma Brombeck offered a particularly unique advantage to those who exercise: "The only reason I would take up jogging is so that I can hear heavy breathing again."

## HEALTH CLUB, HOME, OR RELIGIOUS SETTING

The number of health club members who are over 55 increased by a remarkable 75% from 1987 to 1995 (Johns Hopkins, 1997). Nearly half of all health clubs now offer special exercise classes for members over age 50. Baby boomer membership in health clubs has grown almost as fast during this time with a 61% gain in health club membership among persons aged 45 to 54. In a 7-year period, from 1988 to 1995, health club members aged 45 and over increased from 18% to 29%.

There are many advantages to membership in a health club. Most clubs offer at least one free session from a qualified trainer as part of the membership fee. Weight machines are excellent for beginners because they are easy to use, and they reduce injury by controlling your form and preventing a weight from falling on you. Most health clubs arrange machines in a logical order to promote a balanced approach to strength-building. Free weights are offered as an alternative, and though more likely to produce injury, they involve stabilizing muscles that help you progress faster. Finally, aerobic and yoga classes are commonly offered at health facilities.

The downside is that a fee of approximately $600 a year per individual is typical. Also, many older adults may feel shy or inadequate in a health club with a preponderance of young, fit participants. Finally, if motivation is marginal, some times all it takes is the prospect of a 15-to 20-minute drive to the health facility to put you off.

Before joining a health club, it is wise to visit more than one, to go the same time of day that you intend to exercise, ascertain the qualifications of staff, determine if the classes are reasonable for your level of fitness, and find out if personal training advice is available when you need it.

Exercising in the home setting, on the other hand, is as convenient as it gets. You do not have to worry about how you look, and you do not have to adapt to other people's musical tastes. The investment is a one-time expense consisting of weights, weight machine, treadmill, stair stepper, or other preferred equipment. If money is a barrier, an excellent exercise routine can be devised from using the floor, wall, chair, and your own body weight, or using household items as weights or using a jump rope.

The downside is that you may be distracted by a ringing telephone, the television set, or a family member. You may also lack the peer support of an aerobics class or role models doing strength-building. Home exercise equipment typically lacks the variety of a health club.

If you are going to buy a piece of exercise equipment for your home, consider the low-tech treadmill. One study (Zeni et al., 1996) reported that the walking or jogging machine outperforms a rowing machine, a cross-country skiing simulator, a stationary bicycle, and a stair stepper when it comes to burning calories. Regardless of the home exercise equipment you purchase, check a consumer magazine for recommendations, try out the equipment before you buy, and remember that flimsy, uncomfortable, or noisy equipment is likely to wind up as a clothes rack.

An interesting alternative to the health club or home setting is the faith-based fitness movement. Synagogues and churches are hosting a growing number of fitness programs. A fitness and nutrition program called First Place has been tried in 12,000 churches. Faith-based fitness is more likely to focus on fellowship and community and less likely to be competitive or appearance-conscious. Sometimes an exercise session may end with a meditation or a prayer. Whether religious or not, however, two messages can easily apply to all exercisers regardless of setting: treat your body as your temple, and focus on both inner and outer health.

Two Web sites that relate to exercise and religious institutions are a) www.beliefnet.com, which offers spiritually oriented information on fitness for many faiths, and b) www.jcca.org, to find a Jewish Community Center that provides fitness programs and equipment.

## PERSONAL TRAINER

Is it worth $50 to $75 an hour for a personal trainer? If you can afford it, the answer is yes, both in terms of expertise and motivation. Want to make sure that your instructor is certified? Ask about their certification and call to check on their credentials. Most qualified trainers have been certified by at least one of the following organizations:

- American College of Sports Medicine 317-637-9200
- National Strength and Conditioning Association 719-632-6722
- American Council on Exercise 800-825-3636
- Aerobics and Fitness Association of America 800-446-2322
- International Association of Fitness Professionals 800-999-IDEA
- Cooper Institute for Aerobics Research 972-341-3200
- National Association for Fitness Certification 800-324-8315
- Arthritis Foundation PACE Instructor Training 800-364-8000.

Most exercise certifications are not specific for leading exercises with older adults. Make sure that the personal trainer is experienced with older persons.

There are also a number of online fitness trainers that match your personal health statistics and goals with a predesigned training program. Some sites send the user a daily e-mail prescribing that day's exercises; others display an exercise regimen on a personal monthly calendar that can be downloaded to a handheld computer. Online sites produced by a single trainer tend to be less sophisticated and may merely consist of a training plan with illustrated exercises that are mailed to you.

## THE ROLE OF THE HEALTH PROFESSIONAL

The percentage of inactive older adults would likely decrease if physicians were more inclined to recommend the health benefits of exercise to clients

(Elward & Larson, 1992). Eighty-five percent of adult respondents report that a physician's recommendation would help motivate them to engage in regular exercise (L. Harris & Associates, 1989).

Yet over the past 20 years, physicians have not been so inclined. In 1983, less than half of the primary care physicians surveyed reported routinely asking patients about their exercise habits (Wechsler et al., 1983). A few years later, results from seven surveys of primary care physicians cited that an estimated 30% of all sedentary patients received counseling about exercise (Lewis, 1988). In 1999, a survey of 6,000 older adults aged 50 and older reported that only half of the respondents said their doctor asked about their level of physical activity or exercise during any of their medical checkups over the past year (Kruger et al., 2002). Perhaps due to lower expectations, physicians are even less likely to ask patients age 65 and over to change a health behavior than their younger patients (CDC, 2002; Callahan et al., 2000).

The barriers to physician's counseling older patients include a lack of time, training, teaching materials, knowledge, reimbursement, and confidence in getting compliance from their patients (Kearney, 1998a; Kushner, 1995). Perhaps some of these barriers can be avoided by using other health professionals in the office. There have been examples of nurses being effective with reaching out to patients and encouraging them to exercise. Two nurses, moreover, reported that merely posting a sign by the office elevator giving directions to the nearest stairs is a good way to promote physical activity (J. Jones & K. Jones, 1997). Other nurses have been creative with implementing exercise programs for even the most physically and mentally compromised individuals (Colangelo et al., 1997).

## QUESTIONS FOR DISCUSSION

1. After reviewing the impact that exercise has on several diseases and conditions, why do you think most people still do not engage in regular exercise?
2. Can you think of one way that you could improve upon my community-based exercise class?
3. A client reports to you that friends of his have been injured while exercising, and he heard about one older person who had heat stroke while walking briskly and died. He has decided that it is safer to not exercise. How would you respond?
4. Is it essential that all older persons seek physician approval before participating in any type of exercise program? Explain your answer.

5. Role-play with a partner. Can you counter every excuse that your partner offers for not exercising by suggesting an idea that will encourage your partner to exercise?

6. A client calls you and complains that the surgeon general only recommended moderate exercise like brisk walking and that she is doing a fairly rigorous aerobic class, with strength-building included. She wants to know if she should exert this extra energy if it does not seem to matter. How would you advise her?

7. Has your physician ever talked to you about exercising? If so, did she or he offer guidelines or suggestions, or provide follow-up? Were you satisfied with your physician's involvement—or lack of it—with exercise counseling?

8. Have you tried elastic bands or isometrics for strength-building? If so, what is your opinion of them? If not, what do you think about trying these two options?

9. Why is strength-building more important for older adults than for younger adults?

10. Which do you prefer, the target heart rate or the Borg Technique? Why?

11. An older person wants to know if she should exercise for a longer period of time at a lower intensity level, or a shorter period of time at a higher intensity level. How would you counsel this person?

12. Have you tried one of the more unique exercise options like Pilates or another activity that may be a bit out of the mainstream? If so, what did you think about it? Do you think this option would be appropriate for older adults? Why?

13. What is the primary difference between flexibility exercises and yoga movements?

14. What has been *your* major barrier when it comes to engaging in exercise on a regular basis, and have you attempted to overcome it? If so, how?

15. If you have a regular exercise routine, does it include aerobics, strength-building, *and* flexibility exercises? If not, why?

16. What do you think about the idea of encouraging religious institutions around the country to adopt on-site exercise programs? If you were a member of a religious institution, how would you go about planning, recruiting, implementing, and sustaining an exercise program at your institution? How could you foster a nationwide program of religious-based exercise classes?

# 6

# Nutrition

A dietitian was making a presentation to a group of older adults at a senior citizens center. She began her talk by asking, "Over the long term, what is the single worst food that you can eat?" Immediately, an older woman in the front of the audience stood up and declared, "Wedding cake!"

Older adults may have a sense of humor about their eating habits, but they most definitely take the topic seriously as well. One national study reported that older people are more conscientious about managing their diets than those who are middle age (L. Harris et al., 1989). In this sample, a higher percentage of those over age 65 (approximately two thirds) than of those in their 40s (one half) reported trying "a lot" to limit sodium, fat, and sugar; eat enough fiber, lower cholesterol, and consume enough vitamins and minerals.

If older adults are continuing to pay more attention to their nutritional habits, one can only speculate that they may be motivated by more immediate feedback (heartburn, constipation, and so forth), or feelings of greater vulnerability (higher risk of impairment from disease and of loss of independence). The next cohort of older adults—today's baby boomers—bring more than motivation to the table. They also bring a higher formal education level, including a strong interest in health education.

And advertisers are taking notice of the baby boomers reaching advancing ages. A series of clever television commercials in 1997 targeted the Kellogg's Frosted Flakes that boomers used to eat when they were kids. Sales of this product increased appreciably as boomers combined their former love of this sugary cereal with appreciation for the statement on the cereal box that proclaimed "This product meets the American Heart Association's (AHA) food criteria for healthy people over age 2 when used as part of a balanced diet."

Apparently, the boomers and AHA are paying less attention to the high sugar content on the nutritional label. The AHA criteria for its stamp of approval includes limits on only fat, cholesterol, and sodium content. The AHA does have one more criterion. The willingness of the food manufacturer to pay them for their stamp of approval: $7,500 per product the first year, and $4,500 annually thereafter. Many healthful products made by small manufacturers are unwilling to pay the fee.

Nonetheless, middle-aged boomers and older adults are influenced not only by the AHA's stamp of approval, clever advertising, and an interest in reviving earlier eating habits, but are also influenced by the nutritional content of food products. Sometimes, however, it is difficult to ascertain the nutritional value of food. In 1993, for instance, newspaper headlines and television news announcers proclaimed the importance of bran in the diet but reversed those claims when the findings of a single research project with a small sample size indicated that the importance of bran was questionable.

Before the year was out, a new announcement declared, once again, that bran was an important component of the diet. By 1996 several controlled research studies supported the finding that bran and other forms of fiber reduced the risk of colon cancer and heart disease (*"End of Debate,"* 1996). This was followed a few years later, however, by two impressive studies that used randomization and large sample populations and concluded that a high-fiber diet did not reduce colon cancers (Alberts et al., 2000; Schatzkin et al., 2000). Another large cohort study also concluded that fiber did not lower the incidence of colon cancers (Michels et al., 2000).

The frequent controversies can be confusing and sometimes amusing, but they should not detract from the sensible advice that guides most educated adults. The best recipe for good health is moderation and balance, including ample fiber in the diet, and avoiding excessive fat, sugar, and sodium.

## THE FOOD GUIDE PYRAMID

In the spring of 1991, there were health-related headlines questioning whether the long-standing circle that depicted the four food groups should be changed to a pyramid. This was not merely a question of geometrical aesthetics. The equally divided circle implied that the four food groups— bread/cereal, vegetable/fruit, milk, and meat—were equal in value, whereas the pyramid better portrayed the desirable balance of foods we needed to eat, that is, showing more complex carbohydrates on the bottom of it, and less fat and protein above it.

The pyramid implied a hierarchy of value, with greater emphasis (i.e., space in the triangle) at the base, which is devoted to bread, cereal, pasta, and the like. Higher up are vegetables and fruits, followed by dairy products and meat and, at the narrow apex, the sinful fats, oils, and sweets (see Figure 6.1).

However, after 11 years of study, followed by the launching of the pyramid in 1991 amidst national publicity, the U.S. Department of Agriculture dropped the pyramid and returned to the circle diagram. Many accused the agency of caving in to the dairy and meat industries. Supporters of the retraction denied the political pressure, though not very convincingly (Nestle, 2002). They claimed the pyramid concept overlooked the recent surge of low-fat dairy products and leaner meats that made these foods more acceptable. Also, because we still have to worry about anemia, malnutrition, and calcium deficiency, the claim was made that we should not cut back on milk and meat.

One year later, however, the pyramid concept overcame the dairy and meat industry lobbyists and became the accepted figure for good nutrition. Registered dietitians and nutritionists recommend more daily selections from the bread and cereal group (6 to 11 servings) and the vegetable and fruit group (5 to 9), and fewer daily selections from the milk (2 to 4) and meat (2 to 3) groups than they previously did.

Most Americans, however, fall short of achieving the recommended number of servings in the important bottom parts of the pyramid: grains, cereals, breads, rice, pasta, vegetables, and fruit (Nestle, 2002). These deficiencies occur despite the fact that it is not as difficult to achieve the recommended number of servings in these food groups as many adults think. A pyramid serving is typically smaller than the "average helping" depicted on nutritional labels (to be examined later in this chapter). One slice of bread or half a bagel, for instance, is a pyramid serving; as is one-half cup of cooked cereal, pasta, rice, most vegetables, and cut or canned fruit. The servings on your plate, therefore, often represent more than one serving within a food pyramid group.

## MODIFIED FOOD GUIDE PYRAMID FOR ADULTS AGED 70 AND OVER

Although the food guide pyramid became the standard in 1992, appearing in classes in the public school systems and on shopping bags in

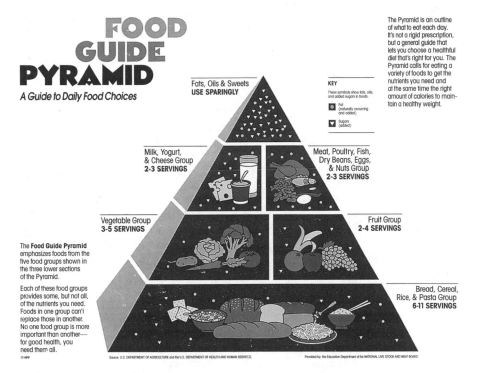

**FIGURE 6.1**    Food guide pyramid.

supermarkets, less than a decade later it began to accumulate considerable criticism. The main problems are that the carbohydrates at the base of the pyramid do not differentiate between the complex and more refined food products; that the protein categories do not differentiate between products that have high saturated fat content, such as red meat, and other products like fish, beans, and nuts; and that the fat category at the top of the pyramid does not differentiate between monounsaturated, polyunsaturated, saturated, and partially hydrogenated fats.

Another line of criticism has to do with not targeting the food guide pyramid to different age groups, particularly to older adults who have been lumped together into the 50 and over category by nutritionists for many decades. The first change in a Modified Food Pyramid for Mature (70+) Adults (Russell et al., 1999) would be to add a new foundation to the pyramid—eight 8-ounce glasses of water (Figure 6.2). Older adults have a reduced thirst mechanism and must consciously think of hydration in order to avoid cardiovascular and kidney complications, as well as constipation. Also, a flag at the top of the pyramid might serve as a

# Modified Food Pyramid for Mature (70+) Adults

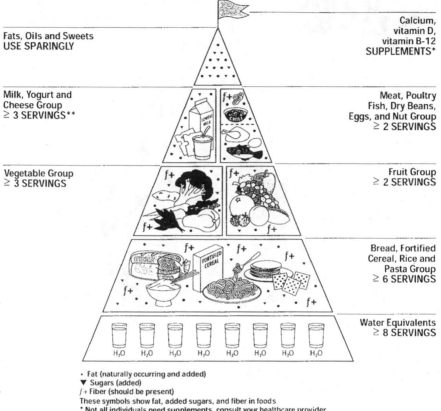

Fats, Oils and Sweets
USE SPARINGLY

Calcium,
vitamin D,
vitamin B-12
SUPPLEMENTS*

Milk, Yogurt and
Cheese Group
≥ 3 SERVINGS**

Meat, Poultry
Fish, Dry Beans,
Eggs, and Nut Group
≥ 2 SERVINGS

Vegetable Group
≥ 3 SERVINGS

Fruit Group
≥ 2 SERVINGS

Bread, Fortified
Cereal, Rice and
Pasta Group
≥ 6 SERVINGS

Water Equivalents
≥ 8 SERVINGS

• Fat (naturally occurring and added)
▼ Sugars (added)
ƒ+ Fiber (should be present)
These symbols show fat, added sugars, and fiber in foods
* Not all individuals need supplements, consult your healthcare provider
** ≥ Greater than or equal to

FIGURE 6.2   Modified food pyramid for mature adults. Reprinted with permission from the Human Nutrition Research Center on Aging at Tufts University.

reminder to older adults that many of them are not able to get adequate amounts of calcium, vitamin D and vitamin $B_{12}$, and that supplements in these areas may be necessary.

Yet even this modified pyramid does not appear to be sufficiently revised. The bottom of the pyramid should be exclusively complex carbohydrates, and the refined carbohydrates should be placed at the top of the pyramid and eaten sparingly. In the protein categories and at the apex of the pyramid there should be a differentiation between fats, with saturated and partially hydrogenated fats at the top and eaten sparingly, and the monounsaturated and polyunsaturated omega-3 fats lower down. In other words, fish, beans, nuts, vegetable oils, and similar products should be consumed in greater amounts than red meat, butter, refined carbohydrates, and sweets.

## THE PERSONALIZED NUTRITION BULL'S-EYE

Nutritionist Covert Bailey may have been the first to develop a replacement for the food guide pyramid, calling it the nutrition bull's-eye (Bailey, 1996). The goal of the bull's-eye is for people to consume the nutritious foods that are listed in the center of it. These foods are low in saturated fat and sugar and high in fiber. They include skim milk, nonfat yogurt, most fruits and vegetables, whole grains, beans and legumes, and water-packed tuna. As you move to the foods listed in the rings farther away from the bull's-eye, you eat more saturated fat, sugar, and low fiber foods. In the outer ring of the bull's-eye, therefore, are most cheeses, ice cream, butter, whole milk, beef, cake, cookies, and mayonnaise.

Unlike the food guide pyramid, Bailey's bull's-eye makes important distinctions *within* food categories. Whole-wheat products, for instance, are in the bull's-eye, while products from refined white flour and with added sugar are placed in the outer circles. Fresh fruits and vegetables are in the bull's-eye, but juiced vegetables and fruit that lose fiber and that concentrate sugars are placed in a ring farther from the bull's-eye. Skim milk, lowfat, and nonfat cottage cheese, and part-skim mozzarella are in the center ring, while whole milk and most cheeses are in the outer circles of the target.

The bull's-eye has been recognized as a useful modification of the food pyramid, and copyrighted alternatives have been developed and published, differing in one aspect or another from the Bailey version. In 1999, for instance, both *Men's Health* and *Prevention* magazines published their own bull's-eyes. The *Men's Health's* adaptation allows the reader to keep score in order to gauge their nutritional state of affairs. Every food or drink that is consumed in the course of a day that is listed in the bull's-eye nets you 5 points; in the next ring, 4 points; and so forth, until you reach the outer ring, which nets you zero points. Add up your points at the end of the day, and find out where you fall on the continuum: from nutritional sainthood to needing to make an emergency telephone call to a registered dietitian.

The *Prevention* rendition has three concentric rings, all of which include healthy foods. In the bull's-eye center are the highest levels of antioxidant-rich foods and beverages, followed by rings of foods and fluids that are lower in antioxidants but rich in other key nutrients. *Prevention* magazine recommends servings in each ring and, similar to the *Men's Health* version, offers you points in each zone. The goal is to achieve 5,000 points a day and, unfortunately for this model, the accumulated points are negatively labeled as anti-aging points. It seems to me that these are *pro*-aging points that allow you to live healthier and perhaps longer.

I offer my own personalized version of a nutrition bull's-eye. In this version, you begin with a blank bull's-eye, and then add food and drink products that you usually consume to each of the rings. The foods and drinks in Suzie Que's bull's-eye (see Figure 6.3) are clearly superior; the second ring is not quite as nutrient dense; the third ring is neutral, products that are not particularly harmful or helpful; and the outer ring includes the least nutritious foods and drinks that should be consumed sparingly.

In the center and innermost ring of the personalized bull's-eye, you also add the foods and drinks that you are not currently consuming, but that you find sufficiently desirable and are considering adding to your diet (in italics in Figure 6.3). The assignment of food and drink products to each of the rings is best done with the aid of a dietitian who can assess their nutritional value.

If motivating, you can add a scoring system to this technique. One system might consist of the following: Give yourself minus 10 points for each food or drink you consume in the bull's-eye, minus 5 points for items in the second ring, no points for items in the third ring, and plus 30 points for items in the outer ring.

Add up your points, which I call pennies (real ones), and at the end of each month (or year), if your point count is on the plus side, send that amount of money to the Center for Science in the Public Interest (CSPI, P.O. Box 9661, Washington, D.C., 20077; or www.cspinet.org), an advocacy organization that has had substantial impact on improving nutrition in America. Because I have not coordinated this effort with the center itself, do not be surprised to find that if your point count is on the minus side, you are unlikely to receive a check from them.

## GOOD NUTRITIONAL HABITS

The principles of moderation, selectivity, variety, and balance are widely believed to be the keys to healthy eating. Reduce the size of portions; consume less sugar, saturated fats, and salt; and consume more fiber, including a balance of vegetables, fruits, and whole-grain breads and cereals. Interestingly, these recommendations are not too different from

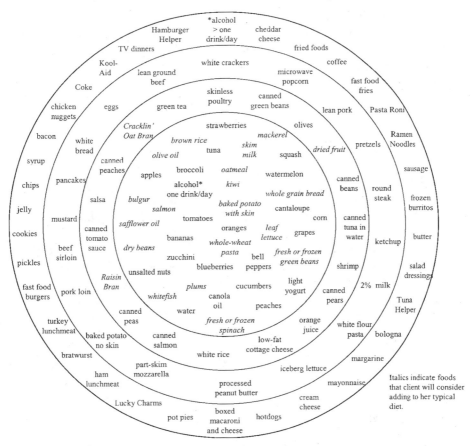

**FIGURE 6.3  Personalized nutrition bull's-eye.**

(Darson Rhodes and Mandy Puckett, graduate assistants at Ball State University's Fisher Institute for Wellness and Gerontology, identified products for Susie Que's personalized nutrition bull's eye).

what the U.S. Department of Agriculture first proposed by way of dietary recommendations in 1917 (Nestle, 2002)!

Although 95% of the American people believe good nutrition is based on these principles (American Dietetic Association, 1990), they find them easier to endorse than to practice. The good news is that some progress has been made. The Department of Agriculture reports that Americans consumed less fat over the past decade. The bad news is that during that time people consumed more calories.

Diet is only one component in the development and exacerbation of disease (heredity, environment, medical care, social circumstances, and other lifestyle risk factors also play a part), but eating and drinking habits have been implicated in 6 of the 10 leading causes of death—heart disease, cancer, stroke, diabetes, atherosclerosis, and liver disease—as well as in several debilitating disorders like osteoporosis and diverticulosis ("Are You Eating Right?" 1992).

## BASIC NUTRIENTS

Nutrients are substances in food that build and maintain body tissues and are necessary for bodily function. Nutrition education helps us learn how to provide our bodies with the more than 40 nutrients they need. Good dietary habits help us feel energetic, whereas poor nutrition contributes to feelings of fatigue and weakness. In addition, good nutrition helps us avoid obesity and other health problems.

The basic categories of nutrients are carbohydrates, fats, proteins, fiber, water, vitamins, and minerals. Carbohydrates—sugars (simple carbohydrates) and starches (complex carbohydrates)—are our main source of energy. Fats provide a reserve of energy. Proteins are needed for the growth and repair of tissues. Fiber aids in the regulation of bowel function. Water—the main ingredient in the body—provides the proper environment for the body's processes, which vitamins and minerals help to control and regulate (Hurley, 1992). Large quantities of fats, carbohydrates, protein, fiber, and water, and small quantities of vitamins and minerals, are needed by the body.

## FATS

The highest percentage of doctor visits, short-stay hospital visits, and bed disability days can be attributed to cardiovascular diseases like heart disease, hypertension, atherosclerosis, and angina. The nation's number one killer, the heart attack, is responsible for 45% of all deaths, or 600,000 per year.

Between 1970 and 1985, the annual number of deaths from heart disease declined by 39%. Between 1981 and 2000, heart disease and stroke death rates have fallen by one third for those aged 65-plus. Public education was given much of the credit for this decline; Americans not only became more knowledgeable about the risk factors for heart disease—smoking, lack of exercise, high blood pressure, sodium, obesity, cholesterol, and fats—but began to do something about them.

The American public became particularly well-informed about fats. In 1984, 8% of Americans considered fats their greatest dietary concern; by

1992, 48% designated it their major concern. Many Americans shifted their beliefs from cholesterol's being their chief health problem in their diet, to fats, which have been implicated in both heart disease and cancer (Hurley, 1992).

Saturated fats have a stronger effect than dietary cholesterol in raising blood cholesterol and increasing vulnerability to heart disease. Dietary cholesterol inhibits to some extent the amount of cholesterol our bodies produce, a compensatory mechanism that helps keep blood cholesterol levels in check. Only 20% of the population is very sensitive to cholesterol-rich diets ("Are You Eating Right?" 1992).

Fat is an essential part of our diet and a major source of energy. It is the most concentrated energy source, with each gram of fat supplying nine calories to the body. Most Americans consume too much of it. According to data from the U.S. Department of Agriculture's food consumption surveys, the average consumption of fat has always been high, reaching 40% in the 1970s, and declining to 33% of total calories in 1994, which is close to the recommended limit of 30%. In recent years, however, fat consumption has leveled off while the recommendation for daily fat intake has declined among some nutritionists to 25% or even 20% (Hoeger & Hoeger, 1997).

The Institute of Medicine (IOM) (see the September 5, 2002, report at www.iom.edu), however, has recommended a range of 20% to 35% of total calories from fat, 45% to 65% for carbohydrates, and 10% to 35% for proteins. The argument is that ranges can be more flexible and useful for dietary planning. The opposing argument is that the IOM ranges include a high-fat and high-protein diet—not to mention high sugar, which we will examine later.

Strong evidence indicates that high-fat diets cause obesity and increase the risk of heart disease and cancer. Yet food manufacturers are not in the business of helping us reduce the fat in our diets. They may, in fact, even be willing to fool us. Foods that were labeled cholesterol-free for many years, for instance, were also high in fat; examples being peanut butter, cookies, nuts, granola, vegetable shortening, and oils.

Another way to fool the public is through partially hydrogenated fats or trans fatty acids that have managed for years to escape detection on nutritional food labels. The hydrogenation process makes the fats artificially hard at room temperature, and appear to raise blood cholesterol about as much as saturated fats ("Trans: The Phantom Fat," 1996). For instance, margarine was considered for a number of years to be a healthy alternative to butter. This belief was compromised, however, when it was discovered that margarine relied heavily on trans fatty acids. It is currently believed that both butter and margarine are unhealthy, perhaps equally so ("Trans: The Phantom Fat," 1996) except for margarines like Promise which are made without trans fat. Other processed foods with trans fatty acids are crackers, cookies, pastries, deep-fried products, candy, cakes, and TV dinners.

The way the public has been fooled is that trans fat is not required to be listed on food labels. The only way to determine if this kind of fat is in a food product is through a chemist in a laboratory.

In 1993, the Center for Science in the Public Interest (CSPI) and other advocacy agencies called for the Food and Drug Administration (FDA) to add trans fat to the nutrition label. Thirteen years after the CSPI petitioned the FDA to require trans fat on nutrition labels (in 2006), the FDA will require it. It will not be added to the saturated fat total, though; nor will it, like other ingredients on the label have to, disclose how much of a day's worth of trans fat a serving of the product contains.

As trans fat gained attention in the public media, McDonald's responded by announcing it would cook french fries in oil with less trans fat. Shortly thereafter, Frito-Lay announced it would eliminate trans fat from its most popular salty chips such as Doritos, Tostitos, and Cheetos, and replace it with corn oil.

## NOT ALL FATS ARE CREATED EQUAL

In 1997 the Mediterranean diet became very popular as Americans discovered that the countries along the Mediterranean had among the lowest rates of coronary heart disease and many common cancers in the Western world. This near-vegetarian diet was high on bread, potatoes, fruit, vegetables, wine, and olive oil, and low on meat, fish, cheese, butter, and margarine.

Surprisingly, the diet was not low in fat, with more than 35% of calories coming from fat, primarily from olive oil, which consists mostly of monounsaturated fat. Thus, Americans began to extol the virtues of olive oil and other monounsaturated and polyunsaturated fats like canola, safflower, sunflower, corn, sesame, soybean, and peanut oils.

Monounsaturated fats are the best type of fat because they appear to slightly lower low-density lipoprotein (LDL) but leave the high-density lipoprotein (HDL) intact or may even raise it a little (Curb et al., 2000; USDA, 1997). Polyunsaturated fats, such as sunflower, corn, and soybean oils, appear to lower LDL, but may be less desirable because they may slightly lower HDL as well.

Saturated fat, solid at room temperature and contained in butter, cheese, and meats, is more damaging than the liquid fats. Saturated fat is converted into LDL, the cholesterol that clogs arteries. It should be noted, however, that all fats are a mix of saturated, monounsaturated, and polyunsaturated fatty acids, so even the best fats contain some saturated fat.

Researchers are beginning to suggest that we should be less concerned about overall fat content and more concerned about what types of fat we eat (Hu et al., 1997). Wolk and colleagues (1998), in fact, conducted animal studies and reported that monounsaturated fat lowered the risk of breast cancer by 45% while polyunsaturated fat raised it by 69%. However, not all polyunsaturated fats are created equal. Omega-6 is abundant in vegetable oils, particularly sunflower, corn, and soybean oils, and is less healthy than omega-3 which is found in fish like salmon, and in nuts, green leafy vegetables, tofu, flaxseeds, and canola oil. Unfortunately, more than 90% of the polyunsaturated fats we consume are omega-6 ("Dietary fat," 2001).

Most nutritional experts fall far short of suggesting that total fat content is now irrelevant, provided we obtain most of it from monounsaturated and polyunsaturated omega-3 fats. They point out that Mediterranean-style cooking is primarily healthy not because it limits saturated fats, but because it relies heavily on vegetables, grains, and beans (de Lorgeril et al., 1999; Trichopoulou et al., 1999). Moreover, the people in the Mediterranean countries have benefited from being traditionally more active than Americans are, and more successful at burning off excess fat (Brody, 1998).

In 1996, the American Heart Association summed it up best when it amended its advice on dietary fat by suggesting that Americans emphasize monounsaturated fats, but also pay attention to total fat. Every tablespoon of olive oil, for instance, supplies 120 calories, and excessive weight raises the risk of heart disease, cancer, and diabetes.

## CALCULATING FAT CONTENT

Fat is more fattening than comparable amounts of protein or carbohydrates; each gram of fat contains 9 calories, compared to 4 in protein and carbohydrates. Ideally, we would calculate fat content by separating out saturated fat and trans fatty acids in our diet, and limiting them to 10% of calories instead of the current level of 15% or 16% ("Dietary fat makes, " 2001). This has been difficult to do because trans fat has only been detectable through chemical analysis. Thus, the emphasis has been on calculating what is easiest to obtain, total fats consumed, and limiting them to 30% or less of total calories.

The formula for computing the percentage of total calories in foods that come from fat is as follows: Multiply the number of grams of fat in a food by 9 (each gram of fat contains 9 calories) and divide the result by the number of calories per serving.

Thus, a food that is advertised as 97% fat free can be much fattier than it implies, depending on the percentage of calories per serving that consists of fat (Hurley, 1992). A cup of whole milk with 8 grams of fat, for instance, may be advertised as 97% fat free. Using the formula, however, 8 grams is multiplied by 9 (72) and then divided by the number of calories per serving (150). Thus, 48% of the calories in whole milk come from fat. In 2% milk, 38% of the calories come from fat (still a high-fat food, despite the low-fat label on the carton), and in 1% milk, 18% of the calories come from fat.

The 30% fat guideline does not forbid the consumption of specific high-fat products. Indulging in high-fat milk or ice cream, for instance, can be balanced by low-fat foods that lower the overall fat intake average to 30% of daily calories. This can be accomplished by eating more fruits and vegetables (which have practically no fat) and fewer foods that are all fat (butter and margarine, for instance). The same is true for celebrating special days like birthdays and holidays, when high amounts of fat are likely to be consumed. A steady diet that stays within the guidelines for fat consumption on other days will help to average out the "exceptional" days.

Using low-fat products can lower fat intake. Many of these products may not be to our taste, but others probably are. In 1990 alone, nearly 1,000 new food products were introduced to the American public ("Are You Eating Right?" 1992). If appetizing low-fat foods cannot be found, fat content can be lowered by avoiding deep-fried foods, choosing lean cuts of meat, trimming visible fat from meat, and baking, broiling, or roasting rather than frying food.

The number of allowable grams of fat per day can be calculated by estimating the *number of calories consumed per day* (2,000 calories, for example), *multiplying by .3* (to reach the goal of 30% of total calories, in this instance, 600), and *dividing by 9* (because each gram of fat contains 9 calories), producing the number of grams (approximately 67 in this example) of allowable fat. A much simpler technique (and much rougher approximation) is dividing your ideal weight, let's say 140 pounds, in half, and allowing yourself that number (70) of grams of fat.

# CHOLESTEROL

Cholesterol is a lipid, a waxy, white, fatty substance that is manufactured by the liver and supplemented through the diet. Excess cholesterol can cling to the interior walls of the arteries and restrict the flow of blood to the heart. Eventually, it can narrow the passage sufficiently so that a heart attack results.

Two types of proteins, called lipoproteins, carry cholesterol: low-density lipoproteins (LDL) and high-density lipoproteins (HDL). Researchers believe that LDL carries cholesterol toward the body cells, leading to plaque buildup, and that HDL carries cholesterol away from the cells to the liver to be further processed and excreted. Saturated fat in the diet increases the LDL lipids in the blood. Exercise and smoking cessation will increase the HDL lipids in the blood (W. Evans et al., 1991).

The American Heart Association recommends a total cholesterol level of less than 200 mg and an HDL of 40 mg or higher. The recommended ratio between the two is 4.2 or less for middle-aged and older persons.

Cholesterol received a great deal of public attention during the 1980s. The Multiple Risk Factor Intervention Trial (MRFIT) added to this attention by evaluating a program that included lowering cholesterol and blood pressure levels among its goals. After 6 years, the men in the treatment group of this sample of 350,000 had lower cholesterol levels than did those in the control group (Stamler et al., 1986). Among the study subjects who lowered their total cholesterol level to under 180 mg, the risk of mortality for heart disease or stroke was 3 to 4 times lower than among those who had cholesterol levels over 245 mg.

In 1985, the National Heart, Lung and Blood Institute (NHLBI) set up the National Cholesterol Education Program (NCEP). The NCEP reported that 60 million American adults, including 24 million aged 60 and over, had borderline or high cholesterol levels. Because heart disease and stroke rise sharply with the cholesterol count, a federal campaign to lower the cholesterol level was launched.

The implications of the research findings on cholesterol for older adults were unresolved in the 1990s. One major limit to the studies that linked heart disease risk to cholesterol level was the lack of evidence determining whether data on middle-aged men can be extrapolated to older persons, and to women in general, who have been studied much less extensively.

Some experts, like P. J. Palumbo, MD, director of clinical nutrition at the Mayo Clinic in Rochester, Minnesota, endorsed the popularly held belief of many health professionals that older persons can tolerate a higher level of cholesterol than the general adult population (*AARP*

*Bulletin,* 1990). Other experts, like William Castelli, MD, director of the Framingham Heart Study in Massachusetts, believed that older adults may be even more vulnerable than others to the effects of a high cholesterol level, and the standards should be more, not less, stringent (*AARP Bulletin,* 1990).

## NATIONAL CHOLESTEROL EDUCATION PROGRAM GUIDELINES: 2001

Under the National Cholesterol Education Program Guidelines that were announced in 2001, the number of Americans who are recommended for cholesterol-lowering drugs will increase from the 13 million designated under the previous 1993 guidelines, to 36 million under the 2001 guidelines. Depending on your perspective, this near-tripling of persons who are now recommended for drugs, either: a) will help many people avoid heart disease, stroke, and other major vascular events, and will customize the clinical decision-making process to treat persons with lipid-lowering drugs, or b) will require the need for a subsidy for many American consumers who cannot afford the drugs, and who can no longer understand the complexity of the clinical decision-making process. In fact, both perspectives are probably true.

The new guidelines clearly represent a more aggressive approach to the treatment of high cholesterol, and a more complicated one as well. In 1993, an LDL of 160 mg/dl was considered the cutoff for treatment for most individuals; now, it can be 160, 130 or 100, depending on a host of other factors like age, total cholesterol level, adult-onset diabetes, blood pressure, abdominal fat, family history, and smoking. The recommended HDL level has not become more complicated, but the approach has become more aggressive. The recommended level used to be 35 mg/dl in 1993; now, it has increased to 40.

During the year prior to the 2001 announcement, U.S. sales of cholesterol-lowering drugs was $10 billion, and many insurance plans had shifted more financial responsibility for medications to the consumer. After the announcement, sales of cholesterol-lowering drugs will undoubtedly increase, though unpredictably, depending on the number of persons who can afford them ("Health guides," 2001). It has been reported, however, that two thirds of people who are already taking cholesterol-lowering drugs are not as compliant as they should be, partly due to the increased financial burden ("Cholesterol-lowering drugs," 2001). This is an example where a medication that is efficacious in a clinical trial may not be as effective in community practice.

The new National Cholesterol Education Program Guidelines reveals that the medical establishment believes cholesterol-lowering drugs are the best solution for cardiovascular risk factors, including for older adults. The issue of primary prevention and the benefit of treating asymptomatic persons older than age 70, however, remains unresolved (Hall & Luepker, 2000).

Although exercise and dietary interventions are also noted in the 2001 guidelines, they are dismissed as not having been effectively introduced into the lifestyle of most Americans. A health promotion policy advocate, on the other hand, would take a small portion of the estimated $300 billion that could be spent on those being recommended for cholesterol-lowering drugs, and set it aside for a new research initiative to examine how clinicians can more effectively counsel patients to improve their nutritional and exercise habits.

## CARBOHYDRATES AND FIBER

Carbohydrates are the starches (complex carbohydrates), sugars (simple carbohydrates), and fiber in our diet. Complex carbohydrates are found most commonly in breads, dry beans, potatoes, grains, pasta, carrots, peas, and corn. Many older adults have subscribed for years to the myth that complex carbohydrates, especially bread and pasta, are fattening. In fact, when carbohydrates are whole-grain they are moderate in calories and rich in fiber and nutrients.

Grains are the seed-bearing fruits of edible grasses. Each kernel of grain has a nutritionally dense "germ" or seed at its core, and a layer of bran that surrounds the kernel itself. When grains are refined into white flour, white rice, and so forth, a process that began in the 1940s, the bran and germ of the whole-wheat kernel are removed through the milling process, losing fiber, vitamins, and minerals, but not fat content.

The term *whole grain* means that the kernels are unrefined, still containing the germ and the protective bran coating. The germ provides fiber, B vitamins, and vitamin E; the bran contains fiber. The most familiar whole grains are wheat, barley, oats, rye, rice, and corn, and the uncooked grains can be added to boiling water or simmering soup. When whole grains are a regular part of the diet, the risk for cancer, heart disease, and adult-onset diabetes declines (Blumenthal, 1996; Liu et al., 2000; Rimm et al., 1996).

However, when grains are ingested exclusively in the form of mashed potatoes, white rice, and other processed foods that have little of their fiber left, the starch converts quickly to sugar. Thus, it is important to pay attention to the nutritional bull's-eye. Just as all fats are not created equal, the same holds true for carbohydrates and other nutrients.

Vegetables and fruits are complex carbohydrates that are low in fat and high in fiber, vitamins, and minerals. The exceptions are items like olives, avocados, salads with high-fat dressing, and vegetables that are fried or seasoned with margarine or butter. Unfortunately, the most popular vegetable is the fried potato, that is, french fries. Not counting the dubious french fry, Americans of all ages tend to eat less than half of the recommended amount of fruits and vegetables. A diet rich in fruits and vegetables protects against cardiovascular disease, cancers, and other morbidities (Van Duyn & Pivonka, 2000).

Fiber is the indigestible residue of food (e.g., the husk, seeds, skin, stems, and cell walls) that passes through the bowel and is eliminated in the stool. It appears to have a positive effect on cholesterol reduction, though scientists do not know exactly how this works. Fiber is a natural laxative that promotes regularity, adds bulk to stool, absorbs water, and reduces the amount of time that stool is in the bowels. A diet that is high in fiber is especially important in later years when constipation is likely to be a problem. Among persons aged 65 years and older, a diet high in fiber will also lower the risk of cardiovascular disease (Mozaffarian et al., 2003).

Nonetheless, only about 5% of American adults follow the National Cancer Institute's recommendation to eat at least 20 grams of fiber a day. This did not stop the Institute of Medicine from issuing new guidelines (Dietary Reference Intakes, September 5, 2002, at www.iom.edu) that raise the recommended amount of fiber grams per day for adult men aged 50 and under to 38 grams of fiber a day! On the bright side, the panel did not make a recommendation for older adults.

Fiber supplements like Metamucil do not contain the essential nutrients found in high-fiber foods, and their anticancer benefits are questionable ("The Many Benefits," 1996). Some older adults still rely on laxatives that are costly and in the long run self-defeating because they create a "lazy bowel." Although laxatives and supplements are not effective complements to fiber, fluid intake is. In fact, fiber needs fluid to be effective and about 64 ounces of water daily is recommended ("The Many Benefits," 1996).

About half of the American diet consists of carbohydrates, and many nutritionists recommend that this be increased to 55% to 60%. We can calculate carbohydrate needs by multiplying the estimated daily caloric intake by 55%, and dividing by 4 (4 calories are derived from each gram of carbohydrate, versus 9 calories from each gram of fat). Thus, if 2,000 calories are consumed per day, 1,100 calories (55%) or 275 grams (divide by four) of carbohydrates are needed. The key of course is to focus most of the 275 grams on complex carbohydrates.

# SUGAR

Sugars (also referred to as fructose, glucose, dextrose, maltose, lactose, honey, syrup, molasses, etc.) are carbohydrates. Some are naturally present in nutritious foods, such as fruit and milk, but a good many are added to foods. Added sugar provides calories that have no nutritional value (i.e., empty calories) while increasing the likelihood of dental caries. Natural sugar in fruit, vegetables, and dairy products differs from added sugar in that it is accompanied by vitamins, minerals, and fiber.

Much of the sugar we ingest is hidden; 29% of Heinz tomato ketchup is sugar, as is 30% of Wish Bone Russian salad dressing, 65% of Coffeemate nondairy creamer, 51% of Shake 'n Bake, and a certain percentage of some unlikely foods like soups, spaghetti sauces, frozen dinners, yogurts, and breads (Hurley, 1992).

The American population consumes more than double the recommended amount of sugar ("Are You Eating Right?" 1992), and the amount of sugar consumed by the public has steadily increased over the past 15 years (Brody, 2000a). The movement toward low-fat foods worsened the situation as many low-fat foods used sweeteners to make up for the lost fat flavor. Many low-fat foods, therefore, result in only a small caloric reduction from their full-fat counterpart.

The Center for Science in the Public Interest petitioned the Food and Drug Administration to change nutrition labels so that sugar can also be included in the percentage of the daily value it represents. At the present time, however, it is listed in grams as a subset of carbohydrates, but it is exempted from the category: percentage of daily value. A nutritionally sound diet should probably derive no more than 10% of its calories from added sugar, a percentage that is almost half of what is consumed by the average American (Neville, 2000).

Recommendations for added sugar range from 8% of calories by the Center for Science in the Public Interest, to up to 25% of calories by the Institute of Medicine (IOM) as part of their September 5, 2002, report. The high end of the IOM's more liberal recommendation is surprising, given that the panel was especially concerned about the rapidly rising number of people who are overweight or obese (see Dietary Reference Intakes, at www.iom.edu).

# PROTEIN

Proteins form antibodies, which help the body to resist disease and enable the growth and repair of body cells—organs, muscles, skin, bones, blood, and hair. Amino acids, the units from which proteins are con-structed, are the end products of protein digestion. Complete protein foods contain, in proper amounts for adults, eight essential amino acids that must be available simultaneously for the body to properly synthe-size protein. Fish, dairy products, and eggs—complete protein foods—contain all the essential amino acids.

Proteins from legumes, nuts, and cereals are incomplete, that is, they lack one or more essential amino acids. Vegetarians, therefore, must combine food sources (such as rice with beans) to meet their need for complete proteins. Proteins obtained from vegetable intake, however, may decrease bone loss and the risk of hip fracture more than proteins obtained from meat and cheese (Sellmeyer et al., 2001). The theory behind this research is that unlike plant protein, animal protein produces an overflow of sulfuric acid into the blood stream and in order for the body to neutralize this excess it must leech calcium from bones.

Protein should account for an estimated 12% to 20% of the total calo-ries in the diet (Moore & Nagle, 1990), and Americans tend to get at least that much. Older adults who are ill, however, are the most likely segment of society to experience protein deficiency. They suffer loss of appetite and oftentimes eat very little if any meat because of the cost, denture problems, lack of ability or desire to cook, or philosophy. Protein defi-ciency in older adults can result in a lack of vigor or stamina, depression, poor resistance to infection, impaired healing of wounds, and slow recov-ery from disease.

# WATER

Although we can get by without most nutrients for several weeks at a stretch, we cannot survive without water, even for a few days. Water is the medium in which all the reactions in cells take place. Water lubri-cates joints, transports nutrients and salts throughout the body, hydrates the skin, promotes adequate blood volume, moistens the eyes, nose and mouth, carries waste, and regulates body temperature. Nevertheless, adults tend to drink only about 3 cups a day, less than half the water they need. This is due in part to reduced thirst percep-tion with age.

Inadequate hydration can have many deleterious effects, beginning with constipation and fatigue, and moving on to hypotension, hyper-thermia, dizziness, breathing difficulties, and irregular heartbeats. Prolonged dehydration can lead to a variety of diseases (Jones & Ross,

1999). It is important, therefore, that older adults with inadequate fluid intake build up gradually to drinking approximately 8 cups of fluids per day, regardless of thirst.

Dehydration in the elderly was responsible for an estimated 1.8 million days of hospital care at a cost to Medicare of at least $1.1 billion in 1991 (Weinberg & Minaker, 1995). The American Medical Association's Council of Scientific Affairs recommended that undergraduate, graduate, and continuing education programs for nurses, allied health professionals, and physicians include the importance of hydration in older adults ("AMA urges awareness of dehydration in elderly," 1995).

Water, juice, and milk meet hydration needs. Additional water required by the body is obtained from foods. More than 80% of many fruits and vegetables, more than 50% of meat, and about one third of bread consists of water. Alcohol, caffeinated tea and coffee, and soft drinks raise fluid level more modestly because of their diuretic effect. One study, however, reported that caffeinated drinks do not dehydrate the body more than noncaffeinated drinks (Grandjean et al., 2000).

Alcohol consumption is not effective for hydration purposes. However, moderate alcohol consumption of one to two drinks per day may lower cardiovascular risk (Baer et al., 2002; Mukamal et al., 2003) and dementia risk (Ruitenberg et al., 2002).

## VITAMINS AND MINERALS

Since 1941 the Food and Nutrition Board of the National Academy of Sciences has published the Recommended Dietary Allowance (RDA) for the majority of vitamins, minerals, and protein that we require, and have updated these recommendations every few years based on research findings. RDAs are the average daily dietary intake level that is sufficient to meet the nutrient requirement of nearly all healthy individuals (97% to 98%) in a particular life stage and gender group.

Tolerable Upper Intake Level was added to warn against the potential for adverse effects. Although the surplus water-soluble vitamins (C and eight of the B vitamins) are excreted in urine, adverse effects can still result from exceeding the upper-level recommendations. The surplus fat-soluble vitamins (A, D, E, and K) are stored in body tissue and excessive amounts can become toxic. The body is especially sensitive to too much Vitamin A and D. Vitamins in the right amounts are needed for normal growth, digestion, mental alertness, and resistance to infection. The body also needs 15 minerals that help regulate cell function and provide structure for cells.

RDAs have been difficult to establish, especially for older adults who have been broadly defined for the past several decades as persons aged 51 and over (Table 6.1). Although we know that increasing age alters nutritional requirements, the Food and Nutrition Board had delayed for many years the establishment of separate categories for adults over 50, based on insufficient research data. The insufficient data has been caused by such problems as inadequate numbers of older adults in research studies, higher nonresponse rates from older adults, and the confounding influence of selective mortality. In addition, vitamin, mineral, and protein requirements for older adults in particular are complicated by physiological changes, living arrangements, transportation access, and disability (Wakimoto & Block, 2001).

As the research base has improved over the past decade, RDAs are being expanded into a broader range of categories, collectively referred to as DRIs (Dietary Reference Intakes) (Trumbo et al., 2001). The most important change embodied within the DRIs regarding older adults is to begin to differentiate persons aged 51 to 70 and persons older than age 70 (see vitamin D in Table 6.1).

A meta-analysis of studies focused on nutrition and age reported that nutritional intake declines with age (Wakimoto & Block, 2001). This is not surprising as energy output and muscle mass declines with age as well. Along with nutritional intake decline, though, potentially important declines in protein, zinc, calcium, folate, thiamin, riboflavin, and vitamins D, E, $B_6$, and $B_{12}$ were observed (see Table 6.2). This raises two questions that cannot yet be answered by research: a) Should nutrient intake *decline* with age, given that energy output declines as well? b) Should intake for some nutrients *increase* with age, given that absorption and utilization efficiency decrease with age?

On the positive side, fruit and vegetable consumption appears to increase with age, especially among older women, along with vitamin A, vitamin C, and potassium intake. And older persons—again, particularly women—are more likely to consume vitamin supplements (Wakimoto & Block, 2001).

To improve the intake of important nutrients, Table 6.3 (p. 178) identifies some of the best food group sources for older adults.

Two minerals of particular nutritional importance for the aging body are sodium chloride (salt) and calcium. Typically, we consume too much of the former and too little of the latter.

## SODIUM AND HIGH BLOOD PRESSURE

Sodium keeps muscles and nerves working properly and attracts water, thereby helping us retain the proper amount of body fluid. Too much

**TABLE 6.1   Recommended Dietary Allowance (RDA) for Selected Vitamins and Minerals by the National Academy of Sciences**

| Vitamin/Mineral | RDA | Upper Level | Food/Drink Sources |
|---|---|---|---|
| Vitamin A | Women: 700 mcg<br>Men: 900 mcg | 3,000 mcg | Liver, fatty fish, carrots, fortified foods |
| Carotenoids | None | None | Fruits and vegetables |
| Thiamin (B$_1$) | Women: 1.1 mg<br>Men: 1.2 mg | None | Breads, cereal, pasta, whole-grain flour |
| Riboflavin (B$_2$) | Women: 1.1 mg<br>Men: 1.3 mg | None | Milk, yogurt, whole-grain flour |
| Niacin (B$_3$) | Women: 14 mg<br>Men: 16 mg | 35 mg from supplements | Meat, poultry, seafood, whole-grain flour |
| Vitamin B$_6$ | Women 50+: 1.5 mg<br>Men 50+: 1.7 mg | 100 mg | Meat, poultry, seafood, fortified foods, liver |
| Vitamin B$_{12}$ | 2.4 mcg[1] | None | Meat, poultry, seafood, dairy, fortified foods |
| Folate | 400 mcg | 1,000 mcg | Orange juice, fortified foods, fruits and vegetables, beans |
| Vitamin C | Women: 75 mg<br>Men: 90 mg | 2,000 mg | Fruits and vegetables, fortified foods |
| Vitamin D | Ages 51–70: 400 IU[1]<br>Ages 70+: 600 IU[1] | 2,000 IU | Sunlight, fatty fish, fortified foods |
| Vitamin E | 33 IU: synthetic<br>22 IU: natural | 1,100 IU<br>1,500 IU | Oils, whole grains, nuts |
| Vitamin K | Women: 90 mcg<br>Men: 120 mcg | None | Green leafy vegetables, oils |
| Calcium | Ages 50+: 1,200 mg[1,2] | 2,500 mg | Dairy, fortified foods, leafy green vegetables, canned fish |

*(continued)*

**TABLE 6.1  Recommended Dietary Allowance (RDA) for Selected Vitamins and Minerals by the National Academy of Sciences** *(continued)*

| Vitamin/Mineral | RDA | Upper Level | Food/Drink Sources |
|---|---|---|---|
| Phosphorus | Age 70+: 700 mg | 3,000 mg | Dairy, meat, poultry, seafood |
| Selenium | 55 mcg | 400 mcg | Seafood, meat, poultry |
| Magnesium | Women: 310 mg<br>Men: 400 mg | 350 mg from supplements | Green leafy vegetables, nuts, whole-grain breads, cereals |
| Iron | Women 50+: 8mg<br>Men: 8 mg | 45 mg | Red meat, poultry, seafood, whole-grain flour |
| Zinc | Women: 8 mg<br>Men: 11 mg | 40 mg | Red meat, seafood, whole grains, fortified foods |

[1] Age 65+ probably need a supplement.
[2] NIH recommends 1,500 mg.

sodium in the system, however, causes the body to retain excess water, increase the blood pressure level, and make the heart work harder.

Americans consume twice the recommended amount of sodium (about 2,400 mgs, or a single teaspoon of salt) each day. Because many foods already contain high levels of sodium (such as potato chips, processed meats, frozen dinners, ketchup, most sauces, and canned foods) and it is hidden in a wide variety of other foods as well, we get plenty of salt (40% sodium and 60% chlorine) in our diet without adding more.

Adding salt to foods has been widely practiced. About half the women who prepared meals used salt when preparing food, and about one third used salt at the table (AARP, 1991). Because sensitivity to flavor and odors decrease with age, the desire to use salt to counteract blandness may increase with age.

Most Americans associate sodium intake with high blood pressure, yet the percentage of Americans whose high blood pressure can be attributed to salt sensitivity is unknown. In the absence of definitive research findings, many registered dietitians recommend that sodium reduction be

**TABLE 6.2   Nutrients and Clinical Manifestation of Deficiency in Older Adults**

| | |
|---|---|
| Protein | Inability to cope with metabolic stress like infection or broken bone |
| Zinc | Impaired immune function, delayed wound healing, lethargy |
| Calcium | Increased risk of fracture |
| Folate | Increased risk of stroke, anemia, appetite loss, fatigue |
| Thiamin | Compromised nervous system, weight loss, fatigue, decreased reflexes |
| Riboflavin | Problems with lips and tongue |
| Vitamin D | Bone pain, fatigue, gait disturbance |
| Vitamin E | Uncertain: perhaps reduction of antioxidant effect |
| Vitamin $B_6$ | Nausea, dizziness, confusion, depression, fatigue |
| Vitamin $B_{12}$ | Nausea, fatigue, depression, memory problems, anemia, neurological disease |

practiced widely. Nevertheless, because it is difficult to determine unequivocally whether an individual is salt sensitive, it may be useful to alternately restrict salt and then remove salt restrictions for specified periods of time, in order to assess its impact on an individual's blood pressure levels.

Salt restriction is recommended for older adults, for people with an elevated blood pressure level, for people with a family history of high blood pressure, and for Blacks, who are more likely to be highly sensitive to excess sodium (U.S. Public Health Service, 1988). The amount of salt used in cooking should be reduced for many people and the saltshaker removed from the table. Some foods that contain large amounts of salt should be avoided altogether. Labels should be read for sodium content, and people should be made aware that sodium content may be indicated by complex names (e.g., monosodium glutamate).

In 1996 two leading medical journals, the *British Medical Journal* (Elliot et al., 1996) and the *Journal of the American Medical Association* (Weinberg & Minaker, 1995), published articles that offered contradictory conclusions. Elliot and colleagues concluded that the traditional association between salt intake and blood pressure is accurate and monitoring salt intake is still important. Moreover, the relationship appears to be stronger in middle-aged persons than in young adults. In addition, other evidence indicated that salt increased calcium excretion, which raised the risk of osteoporosis (Devine et al., 1995).

TABLE 6.3   Good Sources of Nutrition for Older Adults

| To Increase Source Of | Eat More |
| --- | --- |
| Protein, iron, niacin, vitamin B$_{12}$ | Meats |
| Calcium, riboflavin, protein | Milk products |
| B vitamins | Breads and cereals |
| Vitamins C and A, potassium | Fruits and vegetables |
| Vitamin D | Fatty fish |

Weinberg and Minaker, however, concluded that low-salt diets had virtually no effect on people with normal blood pressure, making low-salt diets irrelevant to the majority of the population. This finding supports the skepticism of many physicians. In a study of 418 primary care physicians in Massachusetts, only 13% considered decreasing dietary salt to be very important for the average person (Wechsler et al., 1996).

It probably makes good sense for the time being to err on the conservative side, particularly among older adults with elevated blood pressure. One study, in fact, reported that among postmenopausal women with elevated blood pressure, salt restriction may be more effective than daily walking in lowering blood pressure (Seals et al., 2001). In the future, a so-called salt gene (angiotensinogen) may alert us to who is most likely to develop high blood pressure. It also appears that this gene responds well to a reduced-sodium diet (Johnson et al., 2001).

## CALCIUM AND OSTEOPOROSIS

Calcium is essential for maintaining bone strength. If the amount of calcium contained in the diets of older adults is inadequate, the body takes calcium from the bones and uses it for other purposes. When people lose calcium from their bones, or their body's ability to absorb calcium is reduced (a process associated with age and exacerbated by the excess use of such products as mineral-oil laxatives, caffeine, and alcohol), bones become more brittle and fragile.

This condition, known as osteoporosis, is characterized by low bone mass and an increase in the risk of fracture from ordinary skeletal stress. Over the years, the bones of a person with osteoporosis gradually thin, until some break, causing pain and disability. Almost half of women aged 50 and older have osteoporosis or the condition leading up to it—osteopenia (Siris et al., 2001). Approximately 1.5 million fractures attributable to osteo-porosis occur each year, located most often in the vertebra (700,000), hip (300,000), or wrist (300,000).

Older adult women consume about 500 mg/day of dietary calcium, considerably less than the 800 to 1,200 mg/day recommended for posta-dolescent females (Moore & Nagle, 1990). Postmenopausal women are advised to increase calcium intake to 1,500 mg/day (Heaney, 1993; National Institute on Aging, 1994). Most older adults, however, fall far short of that amount and of the 400 IU to 600 IU of vitamin D recom-mended to help absorb it (Foote et al., 2000; Marshall et al., 2001; Wakimoto & Block, 2001). The most common sources of calcium are dairy products, fortified foods, and dark green leafy vegetables (kale and broccoli, but not spinach).

Weight-bearing exercise helps to maintain strong bones by increasing bone mineral density and reducing calcium loss (Jakes et al., 2001; Kelley, 2001; Rhodes et al., 2000; Vincent & Braith, 2002). The positive effect of exercise on bone strength, however, appears to be lost within a relatively short period of time if the exercise program is discontinued (Fiatarone et al., 1990).

For information and resource materials on osteoporosis, contact the National Osteoporosis Foundation, 1232 22nd St., NW, Washington, DC 20037; 202-223-2226.

## NUTRITION LABELS

The Nutrition Labeling and Education Act passed by Congress in 1990, required that the Food and Drug Administration make food labels more educational and less confusing. The major controversy regarding this law arose from the food industry's reluctance to include the percentage of a daily value for particular nutrients on a label. The industry preferred to inform the consumer that, for instance, a frozen pizza contained 20 grams of fat, rather than that it contained 25% of the total fat that you should consume in a single day ("Are You Eating Right?" 1992). After 2 years of debate and controversy (1990–1992) consumers won out over the food industry. The following rules were implemented in May, 1994:

1.  Terms like *low fat, reduced calorie, light,* and *high calorie* must be based on federal definitions, with uniform serving sizes. Many food labels had implied positive characteristics that were, in fact, mean-ingless (e.g., lite, natural, pure, whole grains). The term *light* could

refer to color or flavor, or something other than fat, such as salt. Now, "light" means a 50% reduction from that which existed in the original product. Additional definitions were provided for "free," "low," "high," "source of," "reduced," and "less."

2. Health or medical claims must be backed by solid research. In 1996, the United States Food and Drug Administration reported that any food containing 13 grams of oat bran or 20 grams of oatmeal can carry a heart-healthy claim, provided that the food did not have other unhealthy ingredients like excessive amounts of fat or salt.

3. All packaged foods must have a standard nutrient chart, with standardized portions to make nutritional and calorie data meaningful. The chart must include information on calories, calories from fat, and the amounts of fat, saturated fat, cholesterol, carbohydrates, protein, and sodium. The label must include the percentage of the total that a person on a 2,000 or 2,500 calorie diet should have for the day.

In 1995, one year after the nutrition labels debuted, 56% of consumers used the new labels often to check nutrients and compare brands. Unfortunately, the public fixated on fat content rather than total calories. As a consequence, from 1995 to 1998 more than 6,500 reduced-fat foods were introduced to the public ("Counting on food labels," 2000), many of which were *not* low in calories. Obesity continued to rise and the interest in nutrition labels began to decline by 1999.

The nutrition labeling law had other defects. Ground beef, for example, accounts for about half of the meat sold in the United States. This one product added more saturated fat to the average American's diet than any other single food. Yet a package of ground beef, which can provide 14 grams of fat in a single serving, can have an "85% *lean*" label on it. This label professes that a serving with 14 grams of fat still can be described as lean.

## MALNUTRITION

Americans are no longer dying of pellagra, rickets, beriberi, or scurvy—due to deficiencies in niacin, vitamin D, thiamin, and vitamin C—thanks largely to the fortification and enrichment of our foods. Nonetheless, malnutrition remains a serious problem. Between 16% and 30% of older Americans are malnourished or at high risk, with higher percentages among older hospital patients and nursing home residents (Beers & Berkow,

2000; "Malnutrition," 1995; "Your Elderly Patients," 1993). These malnourished older adults take 40% longer to recover from illness, have two to three times as many complications, and have hospital stays that are 90% longer.

There are many risk factors for malnourishment in older adults (Table 6.4). The link between malnutrition and social isolation is particularly strong and suggests that "encouraging participation in various activities and clubs, as well as sharing meals with friends or neighbors may be far more effective in improving dietary intake than simple dietary advice" (Horwath, 1991). Men living alone consume fewer fruits and vegetables and have a much greater propensity for selecting easy-to-prepare foods that are high in fat and low in complex carbohydrates than do those who have companions (Horwath, 1989). Loneliness, bereavement, and social isolation are associated with poor dietary intake in late life (Horwath, 1991). An increasing percentage of older adults report difficulty in preparing meals, particularly after age 85 (M. Davis et al., 1985).

Many elderly individuals depend on meals prepared at a congregate nutrition site or meals-on-wheels program. As the demand for services of this type increases along with the number of frail, very old adults, the likelihood that the supply of such services will meet the need is unlikely based on funding trends, and malnutrition may increase.

Nutrition screenings examine characteristics known to be associated with dietary and nutritional problems in order to identify high-risk individuals. One such screening initiative, a collaborative project by the American Academy of Family Physicians, the American Dietetic Association and the National Council on the Aging, resulted in the production of a manual that begins with a checklist "DETERMINE Your Nutritional Health," shown in Figure 6.4.

The manual includes a variety of screening tools on nutrition and related topics, including body mass index, eating habits, functional status,

**TABLE 6.4   Risk Factors for Malnourishment in Older Adults**

| | | | |
|---|---|---|---|
| Inappropriate food intake | Loss of appetite | Decreased thirst | Dental problems |
| Social isolation | Poverty | Dementing illness | Medical disease |
| Physical condition | Alcoholism | Endurance problems | Balance problems |
| Depression | Medication usage | Medication withdrawal | |

*The Warning Signs of poor nutritional health are often overlooked. Use this checklist to find out if you or someone you know is at nutritional risk.*

Read the statements below. Circle the number in the yes column for those that apply to you or someone you know. For each yes answer, score the number in the box. Total your nutritional score.

# DETERMINE YOUR NUTRITIONAL HEALTH

|  | YES |
|---|---|
| I have an illness or condition that made me change the kind and/or amount of food I eat. | 2 |
| I eat fewer than 2 meals per day. | 3 |
| I eat few fruits or vegetables, or milk products. | 2 |
| I have 3 or more drinks of beer, liquor or wine almost every day. | 2 |
| I have tooth or mouth problems that make it hard for me to eat. | 2 |
| I don't always have enough money to buy the food I need. | 4 |
| I eat alone most of the time. | 1 |
| I take 3 or more different prescribed or over-the-counter drugs a day. | 1 |
| Without wanting to, I have lost or gained 10 pounds in the last 6 months. | 2 |
| I am not always physically able to shop, cook and/or feed myself. | 2 |
| **TOTAL** | |

## Total Your Nutritional Score. If it's ---

**0-2**     **Good!** Recheck your nutritional score in 6 months.

**3-5**     **You are at moderate nutritional risk.** See what can be done to improve your eating habits and lifestyle. Your office on aging, senior nutrition program, senior citizens center or health department can help. Recheck your nutritional score in 3 months.

**6 or more**   **You are at high nutritional risk.** Bring this checklist the next time you see your doctor, dietitian or other qualified health or social service professional. Talk with them about any problems you may have. Ask for help to improve your nutritional health.

*These materials developed and distributed by the Nutrition Screening Initiative, a project of:*

 AMERICAN ACADEMY OF FAMILY PHYSICIANS

 THE AMERICAN DIETETIC ASSOCIATION

 NATIONAL COUNCIL ON THE AGING, INC.

**Remember that warning signs suggest risk, but do not represent diagnosis of any condition. Turn the page to learn more about the Warning Signs of poor nutritional health.**

FIGURE 6.4   Determine your nutritional health.

**The Nutrition Checklist is based on the Warning Signs described below. Use the word DETERMINE to remind you of the Warning Signs.**

# Disease

Any disease, illness or chronic condition which causes you to change the way you eat, or makes it hard for you to eat, puts your nutritional health at risk. Four out of five adults have chronic diseases that are affected by diet. Confusion or memory loss that keeps getting worse is estimated to affect one out of five or more of older adults. This can make it hard to remember what, when or if you've eaten. Feeling sad or depressed, which happens to about one in eight older adults, can cause big changes in appetite, digestion, energy level, weight and well-being.

# Eating Poorly

Eating too little and eating too much both lead to poor health. Eating the same foods day after day or not eating fruit, vegetables, and milk products daily will also cause poor nutritional health. One in five adults skip meals daily. Only 13% of adults eat the minimum amount of fruit and vegetables needed. One in four older adults drink too much alcohol. Many health problems become worse if you drink more than one or two alcoholic beverages per day.

# Tooth Loss/ Mouth Pain

A healthy mouth, teeth and gums are needed to eat. Missing, loose or rotten teeth or dentures which don't fit well or cause mouth sores make it hard to eat.

# Economic Hardship

As many as 40% of older Americans have incomes of less than $6,000 per year. Having less--or choosing to spend less--than $25-30 per week for food makes it very hard to get the foods you need to stay healthy.

# Reduced Social Contact

One-third of all older people live alone. Being with people daily has a positive effect on morale, well-being and eating.

# Multiple Medicines

Many older Americans must take medicines for health problems. Almost half of older Americans take multiple medicines daily. Growing old may change the way we respond to drugs. The more medicines you take, the greater the chance for side effects such as increased or decreased appetite, change in taste, constipation, weakness, drowsiness, diarrhea, nausea, and others. Vitamins or minerals when taken in large doses act like drugs and can cause harm. Alert your doctor to everything you take.

# Involuntary Weight Loss/Gain

Losing or gaining a lot of weight when you are not trying to do so is an important warning sign that must not be ignored. Being overweight or underweight also increases your chance of poor health.

# Needs Assistance in Self Care

Although most older people are able to eat, one of every five have trouble walking, shopping, buying and cooking food, especially as they get older.

# Elder Years Above Age 80

Most older people lead full and productive lives. But as age increases, risk of frailty and health problems increase. Checking your nutritional health regularly makes good sense.

The Nutrition Screening Initiative, 2626 Pennsylvania Avenue, NW, Suite 301, Washington, DC 20037
© The Nutrition Screening Initiative is funded in part by a grant from Ross Laboratories, a division of Abbott Laboratories.

FIGURE 6.4 Determine your nutritional health *(continued)*.

cognitive status, and depression. To order copies of this manual, contact Nutrition Screening Manual for Professionals Caring for Older Americans, Nutrition Screening Initiative, 1010 Wisconsin Ave. NW, #800, Washington, D.C. 20007; or access www.aafp.org.

When clients lose their appetite, the following is recommended: eat smaller and more frequent meals; take advantage when you feel good and are hungry, regardless of the time; eat higher calorie foods or consider taking a nutritional supplement; postpone beverages toward the end of a meal; create a pleasant eating atmosphere and find company to enjoy the meal with; and see a physician to either change a medication that is affecting appetite, or add a medication that may relieve nausea, heartburn, or other symptoms that occur when you eat ("Loss of Appetite," 1997).

# MISCELLANEOUS

## PROFESSIONAL INVOLVEMENT

Data on the nutritional counseling of older clients are wanting, but the Healthy People 2000 mid-decade review suggested that about 30% of health professionals offered such counseling to clients in 1992, with no indication that this percentage increased by 1995. Some advocates believe that the percentage is much lower than 30% and question whether federal assessments measure serious attempts by health professionals to analyze clients' diets, or whether they include the offer of a passing comment or two. Michael Jacobson, director of the Center for Science in the Public Interest, estimates that only 5% of physicians offer nutritional counseling to a useful extent.

Dietary counsel by nurses, physicians, allied health professionals, registered dietitians, and nutritionists can be effective in changing the dietary habits of clients (Caggiula et al., 1987). Yet only one in four clients reported a discussion of "eating proper foods" during a routine visit to a health professional in the previous year (NCHS, 1988).

Referrals to qualified nutritionists or dietitians for counseling are also not common (Lewis, 1988). The importance of nutrition referrals by physicians to qualified health practitioners is substantiated by a survey of Massachusetts's primary care physicians. Only 35% reported being very prepared to counsel patients in nutrition and only 7% reported feeling very successful (Wechsler et al., 1983). Wechsler and colleagues' (1996) follow-up survey 13 years later found that physicians were even less attentive to their patients' diets than they had been in the past.

Insufficient training and inattentiveness to patients' diets contributed to the U.S. Preventive Service Task Force 2003 update to conclude that there is insufficient evidence to recommend for or against routine behavioral counseling to promote a healthy diet. If patients have known risk factors for cardiovascular or diet-related chronic disease, however, then counseling by primary care clinicians or by referral to dietitians is recommended.

If diet or health advice is provided by a visibly overweight doctor, nurse, or dietitian, almost half of the Americans (45%) surveyed in a national Gallup poll would either fail to take the advice seriously or be inclined to ignore it (Hurley, 1992).

## ORGANIC FOODS

Although the sales of organic foods are only about 1% to 2% of the total food industry, the growth rate has been 20% per year over the past decade. On October 21, 2002, the first national standards for organic foods were implemented. To earn the organic label, both domestic and imported foods need to be produced without pesticides, hormones, antibiotics, irradiation, or bioengineering. Furthermore, organic farmers must conserve soil and water to enhance environmental quality, and treat animals humanely.

To ensure standards, the U.S. Department of Agriculture uses accredited private companies and state agencies to inspect and certify companies as organic. Companies that illegally state their foods as organic face penalties up to $10,000 per violation.

Foods that are 100% organic can state they are 100% organic, and display the green USDA Organic seal. Foods that are at least 95% organic can state they are organic and use the USDA seal. Foods that are at least 70% organic can state "made with organic ingredients," but cannot use the USDA seal. Foods that are less than 70% organic can state "some organic ingredients," but cannot use the USDA seal.

Organic does not necessarily mean healthy. Organic donuts and organic chips are just as high in fat and calories as the conventional kind. And food labeled natural does not mean organic. Natural means the product contains no artificial ingredient or added color and is only minimally processed.

## ENRICHED AND FORTIFIED FOODS

When nutrients lost through processing are replaced the food is labeled "enriched." When nutrients normally present are added to exceed the natural amount, the food is labeled "fortified." Enriched and fortified foods have made a significant contribution in the reduction of malnutrition in this county, but they are not necessarily good substitutes for other nutrient-dense products. In other words, an orange drink that informs the consumer it is fortified with vitamin C does not report which nutrients from a more nutritious counterpart like orange juice are missing.

## CHOCOLATE

Aside from a few chocolatier entrepreneurs in the state of Pennsylvania—the nation's chocolate capital where 20% of our chocolate is produced—few claim that chocolate is a health food. But there are an increasing number of researchers who are touting the disease-fighting, antioxidant properties of the plant compounds found in dark chocolate ("Is Chocolate Good for You?" 2000). The heart-protecting antioxidants in chocolate are flavonoids, the plant-based compounds that are also found in red wine, tea, and some fruits and vegetables.

On the downside, there are 230 calories and 13 grams of fat in a 1.55-ounce Hershey bar. And if you are like me, you feel bad longer for having eaten it than you feel good during the process of eating it.

## JUNK FOOD AND FAST FOOD

Junk food—also known as energy-dense and nutrient-poor foods in academic circles—provide about one third of the daily calorie intake of adult Americans. Younger adults prefer salty snacks, candy, and soft drinks; older adults prefer fats and desserts (Kant, 2000). In 2001, Americans ate about 6.5 billion pounds of snacks, with potato chips and tortilla chips leading the way. Fast foods, which also tend to be energy-dense and nutrient-poor, are on the rise as well. In 1970, Americans spent about $6 billion annually on fast food; in 2000, over $110 billion.

Older adults often opt for the convenience of prepared, frozen microwaveable meals. These foods, unfortunately, are typically high in fat, sodium, and cholesterol. Healthier options were made available to consumers after ConAgra's CEO, Mike Harper, suffered a heart attack and shortly thereafter created Healthy Choice Dinners. Other companies followed suit.

What are the dietary habits of future cohorts of older adults likely to be? McDonald's, Pizza Hut, Domino's, and other fast food outlets are located in about 30% of public high schools in the United States (Schlosser, 2001). And Ronald McDonald is second only to Santa Claus in familiarity among children ("How McNuggets," 2001).

In 1955, Americans spent 19% of their food dollars on restaurants; today, that figure has increased to 41%. The average American eats out more than 4 times a week, and more than half the time eats at a fast-food restaurant. Restaurant meals contain 20% more fat than home-cooked meals and less desirable in terms of sodium, cholesterol, calcium, and fiber (Brody, 2002).

The most alarming trend in restaurants is an increase in portion size and calorie inflation. An order of McDonald's french fries, for instance, went from 200 calories in the 1960s up to 610 calories in 2000. Muffins and bagels at restaurants have gotten bigger, with calories doubling or tripling. Entrees have gotten bigger also, with portions reaching out to the edges of the plate; and now the plates are getting bigger to accommodate even larger portions.

The good news is that many fast food restaurants offer healthier options, such as a salad bar (though many consumers are imprudent when it comes to adding salad dressing) and the choice of grilled chicken instead of fried meat. Mexican restaurants are offering soft corn tortillas as a substitute for hard taco shells (zero versus 6 grams of fat), and customers can fill up with beans, salsa, and low-fat sour cream. At Chinese restaurants, health-conscious consumers can choose stir-fry fresh or frozen vegetables served over brown rice.

## CONTAMINATED FOODS

Public health officials are concerned about pesticides and other contaminants in the foods that are purchased because they interfere with hormones that regulate how the body functions. Fruits and vegetables are the most likely foods to contain pesticides, with about half of those tested having pesticide residues on or in them ("Pesticide Exposure," 1997). Strawberries are by far the most contaminated fruit or vegetable. When it comes to lettuce and cabbage, washing, peeling skins, and removing the outer leaves are helpful in reducing residues.

Bread and other grain products tend not to have residues because the milling process removes them. Pesticides are more likely to accumulate in fatty meats, fish, and dairy products than in their leaner counterparts. The biggest seafood hazard is raw or undercooked shellfish, which accounts for more than 90% of seafood poisoning cases ("Fishing for Safe Seafood, 1996"). Contaminated seafood causes about 113,000 reported cases of food poisoning each year in the United States, according to the Food and Drug Administration, and countless unreported cases. To find out about meat and poultry food safety issues call the hotline at 202-720-3333, weekdays 10:00 a.m. to 4:00 p.m. EST.

## CAFFEINE

According to the *Mayo Clinic Health Letter* (1997), if you are going to have a vice, coffee is probably one of the least harmful—as long as you drink it in moderation. Caffeine is the stimulant that gives coffee its kick. Evidence that the caffeine in coffee causes serious health problems like cancer, cardiovascular disease, osteoporosis, and fibrocystic breast changes is weak, and if health problems are found at all, they occur only at very high levels of coffee consumption.

Less harmful, but nonetheless annoying, problems such as irritability, heartburn, and bladder or stomach ulcer irritations tend to occur only when large quantities of coffee, perhaps eight cups or more, are consumed during the day. To reduce consumption, it is best done gradually to avoid withdrawal symptoms such as headaches, or even nausea or depression.

For those who do not like coffee but want a bad alternative, there is caffeine-spiked water like Aqua Blast and Water Joe or juice drinks like Java Juice and Energy Booster. These products contain from 60 to 125 mg of caffeine, compared to an 8-ounce cup of coffee that has 135 mg of caffeine.

## SENSORY DECLINE

An age-related decline in the sense of smell (not taste) directly affects a person's ability to taste or enjoy food (Greeley, 1990). Older persons have more trouble identifying pureed foods, for instance, than do younger persons. If younger persons held their noses while eating, their ability to identify foods would drop to the level of older adults.

To enhance food aromas for older adults, herbs and spices are encouraged. Adding flavors and sweeteners also can enhance taste. Another technique for stimulating appetite is a combination of different textures, for example, adding granola to yogurt.

## QUACKERY

The following examples can help to distinguish between a certified health professional and a quack. Dietitians and nutritionists individualize a nutrition plan and make sure that fat is limited and complex carbohydrates and fiber emphasized. They encourage lifelong changes that include regular exercise, ongoing behavior management techniques, and identifying sources of emotional support in order to help clients sustain changes in their eating habits. They advocate for the consumption of a wide variety of foods and suggest supplements primarily when needs cannot be met through diet. They do not promise cures, and they do consult with physicians. They are also more likely to have earned a nutrition-related degree from a 4-year accredited college or university or are registered dietitians (RD) which requires passing a national exam.

Quacks, on the other hand, rely on testimonials, are not shy about promising to cure a disease, typically foresee quick results, often emphasize one or two food groups, frequently encourage megadoses of vitamins, and repeatedly denigrate other people's ideas, even those based on scientific evidence.

Want a qualified nutritionist to design a healthy eating plan? Call the Nutrition Information Line of the American Dietetics Association, at 800-366-1655 to find an adviser in your area.

## Socioeconomic and Cultural Sensitivity

In addition to the physiological changes that occur with age, health professionals need to be sensitive to the socioeconomic and cultural factors that influence their clients. For example, health professionals ought not to try to increase the protein consumption of clients who have low-income by recommending diets that contain expensive lean meat, fish, or poultry. Nor should health professionals recommend diets that completely ignore the food preferences of members of particular ethnic groups. Ethnic foods are a source of pride, identity, and fond memories. Every effort should be made to incorporate food preferences in nutritional planning.

## Advocacy

The Center for Science in the Public Interest (CSPI) is an educational and advocacy organization. Its educational component consists of the *Nutrition Action Healthletter*, published monthly, which informs more than 800,000 subscribers, including this author. The organization is best known, however, for its advocacy accomplishments, under the leadership of its executive director and cofounder (in 1971), Michael Jacobson.

Jacobson and CSPI staff, for example, have led the fight for nutrition labels on food items in the supermarket; for exposing the hidden fat in Chinese, Mexican, Italian, and delicatessen food; for pressuring movie theatres to stop cooking popcorn in artery-clogging coconut oil; for warning labels on Procter & Gamble's fake fat, Olean, which may interfere with the absorption of nutrients and cause loose stools and cramping; for more accurate labeling of ground beef in supermarkets; and for the listing of trans fat on nutrition labels.

For more information, contact the Center for Science in the Public Interest, 1875 Connecticut Avenue, NW, Suite 300, Washington, DC 20009; 202-265-4954 (fax); or connect to www.cspinet.org.

## NEWSLETTERS

To obtain a newsletter on nutritional topics, contact one of the following:

- Center for Science in the Public Interest, *Nutrition Action Health Letter,* 1875 Connecticut Avenue, NW, Suite 300, Washington, DC 20009; 202-265-4954 (fax); www.cspinet.org
- *Environmental Nutrition: The Professional Newsletter of Diet, Nutrition and Health,* 2112 Broadway, New York, NY 10023; 800-829-5384
- Mayo Foundation for Medical Education and Research, *Mayo Clinic Nutrition Letter,* 200 1st Street, SW, Rochester, MN 55905
- Diet, Nutrition and Cancer Prevention, National Cancer Institute, Building 31, Room 10A24, Bethesda, MD 20892; 800-4-CANCER
- National Center for Nutrition and Dietetics, 216 W. Jackson Boulevard, Suite 800, Chicago, IL 60606-6995
- Consumer Nutrition Hotline 800-366-1655
- *Tufts University Diet & Nutrition Letter,* P.O. Box 57857, Boulder, CO 80322-7857; 800-274-7581
- University of California Berkeley Wellness Newsletter, P.O. Box 420148, Palm Coast, FL 32142; 800-829-9170

## WEB SITES

- www.usda.gov/cnpp—USDA's online Interactive Healthy Eating Index helps you assess the quality of your daily diet.
- www.cyberdiet.com—Commercial site that provides nutritional information and support for a better diet and healthier lifestyle.

# QUESTIONS FOR DISCUSSION

1. What are some differences to consider when attempting to motivate an older adult to change an eating habit, versus a younger adult?

2. Research suggests that older adults are more conscious of their nutritional habits than younger adults. Conduct your own survey of five older adults and five younger adults, asking them to rate how much attention they pay to eating what is good for them, using a scale of 1 (not very often) to 10 (all the time). Does your convenience sample corroborate the positive relationship between age and good nutritional habits?

3. Can you give three examples in which changing a dietary habit might be an acceptable alternative to taking a medication for a health problem?

4. How would you improve nutrition labeling?

5. Ask someone about an important change they made in their eating habits. What difficulties did they encounter making the change, and how did they overcome them?

6. Offer five tips to someone who eats often at restaurants, but wants to eat more nutritiously.

7. Not all fats are created equal. Can you explain the differences?

8. Is 2% milk low-fat? Why?

9. What does the author have against the National Cholesterol Education Program Guidelines of 2001? Make an argument that the Guidelines do more good than harm.

10. Not all carbohydrates are created equal. Can you explain the differences?

11. Should most older Americans be concerned about the amount of sodium in their diet? Why?

12. Should we *routinely* counsel older adults to supplement their dietary calcium and vitamin D, or should we target older adults who are most likely to be at risk? Why?

13. What are four ways to improve bone strength?

14. Which RDAs have acknowledged age differences?

15. Create your own nutrition bull's-eye, filling in the foods and drinks that you consume or might consider consuming. Use it for a week to guide your eating choices. Take a list of the food products in the center of your bull's-eye to the supermarket with you. Did you find this technique to be helpful?

# 7

# Weight Management

## TRENDS IN WEIGHT GAIN

According to the Centers for Disease Control and Prevention, between 1988 and 2000, the percentage of overweight American adults aged 20 to 74 rose from 56% to 65%, and the percentage of obese adults increased from 22% to 31%. The highest percentage of obese adults are in the age group 50 to 69, with those aged 70 to 79 the next most obese (Squires, 2002).

This surprising epidemic has escalated despite the fact that Americans spend about $40 billion a year on diet products and programs; that excess weight is widely known to be a risk factor for disease and death; that obesity is a social stigma in our society and continues to offend most people's personal vanity; and that a health revolution has supposedly occurred in America.

It does appear that some type of health revolution occurred in America during the past 25 years. Cigarette smoking declined significantly during that time; alcohol abuse was identified as a common risk factor, and steps were taken to curtail it, especially among automobile drivers; seat belt use has risen steadily; brisk walking, jogging, aerobic dancing, and other exercises have attracted tens of millions of new participants; and the use of low-fat food alternatives has proliferated. How could the nation have grown fat while all of this was happening?

Some health analysts believe that the fitness revolution was limited to only a segment of the population, perhaps 20%, with the majority of Americans still sedentary and consuming more calories than ever. Others theorize that significant numbers of Americans have been responding to the computer age by relying on their computers rather than physical activities for entertainment as well as work. Another theory is that many people in this highly stressful era have been using food as a coping device to combat the anxiety and depression caused by violence, job reductions, divorce, and so forth. It has also been suggested that while many Americans have been preoccupied with fat reduction, they were not as vigilant with calorie reduction. Yet another theory is that legions of ex-smokers have turned to overeating.

Each of these ideas contains some elements of truth, yet I favor still another theory. Our society is aging. As noted in chapter 1, the familiar population pyramid, with a few old people at its top and many young people at its base, is fast becoming a rectangle. This population rectangle, which has been taking shape over the past 20 years, will complete its metamorphosis over the next three decades. In 1980, nearly three times as many persons were under age 18 as were over age 65 (28% vs. 11%). By 2030, slightly more people will be over age 65 than are under age 18 (22% vs. 21%).

As we age, our metabolism—the chemical processes that build and destroy tissue—gradually slows. When it comes to eating, our fat oxidation or fat-burning rate slows down about 30% with age (Roberts et al., 1996). The metabolism that breaks down food components releases them in the form of energy and heat more slowly. Thus, the number of calories that were required to maintain our weight when we were young no longer maintains our weight, but increases it. Also, chronic conditions—most notably arthritis—that accompany the aging process can place limitations on our ability to stay active. Activity is a crucial factor in long-term weight management.

According to the Harris poll and the National Health and Nutrition Examination Survey, obesity reaches a peak among people in their 50s. More specifically, obesity peaks between the ages of 45 and 55 for men, and between 55 and 65 for women (Van Itallie & Lew, 1990). Between the ages of 25 and 55 the average American gains 30 pounds of weight, about a pound a year. Moreover, during this time period most Americans are sedentary and *lose about 15 pounds of muscle mass,* so the 30-pound weight gain actually translates into a 45-pound *fat* gain.

Between the ages of 60 and 70, weight tends to be maintained, and around age 75 there begins to be a tendency to lose weight. Unfortunately, this weight loss is due more to lost muscle than lost fat, and older persons not only become thinner, but weaker and less functional as well.

Obesity is more prevalent among low-income minority women. In 1980, 25% of women above the poverty level were overweight, while 37% of women with incomes below the poverty level were overweight (U.S. Public Health Service [USPHS], 1988). In 1999–2000, Mexican

American women were 40% obese compared to 29% for Mexican American men; African American women were 50% obese compared to 28% for African American men (Flegal et al., 2002; Squires, 2002). Using the less rigorous criterion of being overweight, more than 80% of African American women aged 40 years or older were overweight (Flegal et al., 2002).

Just days prior to leaving his post in 2002 to work at Morehouse University's School of Medicine, U.S. Surgeon General David Satcher declared overweight to be of epidemic proportions in America. He then released a Call to Action to Prevent and Decrease Overweight and Obesity. This document contends that weight-control activities should be a national priority for immediate action, and that all sectors of society should participate.

It remains to be seen, however, whether the current surgeon general, Dr. Richard Carmona—a trauma surgeon with battlefield medical experience—will take up the challenge to fight obesity, or whether his focus will more likely reflect his combat background and target another national priority: the fight against terrorism.

## OBESITY AND OVERWEIGHT

The terms commonly used to refer to people who weigh more than recommended are *overweight* and *obese*. One way to define these terms is that people who exceed the desirable range by 10% are classified as overweight, and by 20% or more, obese.

The body mass index (BMI) also provides a simple and roughly accurate method for determining population overweight and obesity. BMI can be calculated easily by multiplying weight in pounds by 700, divided by height in inches, and then dividing by height again; or if you have a pocket calculator, divide body weight (kg) by height squared (m²). Persons who have a BMI between 25 and 29.9 are overweight, a BMI between 30 and 39.9 are obese, and a BMI of 40 or over are extremely obese. According to this criterion, almost two thirds of adult Americans are overweight, almost one third are obese, and about 5% are extremely obese.

The BMI is a useful tool for screening the general population but, similar to height/weight charts, fails to differentiate fat from lean body mass. Thus, the BMI has three weaknesses when it comes to individual assessment: a) Persons with a large amount of muscle mass can appear to be overweight and erroneously fall into the high-risk category. b) There is no differentiation between the centrally obese apple-shape body (a heart risk factor) and the pear-shape body (less of a risk factor). c) Older adults at high risk of excess weight are likely to be underestimated because many have excess body fat that is counteracted by a loss of muscle mass with age. The net result can be a BMI under 25 despite the excess body fat.

One study reported that even being modestly overweight increases the chances of developing heart failure. This study of almost 6,000 adults reported that while the risk of heart failure is double in obese people, it is still a substantial 34% higher in those who are only overweight (Kenchaiah et al., 2002). For each increment of one unit on the BMI scale, the risk increased 5% for men and 7% for women.

Obesity is associated not only with heart disease, but also with hypertension, late-onset diabetes, hypercholesterolemia, gallbladder disease, cancers of the breast, colon, and prostate, osteoarthritis of the weight-bearing joints, and premature mortality (Calle et al., 1999; Calle et al., 2003; Maison et al., 2001; USPHS, 1988). Moreover, obesity itself appears to be a cause of heart failure, even beyond its association with other cardiac risk factors like hypertension, diabetes, and hyperlipidemia (Kenchaiah et al., 2002). A follow-up of the Framingham Heart Study reported that obesity decreased life expectancy by 6 to 7 years, and the difference in life expectancy between obese and normal-weight adults is similar to that between smokers and nonsmokers (Peeters et al., 2003).

Surprisingly, a national survey of seriously overweight persons reported that 70% did not view their excess pounds as a health concern ("Most patients," 1999). Although most respondents were not in denial about being overweight or about the stigma associated with their appearance, they were in denial about the health consequences of their excess weight.

# GENETICS, LIFESTYLE, AND ENVIRONMENT

## GENETICS

Although genes do not destine you to become fat, a family history of obesity increases your chances of becoming obese by about 25 to 30% ("Weight Control," 1994). Moreover, if you carry the extra weight primarily around your waist (apple-shaped), you are at higher risk for heart disease, hypertension, stroke, and diabetes than the noncentrally obese (pear-shaped) (Young & Gelskey, 1995). A reasonably accurate way of gauging central obesity is to divide the measurement of your waist at the narrowest point by the measurement of your hips (over your buttocks) at the widest point. If you are a woman, a waist-to-hip ratio greater than .85 indicates a health risk; for a man, above 1 (American College of Sports Medicine, 1995).

The set-point theory states that the body has what amounts to a genetic thermostat for body fat, which maintains a fairly constant weight. If body weight decreases through dieting, the set-point either triggers appetite or makes the body conserve energy (lowers the basal metabolic rate) to maintain the fat cells and a set weight. Research supports the idea that the body burns calories more slowly than normal when weight is lost (Leibel et al., 1995). When fewer calories are consumed, the thermostat is lowered to conserve energy. This is a useful compensation when sources of food are unpredictable or possibly scarce.

This set-point theory needs more empirical support, as does its corollary: though the thermostat setting for fat cells and weight is resistant to dieting, exercise appears to speed up metabolism and lower the set-point. Muscle has a higher metabolic rate than fat tissue, and exercise increases the muscle-to-fat ratio (Wood et al., 1988).

## LIFESTYLE

Although genetics is a contributor to the development of obesity, the primary reason that an individual becomes overweight or obese is related to lifestyle (Howley & Franks, 1997). By limiting the types of food and how much one eats and increasing daily energy expenditure through physical activity and exercise, one has the ability to make a significant impact on body weight.

The National Weight Control Registry is an ongoing study of 800 persons, average age 45, who shed at least 30 pounds and have kept the weight off for at least 5 years (Klem et al., 1997). Weight loss was confirmed in a variety of ways, including documentation from physicians, interviews with family members or friends, and photographs. The researchers concluded that persistence was one of the most important components of successful weight loss. The average person failed half a dozen times before success was obtained.

Moreover, there was no single magical way to achieve success, unless you count modifying eating and exercise habits as magical. Most of the participants lost weight on their own, with the second most frequent intervention a consultation with a physician, psychologist, or nutritionist. About 44% limited their food portions, 40% counted calories, 33% limited fat intake, and 25% kept track of fat grams. Only 4% relied on diet drugs, though the study results were obtained prior to a new wave of diet drugs on the market.

Most of the registry's participants had been overweight since childhood, nearly half had at least one overweight parent, and more than a quarter had two overweight parents. Genes may predispose some toward obesity, but apparently lifestyle changes can initiate and sustain weight loss. On average, the participants reduced their body weight by 29% and successfully moved into the normal weight range.

A similar study with a smaller sample size (n = 160) was conducted earlier by Anne Fletcher (1994), a registered dietitian, and reported in her book, *Thin for Life.* Fletcher distilled her strategies for success from persons who kept off at least 20 pounds (average weight loss was 63 pounds) for a minimum of 3 years (most achieved their weight loss for more than 5 years). The successful strategies employed by this sample of adults included:

1. focus on what you can eat, not on what you cannot eat;
2. do not deny yourself your favorite foods and do not worry about periodic slip-ups;
3. identify and then avoid high-risk situations and emotional eating;
4. find a way to incorporate exercise into your weekly routine; and
5. identify when you need to seek outside help.

These strategies were later corroborated by a larger sample size employed by the National Weight Control Registry study.

## ENVIRONMENT

Most Americans are overweight. Is it our genes, or do we lack will power? Or is there something else also at play? Perhaps our environment is a major contributing factor. Our society produces an abundance of food; food that is high in fat, sugar, and salt, and much of it is processed and packaged for our convenience; food that is advertised by tens of billions of dollars per year; and food that is available everywhere—gas stations, drugstores, food courts in shopping malls, and vending machines located just about everywhere, including in 98% of our high schools.

Also, during the last 25 years Americans have doubled the amount they eat at restaurants; and when they eat out, they eat more. In a busy society, consumers seek the convenience that restaurants provide. Consumers also have been seeking greater value at restaurants. Profit-seeking restaurant owners have come to the realization that the food itself is the least costly ingredient of a food product, compared to the costs of labor, packaging, and marketing. Thus, restaurant owners are providing ever-larger portion sizes at small increases in cost.

Food is low-cost and overproduced in the United States. According to Marion Nestle, chair of the Department of Nutrition and Food Studies at New York University, there are 3,800 calories produced per person per day in the United States, and we only need about half of that (Nestle, 2000). Food is abundant, ubiquitous, cheap, and fattening, and it is promoted everywhere, all the time.

## SHOULD WE GAIN WEIGHT WITH AGE?

Although the answer to this question is controversial, many argue that gaining a few extra pounds with age may be not only common in America, but healthy. Dr. Reubin Andres, clinical director of the National Institute on Aging, conducted a series of long-term studies and found that people in their 60s who are somewhat overweight—according to the Metropolitan Life Insurance charts—but not grossly obese had a better chance of living into their 80s and 90s than those whose weight is "normal." Thus, he created age-specific weight tables that generally have upper weight limits that are 10 to 20 pounds higher than the insurance-based tables (Salon, 1997).

A study by the Cooper Institute for Aerobics Research (C. Lee et al., 1999) appears to support Andres' contention that we need to be more lenient with recommended weight ranges, especially among persons who maintain their fitness. Men who gained significant amounts of weight over time but remained moderately or very fit had lower death rates than men who were in the average weight rate for their group but were unfit.

The chief opponent of Dr. Andres' theory, Dr. Roy Walford at U.C.L.A. School of Medicine, practices what he preaches, and has placed himself on a lifelong diet of 1,500 calories a day. Dr. Walford's animal research has shown that underfed rats live one-third longer than well-fed rats. Critics of his research, however, are concerned not only with his extrapolation from rodents to humans, but also with whether longer life on an "eat less" diet, even among the rats Dr. Walford studied, is associated with stunted growth and lower energy levels (Finn, 1988).

Comedians are also critical of Dr. Walford's diet, lamenting that eating less may not really lengthen life, it may just make life *seem* longer.

Though Dr. Andres' extra-weight theory has been supported by some studies (Finn, 1988), it has not been corroborated by others (Tayback et al., 1990; Van Itallie & Lew, 1990). Critics note that Andres' sample is biased toward the affluent elderly who can pass life-insurance medical examinations, and that he ignores health problems like diabetes, hypertension, and hyperlipidemia that are often unfavorably influenced by weight gain.

The Nurses' Health Study also suggests that the increasingly permissive weight guidelines may be unjustified. The researchers tracked the health status of 115,000 female nurses for 16 years and discovered a direct correlation between weight and susceptibility to stroke (Rexrode et al., 1997). Women whose BMI score rose into the 27 to 31 range during the 16 year period were 1.7 times more at risk for stroke; women who rose to a BMI of at least 32 more than doubled their risk.

## BODY COMPOSITION

Body composition is a better measure of health and fitness than body weight. Improving your fat-to-muscle ratio helps protect you from serious ailments and improves your fitness. No one, however, has been able to evaluate the ideal percentage of body weight that should be fat versus lean tissue. Researchers have attempted, though, to develop broad guidelines for body fat ranges for men and women. Table 7.1 has been derived from data provided in an article by Gallagher and associates (2000).

Another study reported that middle-aged and older men with more than 24% body fat, and women with more than 31%, are at increased risk for heart disease, stroke, various cancers, high blood pressure, diabetes, and degenerative joint disease (Howley & Franks, 1997).

There are several ways to measure body fat. The gold standard is hydrodensitometry, or underwater weighing, and is based on the principle that fat is less dense than water and that overweight individuals weigh less in water. After air is exhaled from the lungs, the body is immersed into a tank of water and the underwater weight is registered on a scale. This technique is very accurate but expensive and time consuming (about 30 minutes).

Skin-fold caliper is the most commonly used method because it is quick and reasonably accurate. Fat is pinched and measured in several areas, including the triceps, suprailium, and thigh for women; chest, abdomen, and thigh for men. Using fewer sites or employing technicians with inadequate training lowers the accuracy. Even more problematic, however, is that this technique came into use in the 1950s when people were leaner than they are at this time. Now, nearly 25% of women in their 50s have too much body fat to be measured with the traditional 2-inch calipers, and they are being excluded from research samples (Himes, 2001).

Bioelectrical impedance is another standard way of measuring body fat. One electrode is attached to an individual's foot and another to the

**TABLE 7.1   Age and Recommended Body Fat Ranges**

| Age | Men | Women |
|---|---|---|
| 18–39 | 9%–19% | 22%–32% |
| 40–59 | 12%–21% | 24%–33% |
| 60–79 | 14%–24% | 25%–35% |

hand, and a weak electrical current (that is safe and painless) is sent from one electrode to the other. The technique is based on the premise that the signal will travel faster through muscle because water conducts electricity and muscle is 70% water. Fat, in comparison, is about 9% water. Readings, however, can be affected by recent vigorous exercise, a recent bath or sauna, or by alcohol or water intake

Another technique is the Bod Pod, which works on the premise that a muscular body is denser and takes up less space than one that has more fat. The pod has a built-in computer that uses your weight and how much volume you take up and then converts it into a percentage of your body that is fat. Preliminary tests report that this technique and the dual energy X-ray absorptiometry machine (better known for measuring bone density) are nearly as accurate as hydrodensitomtry, but not as demanding on the participant (Miyatake et al., 1999).

# EXERCISE

It has been said that man does not live by bread alone. It can also be said that man does not control his weight by nutrition alone. Restricting the number of calories consumed without exercising can result in quick, dramatic weight loss. Unfortunately, it can also result in quick, dramatic regaining of weight. About half the initial weight loss will be water, which will be regained, and muscle, which will make us weaker. Dieting without exercise also lowers our metabolic rate (the amount of energy used for physiological processes) causing a reduction in our fat-burning capacity. This not only slows weight loss, but when the dieting ends, the weight is gained back faster than ever.

Exercise, in contrast, assures that weight loss will come primarily from fat, not water and muscle. Exercise also increases metabolic rate so that our body burns calories more efficiently and over a longer duration. Because muscle tissue is metabolically more active than fat, it burns more calories.

A study of more than 8,000 dieters who lost 10% of their starting weight and kept it off for at least a year reported that their number one successful weight-loss maintenance strategy—cited by 81% of respondents—was exercise ("Dieting," 2002). The most common form of exercise was walking, followed by increasing physical activity in one's daily routine. A surprising finding from this study was that an unexpectedly high 29% of respondents reported that they added weight lifting to their exercise regime.

The vital role of exercise, however, appears to apply more to the maintenance of weight loss than to losing weight in the first place, where changing your eating patterns is the most important behavior change ("Dieting," 2000). A meta-analysis of U.S. studies on long-term weight-loss maintenance concluded that exercise or a high level of physical activity is one of the two most important ingredients of maintaining weight loss (along with restricted caloric intake) (Anderson et al., 2001). The researchers reported that their findings were in agreement with the National Weight Control Registry study (Klem et al., 1997): exercise and physical activity are essential for most people in maintaining substantial amounts of weight loss over the long-term.

Exercise as a weight maintenance strategy, however, may become less effective as we age. Researchers monitored the fat and carbohydrate breakdown for older and younger participants who pedaled 60 minutes on stationary bikes. Measurement of oxygen consumption indicated how hard they were able to exercise. Then the study subjects pedaled at speeds that made them consume identical amounts of oxygen. Older participants oxidized less than a third as much fat as their younger counterparts (Klein, 1997). In other words, older adults appear to burn less fat doing equivalent exercise than younger adults. Paul Williams (1997) of the Lawrence Berkeley National Laboratory provisionally concluded that runners would have to increase the amount of mileage they run each decade in order to stay at the same weight.

The best exercises for weight control are a combination of aerobics and strength-building. The aerobic activity should involve the large muscle groups like the quadriceps. Longer durations and higher-intensity levels accelerate progress, but are also likely to increase the likelihood of dropping out of an exercise routine. Strength-building increases muscle mass and boosts the metabolic rate, which allows the individual to burn calories longer, not just when exercising.

Can we be fit and fat? Yes, according to the research of Stephen Blair and his colleagues at the Cooper Institute for Aerobics Research. Their data reveal that exercise can reduce disease risk even if body weight remains high. There is lower cardiovascular risk among persons who are overweight and fit, versus those who are normal weight and unfit (Blair et al., 1996; C. Lee et al., 1999).

Unfortunately, many Americans believe you can get fit without much physical effort, as proclaimed on commercials and infomercials on television. Instead of accenting the physical effort it takes to lose weight, viewers learn that weight reduction is the consequence of buying a particular product that does not require much physical exertion to use. For the past several years, for instance, electrical muscle stimulators have been a popular product purchased by consumers. By passing currents through electrodes applied to the skin you contract muscles and, allegedly, can either build them or reduce them. These devices tended to focus on the abdomen. By placing an electronic "exercise" belt around your waist and pushing a button you develop "washboard abs." After more than $100 million worth of the devices were sold during 2002, the Federal Trade Commission took three of these companies to court.

Adults also spent $2.5 billion on exercise equipment for home use in 1996 (Jackman, 1997). For a large but unknown percentage of persons who purchase exercise equipment to use while watching television, television viewing rather than the exercising continues to be the leisure activity of choice (Buchowski & Sun, 1996).

## HIGH-PROTEIN AND LOW-CARBOHYDRATE DIETS

Miracle weight loss diets like the Rotation Diet, the Beverly Hills Diet, and the Scarsdale Diet have been with us for many years and there is no sign that the popularity of these types of diets is waning. The diets have tended to reduce weight in the short run (due primarily to loss of water and high short-term motivation) but invariably proved ineffective in the long run. Typically, the diets were condemned by nutritionists and researchers because of lack of supporting data from peer-reviewed studies. But diets in general do not lose their popularity, because lo and behold, along comes another one that this time "really works!"

The latest diet craze—actually one that has resurfaced from the early 1970s—is the high-protein, low-carbohydrate diet described in the best-selling books of Robert Atkins, MD (*Dr. Atkins' New Diet Revolution;* Atkins, 1997), Barry Sears (*Mastering the Zone and Entering the Zone,* 1997 and 1995), H. Leighton Steward and colleagues (*Sugar Busters,* Steward et al., 1998) and several others. What makes this type of diet unique, though, is not only the longevity of its popularity but also the fact that it may really help people lose weight—much to my surprise. It may work, however, for reasons other than the one offered by its proponents.

Dr. Atkins, who began publishing his work in the early 1970s, and his more recent dietary disciples believe that obesity is increasing in America because we consume too many carbohydrates. If carbohydrates are restricted, blood-sugar levels will be restricted and the pancreas will produce less insulin. With less insulin, the body is forced to burn fat reserves for energy.

Opponents of this theory say it is speculative at best. They argue that the real theory behind this diet is that dieters eat fewer calories, both by consuming fewer carbohydrates and by eating a monotonously high-protein diet that curbs their appetite. Despite the bacon and other high fat foods that are permitted on this diet, the typical Atkins dieter amasses only 1,500 calories a day (or about 1,700 with the Zone diet).

The differences between these two high-protein, low-carbohydrate diets and the recommendations of the American Heart Association are summarized in Table 7.2. (I provide the average of two different estimates of Dr. Atkins' plan, from the *Nutrition Action Healthletter,* March 20, 2000 issue, page 6; and *Health* magazine, the January/February 2001 issue, p. 94):

Protein and fat are doubled in the Atkins diet compared to the American Heart Association recommendations, and carbohydrates are drastically reduced. The Zone and other high-protein/low-carbohydrate disciples—like *Sugar Busters* (Steward et al., 1998)—are less extreme.

The Atkins diet is beginning to be scrutinized through randomized controlled trials at major health science centers. And the results have been surprising! The Atkins diet, compared to a conventional low-fat, low-calorie diet, produced favorable results after 6 months. Not only did participants lose considerably more weight than the low-fat, low-calorie diet, but there were also improvements in HDL and triglycerides (Foster et al., 2001; Yancy et al., 2001). Another 6-month study, limited by the lack of a control group, reported an average 10% weight loss among the 41 participants who completed it, along with a decrease in fat mass, LDL cholesterol, and total cholesterol/HDL ratio (Westman et al., 2002).

Before the reader runs out and buys a copy of Dr. Atkins' diet book, two cautions need to be noted. Six months does not prove that Dr. Atkins is proposing a healthy diet. The negative results of elevated dietary fat may not appear within that time period. In fact, one study reported that high-protein, low-carbohydrate diets deliver a marked acid load to the

## TABLE 7.2 High-Protein and Low-Carbohydrate Diets

| Weight Loss Plan | Protein | Fat | Carbohydrate |
|---|---|---|---|
| American Heart Association | 15% | 30% | 55% |
| Dr. Atkins | 27% | 61% | 12% |
| The Zone | 30% | 30% | 40% |

kidney after only 6 weeks, increasing the eventual risk for stone formation. There was also a detrimental effect on calcium levels that may increase the eventual risk for osteoporosis (Reddy et al., 2002).

Moreover, the vitamin and mineral supplementation that Dr. Atkins recommends with his diet may not be an effective substitute over the long term for the vitamins and minerals that are usually obtained through food. The Atkins diet appears to be shy on the B vitamins, as well as on vitamins A, C, and D.

Also, the high-protein/low-carbohydrate diet builds up a compound called ketones, which curbs appetite, but also makes you nauseous and causes bad breath. About two thirds of one sample on this type of diet reported halitosis and constipation after 6 months (Westman et al., 2002). In addition to these nasty side effects, the narrow range of the diet is likely to become monotonous. This probably is the major contributor to the low 1,500 mean daily caloric intake that the Atkins dieters tend to hover around, despite the fact that caloric intake on this diet is not limited. *After* 6 months, though, it is not clear to what extent dieters crave more carbohydrates and how likely dieters are to cycle off of it.

On the positive side of the ledger, the Atkins diet may be teaching us a legitimate dietary lesson. Most of the carbohydrates that Americans eat are refined rather than high-fiber. These fast-acting carbohydrates unleash a surge of insulin that lowers blood-sugar levels below normal, and low blood sugar levels make us feel hungry. Conversely, the high protein content of these diets slows the absorption of food and decreases hunger.

Perhaps the answer is not to reduce carbohydrates, a la Atkins, but to encourage the consumption of more high-fiber complex carbohydrates that satisfy our hunger. And, in a similar vein, we may need to increase lean protein, monounsaturated fats, and polyunsaturated omega-3 fats (avocados, walnuts, salmon, etc.) to satisfy our hunger as well. The secret strategy to Dr. Atkins diet—curbing hunger—may be achieved in healthier ways over the long term.

As the comedian and quasi-nutritionist Art Buchwald is fond of saying, the word *diet* comes from the verb to *die*. Or stated another way, the best diet is not something special that you go on for a period of time, but one that you can maintain over a lifetime, without feeling deprived. When accompanied by a feeling of deprivation, dieting becomes a never-ending cycle of starting and stopping, a cycle that is not only unsuccessful for weight loss and maintenance, but also is likely to stress the cardiovascular system with unhealthy consequences (Olson et al., 2000).

## OTHER WEIGHT LOSS PROGRAMS

Americans spend about $40 billion a year attempting to lose weight (Hoeger & Hoeger, 1997). Despite this investment, 95% of people who lose weight regain the weight in 5 years ("Weight Control," 1994) and the percentage of overweight American adults continues to increase. Repeatedly losing and gaining weight, or yo-yo dieting, may increase the risk of coronary artery disease and a higher death rate (Olson et al., 2000).

About 8 million Americans enroll in a commercial weight-loss program each year. In 1993, *Consumer Reports* completed the first large-scale survey (n = 19,000) of people who joined one or more of the nation's five largest diet programs: Diet Center, Jenny Craig, Nutri/System, Physicians Weight Loss Centers, and Weight Watchers. Three fourths of the participants in these commercial diet programs were *not* able to keep off the weight they had lost for 2 years.

Respondents reported, on average, that they stayed in a program for 6 months, lost 10% to 20% of their starting weight, but gained back half of it in 6 months. Almost half of Jenny Craig and Nutri/System participants (but only 7% of Weight Watchers) reported higher costs than they were led to believe.

*Consumer Reports* (1993) also surveyed participants in three very-low-calorie liquid diets: Optifast, Medifast, and Health Management Resources. Although the participants lost weight more rapidly than regular diet programs, they regained it more quickly as well. Crash diets or very-low-calorie diets depend on rapid weight loss from loss of water and lean muscle tissue and are usually regained quickly (Caterson, 1990; Stunkard, 1987). The loss of lean muscle tissue can translate into a higher fat ratio, even as we lose weight. In addition, because the metabolic rate has slowed, we easily regain weight that returns mostly as fat, because it is easier to gain fat than lean body mass. Dietitians and nutritionists, therefore, prefer that individuals consume sufficient calories (at least 1,200 for women per day and 1,500 for men) to prevent the metabolic rate from slowing too much.

Christian weight-loss programs began in 1957 when Presbyterian minister Charles Shedd urged his readers to pray their weight away. During the 1990s, Christian diet books and church-based weight loss programs began to proliferate, combining evangelical theology, psychology, and nutrition education. Critics have expressed concern about the accuracy of the nutritional advice and the questionable association between losing weight and gaining God's approval.

One of the more successful Christian diet books is Gwen Shamblin's (1997) *The Weigh Down Diet.* This book sold more than a million copies and was followed up with a second book, *Rise Above* (Shamblin, 2000). One concern with her advice is that despite her background as a registered dietitian with a master's degree in food and nutrition, Shamblin advocated that even people with serious weight problems, such as from anorexia, should turn to God rather than to medical professionals. The other concern is her attitude toward exercise: "Trust God, not exercise. The only exercise you need is getting down on your knees to pray."

It is unclear whether incorporating religious ideology into weight loss or a weight management program is widely practiced, or even whether it is helpful to participants in terms of motivation or other factors. Regardless of ideological content, however, program participants in synagogues and churches can take advantage of the fellowship, trust, and support that typifies these settings.

Most commercial weight-loss programs have been tardy in their inclusion of exercise. As the authors of the *Consumer Reports* (1993) study concluded, "None of the diet programs we investigated give top priority to increasing physical activity, a change that researchers now unanimously agree is critical to lasting weight loss. If you use one of these programs, you should be prepared to find a way to exercise on your own." Since that time, however, most commercial weight-loss programs have begun to stress the importance of exercise.

The commercial weight-loss program that tends to get the most praise is Weight Watchers. Under the plan, each food is assigned a point value based on its calories, fat, and fiber content. The participant is allocated a range of total points each day, which can be "spent" anyway they like. The dieter is encouraged to seek a more rigorous 20% of total calories from fat, rather than the more widespread recommendation of 30%. The organization also encourages participation in a weekly support group meeting. One study reported that it was more effective than a brief counseling and self-help program (Heshka et al., 2003).

A more radical weight loss strategy is surgical modification of the gastrointestinal tract, or bariatric surgery. Due to a high incidence of complications and subsequent dietary restrictions, this technique is usually reserved for clients with extreme obesity—those with a BMI of 40 or more who have attempted nonsurgical weight loss without success.

In 2002, nearly 60,000 people had received bariatric surgery, an increase of 50% over the number of surgeries performed in 2000. This increase in surgeries parallels the increase in the number of American adults with extreme obesity. Between 1990 and 2000, for instance, the number of persons with a BMI of 40 or more had tripled (D. Freedman et al., 2002).

The most unique weight loss program (appealing to my eccentric personality) is labeled "fidgeting," or what researchers so eloquently refer to as "nonexercise activity thermogenesis." Spontaneous fidgeting can make a significant contribution to daily energy expenditure, while nonfidgeters may experience a 10% additional weight gain (J. Levine et al., 1999).

Along this same vein was a purported study (no reference provided) in *Health* magazine that reported on gum-chewing. Chomping for an hour on a big wad of sugarless gum raises the metabolic rate 19% and burns 11 extra calories. The researchers alleged that chewing gum every waking hour can knock off 10 pounds a year. It would seem to me that chewing gum every waking hour and missing three meals a day would result in a weight loss of more than 10 pounds a week—until there was no more you. (See Figure 7.1 for another fanciful diet).

## CALORIC INPUT AND EXPENDITURE

Lifestyle changes gradually implemented are the key to successful weight management. These changes should involve both eating and activity habits. People who successfully lose or maintain weight have a favorable balance between caloric input and caloric expenditure.

Calories are a measure of the energy contained in food. Calories tell us how much work our body can do with the energy it gains when we eat specific foods. If we consume more calories than needed for our particular activity level, we gain weight; if we consume fewer calories than needed for our activity level, we lose weight.

A nutritionist can prescribe a specific number of calories for an individual to consume each day that is based on weight, age, and level of physical activity. An older adult woman, for instance, who is trying to lose weight but is not physically active might be prescribed a diet of 1,800

## TEN CALORIE DIET

| | | |
|---|---|---|
| MONDAY | Breakfast: | Weak tea |
| | Lunch: | 1 bouillon cube in 1/2 cup of diluted water |
| | Dinner: | 1 pigeon thigh and 30 oz. of prune juice (gargle only) |
| TUESDAY | Breakfast: | Crumbs scraped from burned toast |
| | Lunch: | 1/2 dozen doughnut holes |
| | Dinner: | 2 jellyfish skins |
| WEDNESDAY | Breakfast: | Boiled-out tablecloth stains |
| | Lunch: | 1/2 dozen poppy seeds |
| | Dinner: | Bee knees and mosquito sauteed in vinegar |
| THURSDAY | Breakfast: | Shredded egg shell skin |
| | Lunch: | Belly buttons from navel oranges |
| | Dinner: | 2 eyes from Irish potatoes |
| FRIDAY | Breakfast: | 2 lobster antennas |
| | Lunch: | 1 guppy fin |
| | Dinner: | 1 filet of softshell crab claw |
| SATURDAY | Breakfast: | 4 chopped banana seeds |
| | Lunch: | Broiled butterfly liver |
| | Dinner: | Jellyfish vertebrae |
| SUNDAY | Breakfast: | Pickled hummingbird tongue |
| | Lunch: | Prime rib tadpoles |
| | Dinner: | Aroma of empty custard pie plate, tossed paprika and 1 cloverleaf |

The first week you lose 50 pounds, the second week you lose another 50 pounds, and the third week we lose you.

FIGURE 7.1   10-calorie diet.

calories per day. This fairly rigid calorie limitation does not allow for many empty calories, that is, junk or luxury foods that contain plenty of sugar, salt, or saturated fats and not many important nutrients. The more this older person increases her physical activity, however, the more leeway she can have with her diet.

As a general rule of thumb, daily caloric intake should be 15 times your desired weight, 10 times your weight if you have a light activity level, or 20 times if you have a heavy activity level. Thus, if you engage in a moderate activity level and wish to weigh 160 pounds, your daily caloric intake will be approximately 2,400.

It takes a reduction of 3,500 calories a week from the normal calorie level to lose a pound of fat. If you reduce food intake by 500 calories per day, a loss of one pound per week will result. If you reduce food intake by 200 calories per day, a loss of two pounds per month will result. These modest goals are more likely to lead to permanent changes in eating patterns than are more ambitious weight loss goals.

## PORTION CONTROL

As the number of low-fat foods have proliferated, the percentage of Americans who are obese has increased. This may not be a coincidence. Low-fat foods have calories (sometimes a substantial amount from sugar), and the more low-fat foods eaten, the more calories consumed. The average consumption of fat was 33% of total calories in 1994, down from 40% in the late 1970s; but people still managed to eat between 6% and 15% more calories over this period of time (Food and Nutrition Research Briefs, 1996; Harnack et al., 2000).

Nutritionists contend that one of the main problems people have with maintaining or losing weight is portion control (Marston, 1996a). A major contributor to this problem is that Americans are eating more meals outside the home, relying more on convenience foods, and consuming larger food portions. The Center for Science in the Public Interest, for instance, investigated dinner-house restaurants and discovered that many serving sizes are at least twice that recommended by the U.S. Department of Agriculture (Liebman & Hurley, 1996). A side order of french fries or a muffin ordered at a restaurant, for example, is typically equivalent to 2 serving sizes.

To get the equivalent of a single drink serving, a customer must drink only two thirds of a soft drink can; instead, that person might drink the 7-Eleven Double Gulp, which is equivalent to 8 serving sizes. Steak portions are typically 5 times what is recommended. Tuna salad sandwiches are almost 3 times the recommended size.

In the 1960s, McDonald's offered one size of french fries, and it contained 200 calories. In the 1970s, the original fries became a small size, and a 320-calorie large size was introduced. In the 1980s, the previous large size became a medium, and a new large size contained 400 calories. In the 1990s, they increased the large size to 450 calories and added a super size with 540 calories. By 2000, the large size became a medium, the super size became a large, and a new super size increased to 610 calories ("Diet & Health," 2001).

One study reported that the amount eaten is related to the size of the portion placed in front of the person. Subjects consumed 30% more calories when offered 1,000 gram lunches than when offered 500 gram lunches, regardless of whether the portion was offered on a plate or was placed in a serving dish (Rolls et al., 2002).

Adults may have difficulty with portion control because they are unfamiliar with what constitutes an official serving size and underestimate what they eat. Even when told what an official serving size is, adults have trouble visualizing it. Many nutritionists compare a serving of meat to a tape cassette, rather than stating it is 3 ounces. They compare a cheese serving to a pair of dice, instead of stating it is 1 ounce. Other visual comparisons are a small fistful of french fries, a baseball-size salad with 2 tablespoons of salad dressing, and a fist of pasta, rice, or mashed potatoes.

Complicating the problem of portion control is not only the fact that restaurant serving sizes have gotten increasingly large, but that between 1955 and 1996, Americans doubled the number of meals eaten at restaurants (Food and Nutrition Research Briefs, 1996; Marston, 1996a).

These meals tend to be not only supersized, but also high-fat, with an increase in popularity of quesadilla, chile relleno, cream-based sauces, fried rice, breaded dishes, and sandwiches with mayonnaise.

Americans, however, are not just supersizing their portions in fast-food restaurants, but they are serving larger portions in their own homes (Nielsen & Popkin, 2003). This may be due to the increasing likelihood of encountering large portion sizes, and perceiving them as normal size.

## MEAT AND MILK

The two largest contributors of fat to the American diet are hamburger meat and milk. Unfortunately, extra-lean and low-fat versions of these products are neither lean nor low-fat. Using the formula for calculating the percentage of calories from fat (grams of fat x 9/total calories), extra-lean ground beef is really 48% fat calories, and low-fat 2% milk is really 38% fat calories.

Why is there confusion on this matter? Because calculating fat as a percentage of the overall weight of the food product disregards the fact that more than half of the content may be water. Take 90% *lean* meat, for example. Sounds healthy, right? Wrong. It is the percentage of fat by weight, not the percentage of calories from fat. Remove the 50% or more of water content which has no calories, and we find that 51% of calories comes from fat. Eighty percent *lean* meat? A whopping 70% of calories comes from fat! That is considerably higher than the recommended 30% level.

## HOLIDAY GAIN

The good news is that many Americans may gain only four fifths of a pound during the mid-November to mid-January holiday period. The bad news is that this gain may not be reversed during the rest of the year and this translates to a 24-pound weight gain over 30 years of celebrating the end-of-year holidays (Yanovski et al., 2000).

# TEN TIPS FOR WEIGHT LOSS OR MAINTENANCE

Applying the Ten Tips model from Chapter 4 on Health Behavior to weight loss or weight maintenance produces the following list of suggestions:

1. *Motivation.* Two general categories of motivation when it comes to behavior change are improved function and disease prevention. Is the client motivated by functioning better, that is, more energy, better mood, and so forth? Or is he or she motivated by avoiding, or reducing his or her chances for, heart disease, cancer, and so forth? With the topic of weight loss or weight maintenance, though, there is another motivational source: appearance. Does the client want to look good, fit into his or her clothes, and garner the approval of others? The challenge is to find out which motivation works best for the client, and then encourage repeated reminders.

2. *Modest.* Clearly a 1 pound weight loss each week is more achievable than a 40-pound weight loss goal with no particular time frame in mind. An even more modest goal is to avoid a focus on poundage and to focus instead on improved nutrition and exercise. That is, establish a goal to eat one additional fruit and vegetable each day, to substitute one whole-grain product for a refined one each day, or to walk briskly an additional time or two each week.

3. *Measurable.* Make sure that the client's goal is measurable, and that it is also for a measurable and modest period of time, perhaps a week or a month. What will the client accomplish at least 3 days during the upcoming week? A brisk 30-minute walk? One additional vegetable serving? And does the client's measurable goal modestly allow him or her to have days during the week when the goal does not have to be met?

4. *Memory.* Can the client place a subtle, or not-so-subtle, sign on the refrigerator? Can a list be made before food shopping? Does the client

need a friend to call regularly to remind and motivate them? Does the client need to associate a brisk walk with an existing habit that will rarely if ever be missed—like walking just before or after dinner?

5. *Positive thoughts.* It is hard to nurture positive thoughts when it takes the average person several failed attempts before they succeed at weight loss. Hard, but not impossible. Encourage the client to be persistent, until positive thoughts finally match positive deeds.

6. *Reinforcement.* Losing weight or maintaining a desired weight tends to be reinforcing in its own right. But if the client needs additional external reinforcement, just about any reinforcement not involving food will do.

7. *Environmental support.* If at all possible, keep the junk food out of the house. Have a jar of healthy snacks handy. Keep another jar of water in a prominent place in the refrigerator, and make sure it is always stocked with carrots or celery. Place health magazines around the house. Keep enjoyable activities (crossword puzzle, letter-writing, organizing a photo album) at strategic locations in the house, as a substitute activity for snacking.

8. *Stress management.* This is particularly important with weight loss or weight maintenance, because emotional disturbances can lead to poor eating habits. One of the best stress managers is also the best technique for long-term maintenance of weight loss—exercise. For most people, timing exercise before meals decreases appetite; or timing it between meals, when you are most likely to snack, can take your mind off eating. Other techniques, such as deep breathing or progressive muscle relaxation, may also work.

9. *Social support.* Someone who used to be overweight and has kept the weight off makes for a particularly effective social support person. But just about any person who genuinely cares for the client will do. And multiple sources of support are preferable to reliance on a single person.

10. *Problem-solve.* The typical client can examine several failed previous attempts at achieving a desired weight, or anticipate new problems likely to emerge in the future. Another problem-solving strategy is to keep a record of what you eat, where you eat, and who you eat with, and try to reduce unhealthy eating patterns triggered by emotions.

## OTHER WEIGHT MANAGEMENT TOPICS

### FAT SUBSTITUTES

In 1995 the Food and Drug Administration approved a fat substitute called olestra (manufactured by Procter & Gamble and sold under the brand name Olean). Olestra tastes like fat and in fact is a fat-based product made from vegetable oil and sugar. It is engineered so that it is too large to be absorbed and passes right through the digestive tract. The downside is that it is associated in some people with cramps, gas, and diarrhea.

In addition, though olestra is fortified with the vitamins A, D, E, and K that it removes from the foods it is eaten with, it is not fortified with the carotenoids that it removes, because its nutritional role is not clear. Some studies have suggested a relationship between high blood levels of carotenoids and low rates of some cancers and heart disease ("Olestra-Fried Snacks," 1996).

Not surprisingly, after an initial period of popularity, sales plummeted more than 60% over a 5-year period. The FDA received reports of digestive problems from 20,000 people. Proctor & Gamble's plan was abandoned to expand fake fat from its potato chip products, to french fries, cheese, and ice cream.

## DIET DRUGS

In the 1960s and 1970s, the drug of choice for desperate dieters was amphetamines, or speed, which promoted weight loss by boosting metabolism. Unfortunately, the drugs caused more problems than they solved, not the least of which were addiction and serious side effects. In the 1990s, two new drugs were introduced to Americans: fen-phen (fenfluramine and phentermine) and Redux (dexfenfluramine).

With one third of Americans seriously overweight and a majority of them unsuccessfully attempting to reduce to a healthier and more socially acceptable weight, it was not surprising that fen-phen and Redux became best-selling diet drugs. New prescriptions for fen-phen increased by 6,390% in the 4 years before fenfluramine was taken off the market in 1997, and similar statistics were unofficially estimated for Redux, which had been sold in this country for 16 months prior to its withdrawal from the market in 1997.

In total, these two diet drugs were prescribed to more than 50 million people in the United States (60 million worldwide), with 18 million prescriptions filled in 1996 alone. The drugs worked by curbing people's appetites, and studies reported the average weight loss to be about 20 pounds in a year's time. Unfortunately, the drugs had been linked to heart-valve abnormalities (H. Connolly et al., 1997), life-threatening pulmonary hypertension (Mark et al., 1997), and long-lasting brain cell damage in animals. Brain cell damage may also occur in humans because short-term memory loss had been reported in 13% of the people who had taken fen-phen.

Defenders of diet drugs proclaim that the hazards from serious obesity is a far greater risk, resulting in 300,000 deaths a year from heart disease, diabetes, kidney disease, and stroke. Many people who had taken the diet drugs, however, were not obese and were taking them from commercial weight-loss clinics without a physician's supervision.

The next generation of antiobesity drugs (such as Meridia, Xenical, leptin, and neuropeptide-Y blockers) were moving from the strategy of appetite suppressant to absorption blockage. Meridia was approved by the FDA in 1997 and came on the market in 1998. Trial results had indicated that dieters using this drug lost about 10 pounds more than mere dieters and at the same time did not pose the risk of heart valve damage that forced the ban on Redux and fenfluramine. Meridia, however, can elevate blood pressure and pulse rate even as patients are losing weight, and it is also believed to be psychologically and physically addictive.

On March 19, 2002, a consumer group called Public Citizen petitioned the FDA to take the popular weight-loss drug Meridia off the market after 19 deaths were reported as possibly related to this prescription medication. The group argued that the small benefits (loss of 6 to 8 pounds), usually achieved within the first year of taking Meridia but not thereafter, do not justify the substantial risks that may be involved.

Xenical was approved by the FDA in 1999. When taken before, during, or after the meal, it prevents the digestion, and thus absorption, of about 30% of the fat in that meal, and it is then excreted itself. Trial results had indicated that those taking Xenical lost 14 pounds during the first year; those getting a placebo, however, lost 8 pounds. For a 6-pound weight loss, therefore, the consumer paid $6 a day, had to take a multivitamin pill that may or may not have compensated for the fat-soluble vitamins that were blocked by the drug, and experienced unpleasant gastrointestinal side effects. If that wasn't discouraging enough, all of the weight loss occurred during the first 8 months; after that, subjects started to regain weight ("The new diet pill," 2000).

In the last several years, herbs have grown popular for promoting weight loss. St. John's wort, taken for years in Germany to lift sagging spirits, has been used for weight loss in America. Repackaged with names similar to the unavailable fen-phen, like Herbal Phen Fuel and Diet Phen, this herb has not been tested for weight loss.

An herbal mixture used at Nutri/System weight loss centers was called Herbal Phen-Fen, a combination of St. John's wort and ephedra. Ephedra, an herb that is also known as *ma huang,* is a major constituent in many herbal weight-loss products and appears to work in the short run. But ephedra is also the likely culprit in approximately 800 health problems reported to the FDA, including more than 40 deaths (Haller & Benowitz, 2000; "Are Natural Fen-Phens Safe," 1998).

Yet another popular alternative to fen-phen is phen-pro, a mixture of phentermine and Prozac. Although Eli Lilly, the makers of Prozac, once considered marketing this antidepressant for weight loss, the data were never strong enough to win the approval of the Food and Drug Administration. Officials of Lilly wrote the Nutri/System Weight Loss Centers warning them against the use of Prozac for weight loss ("Lilly Issues Warning," 1997).

Finally, *Consumer Report's* large-scale survey of people who joined one or more of the nation's five largest diet programs reported that *less than 5%* of those who had tried the most popular over-the-counter appetite suppressants at that time (Acutrim and Dexatrim) were very satisfied with how well these medications helped them to lose and keep off weight.

## PSYCHOLOGICAL ASPECTS OF DIETING

A study of 183 overweight older adults reported that those individuals who exhibited the most effective dieting behaviors might also be particularly vulnerable to an emotional vacuum that can worsen with the loss of desired foods in their diet (Rosendahl & Kirschenbaum, 1992). Dieting may also be especially difficult for older adults who may become discouraged by the inevitably slow progress that results from slow metabolic rates.

A program called The Solution encourages older dieters to add aerobic exercise and social support to the changes undertaken in their eating patterns, and to focus attention on counteracting a tendency to seek love and comfort from food or drink. These interventions may help to offset the emotional distress and discouragement that can result from dieting (Mellin et al., 1997).

Aerobic exercise as a component of a weight loss program may not only enhance the ability to achieve dieting goals, but may also improve mood, reduce depression, decrease somatic symptoms, and reduce muscle tension (McNeil et al., 1991). Though mixed, evidence on the impact of exercise on psychological function is promising (Blumenthal et al., 1991).

A social support component of weight loss programs may be especially important to older dieters who are vulnerable to emotional distress while dieting. The positive and independent effects of exercise and social contact on depressive symptoms was reported by McNeil and colleagues (1991). Social support may be provided by sharing experiences with peers or by seeking it from a spouse or health professional. In one study, two thirds of people who received strong support from friends, both within and outside of a weekly weight-loss meeting, sustained their weight loss for at least 10 months, compared with just one fourth of those who attended the meetings without such support (Wing & Jeffery, 1999).

## THE TERMINATOR AND IMPLICATIONS FOR ADVOCACY

Given America's fixation on food and on competitive events, it was not surprising to find out that there is an International Federation of Competitive Eating, and most of the events take place in America (Hesser, 2002). One of the more popular competitive eating events is hosted by Nathan's, known for its hot dogs.

Steve "the Terminator" Keiner ate 20 hot dogs in 12 minutes at Nathan's 84th Annual Hot Dog Eating Contest. Keiner used what he called a very American strategy—a pile driver approach—keeping hot dog and bun together as he rammed them down his throat. In contrast, a Japanese competitor separated the bun, dipped it in water to condense it, and ate it separately.

When explaining his eating philosophy the Terminator said he had an advantage by being able to combine the American pile-driving strategy with a Zen philosophy to achieve his victory: "I went down a path that the hot dog was one with me and I was one with the universe."

There is something sad and funny about this anecdote. Sad, because many Americans have an unhealthy relationship with food. And besides the excess weight, gorging on food can pose immediate health dangers. Funny, because Americans are a diverse and tolerant lot, and perhaps we do not need to get the Wellness Police to shut down a New York tradition of several decades. (In the interest of reportorial candor, I should note that Nathan's hot dogs were one of my favorite foods growing up in Brooklyn about a half century ago).

There is a similar conflict in attitude regarding obesity. Most persons would argue that obesity is unhealthy and we need to do as much as possible to reduce this epidemic. Yet a growing number of health-promoters advocate a more laissez-faire approach, because some overweight Americans are fit and should be left alone, and others are not helped by the stigma and rejection that add to their burden.

A more laissez-faire approach toward overweight individuals, however, does not necessarily mean a do-nothing approach. The food industry spends $30 billion on marketing food each year, and the government spends only a tiny fraction of that on nutrition education. What should be done to address this imbalance?

Should we tax junk food to subsidize nutrition education? Should soft drink advertising be banned in public schools? Should restaurants be required to provide information on the nutritional content of their food servings? Should a breakfast cereal that has as much sugar as a candy bar be required to display a label that it is breakfast candy rather than a cereal? Should "lean" beef be redefined?

The general issue of health advocacy, including advocating for better nutritional habits in this country, is discussed in more detail in chapter 14 on Public Health.

### SURFING FOR SLIMNESS

Here are three computer-related strategies for losing weight:

1. www.eDiets.com—This Web site claimed that its 800,000 registered members had lost a total of 1,744 tons as of June 2002.
2. www.HealthandAge.com—This Web site does not make claims for weight loss, but it does provide interesting articles. And it also provides its older surfers with a choice of normal, large, or extra-large font size for their reading pleasure.
3. And the last strategy for losing weight is, ironically, to spend less time sitting in front of your computer.

## QUESTIONS FOR DISCUSSION

1. Do you believe that gaining some extra weight with age is healthy? Support your view.
2. For an older person who wants to follow the American Heart Association's recommendation for fat as a percentage of total calories, how many grams of fat should be consumed with an average daily caloric intake of 2,100 kcal?
3. A 70-year-old woman has been unsuccessful with losing weight, despite watching her caloric intake and increasing her activity level. She wants to try a high-protein/low-carbohydrate diet. What is your advice to her?
4. What role does exercise play in weight management?
5. If you had developed your own effective weight loss program and you wanted to implement a program with older adults in your community, where do you believe would be the best place to locate it: a physician's office, a church, or another community location? Explain your answer.

6. Regarding weight management, which is more important: lifestyle counseling or environmental change? Explain your answer.
7. Without regard to political correctness, or health correctness for that matter, which diet discussed in this chapter intrigues you the most, and why?

# 8

# Complementary and Alternative Medicine

## NATIONAL CENTER FOR COMPLEMENTARY AND ALTERNATIVE MEDICINE

The Office of Alternative Medicine existed between 1992 and 1998 as the newest and the smallest of the institutes of the National Institutes of Health. In 1998, it was renamed the National Center for Complementary and Alternative Medicine (www.nccam.nih.gov) and given a budget increase to $50 million, up from an initial budget of $2 million in 1992. In 2000, the budget was further increased to $70 million. The 35-fold increase in the budget for complementary and alternative medicine over this 8-year period confirms the growing significance that the United States Congress has attached to this movement.

At the same time, the federal government appeared to resolve the conflict over the labeling of this movement, settling on the National Center for Complementary and Alternative Medicine (CAM). The original name—Office of "Alternative Medicine"—was probably considered too adversarial, as if the consumer must choose between it and more conventional medicine. Another popular term, complementary medicine, suggested that these types of activities are used only in conjunction with more traditional allopathic medicine. The compromise term, CAM, indicates that consumers sometimes use it as an alternative to mainstream medicine and sometimes along with it.

Two other terms that are used often are "integrative medicine" and "holistic health care." However, the use of the term CAM has become the most popular alternative since the United States Congress gave it its blessing with the renaming of the national center.

The purpose of the National Center for Complementary and Alternative Medicine (NCCAM) is to sponsor research on nontraditional topics like mind-body medicine, manipulative and body-based therapies, energy therapy, dietary supplements, and other modalities that are off the beaten research path. The primary goal of the NCCAM is to begin to separate research fact from practitioner and consumer fancy and to answer the question: Do these therapies work?

This question is not unique to CAM, as the movement for more evidence-based medicine in mainstream medicine attests to. And the safety of CAM services is not necessarily more of an issue than it is in traditional allopathic medicine. The Institute of Medicine reported in 1999 that medical mistakes in mainstream medicine caused between 44,000 and 98,000 deaths per year.

The characteristics in Table 8.1 are typically associated with CAM versus the biomedical (or allopathic or mainstream) model of health care.

## PREVALENCE OF CAM

In 1997, 40% of American adults used some type of complementary or alternative care (Astin, 1998), an increase from 33% of American adults in 1991 (D. Eisenberg et al., 1993). The 1991 survey conducted by Eisenberg and colleagues reported that the number of visits to providers of CAM exceeded the combined number of visits to all U.S. primary care physicians by 37 million. Visits to complementary and alternative healers resulted in the expenditure of nearly $14 billion that year, with only 25% of the cost covered by health insurance.

One study reported that the highest use of complementary and alternative healing, 50%, was in the baby boomer group, ages 35 to 49 (D. Eisenberg et al., 1998); but another study reported that the highest use was between ages 50 and 64 (Astin, 1998). Yet another study reported widespread usage of complementary and alternative medicine among older adults, reaching almost two thirds of persons aged 65 and older (Sierpina, 2001). An additional study reported that 61% of older White Americans and 47% of older African Americans utilized CAM (Flaherty et al. 2001).

It is not clear when CAM usage peaks over the lifecycle and this is due to the differing definitions of CAM and the variability in sample selection. Although we may not have reached a consensus on CAM utilization patterns over the life cycle, it should be noted that these techniques are primarily utilized for chronic conditions—conditions that increase both in number and severity with age.

**TABLE 8.1   Characteristics of Complementary and Alternative Medicine and the Biomedical Model**

| Complementary and Alternative Medicine | Biomedical Model |
| --- | --- |
| Patient responsibility | Health professional responsibility |
| Mind/body/spirit | Body and mind separate |
| Healer serves as guide | Physician in charge |
| Holistic | Specialized |
| Promoting health | Fighting disease |

Among all age groups there is a failure among clients of CAM to notify their physicians about their treatments (Astin, 1998). One study reported that more than three quarters of the clients of CAM therapies neglected to communicate with their physicians. In another study, among older adults, 52% of White Americans and 58% of African Americans failed to communicate with their physician (Flaherty et al., 2001). Among Medicare recipients in yet another study, 58% did not discuss CAM use with their physicians (Astin et al., 2000). Regarding dietary supplement usage, one study examined the medical charts of 182 older adults; only 35% of self-reported dietary supplements were documented in the medical charts (R. Cohen et al., 2002).

There are several reasons why CAM users may not want to communicate with their physicians. They may believe their physicians do not approve their activities, do not understand their motivations, or do not have the expertise to contribute to their own CAM knowledge. The consequences of this lack of communication, however, can be serious. For instance, over-the-counter herbal therapy—plant-derived preparations to improve function, prevent illness, or counteract pain—can diminish or alter the effects of prescription drugs.

## TYPES OF CAM

Exactly what constitutes complementary and alternative medicine (CAM) has never been clearly established. Reinforcing this assertion, the National Institutes of Health is known for providing a definition of CAM that describes what it is not, rather than what it is: "Those treatments and health care practices not taught widely in medical schools, not generally used in hospitals, and not usually reimbursed by medical insurance companies."

Despite the imprecision, some practices have been consistently associated with CAM. Herbal medicine and other dietary supplements fit into the CAM bailiwick, for instance, and will be given considerable space in this chapter. A collection of techniques, referred to as mind-body medicine, falls within CAM and might include such modalities as meditation, visualization, prayer, humor, tai chi, yoga, and support groups.

Another set of techniques associated with CAM, and often referred to as manipulative and body-based therapies, includes chiropractic, massage therapy, postural restructuring, and osteopathic medicine. Energy therapies refer to yet another group of CAM methods that include healing touch, reiki, magnetic field therapy, and laying on of hands.

Many CAM techniques are hard to categorize, like acupuncture (small needles inserted into a variety of points along the body's "meridians"), homeopathy (highly diluted substances with little or no active chemical content, but that leave an "energy signal"), and chelation therapy (intravenous infusion of ethylenediamine tetraacetic acid to bind heavy metals in the bloodstream).

There are also activities like nutrition education and exercise, which are sometimes included in CAM. Nutrition and exercise, however, are claimed by many different types of practitioners to be a part of their purview—including the practitioners of allopathic medicine, though oftentimes it is only included as an add-on strategy that is superficially presented to a patient.

# POPULAR CAM TECHNIQUES

## DIAPHRAGMATIC BREATHING

One symptom of stress is shallow and rapid breathing. One way to counteract this stress is through diaphragmatic breathing, also called belly breathing, deep breathing, or yoga breathing. This technique is seemingly easy, convenient, and has face validity for most adherents. In other words, people feel better quickly. From a research perspective, however, the technique's short or long-term effect on stress management is largely untested, and the results with disease management are mixed (Cahalin et al., 2002; DeGuire et al., 1996).

This technique is not easy for most older adults to learn (based on my personal experience teaching it). The imagery I use to facilitate learning is to imagine your stomach and chest as a pitcher to be filled with air. Place one hand on your stomach and the other on your chest, and inhale for about 6 seconds through the nose (this warms and moistens the air and screens impurities). Allow the lower hand to move out as the air fills up the bottom of the pitcher, then the upper hand as the top of the pitcher is filled. Exhale for about 8 seconds, with the upper hand moving in first as the top of the pitcher is emptied; then draw in the abdomen as the bottom of the pitcher is emptied last and the lower hand moves in. The placement of the hands on the stomach and the chest help to clarify this breathing procedure (see Figure 8.1).

Because most persons are shallow chest-breathers, light-headedness may occur. To reduce or avoid light-headedness, decrease the length of the inhalation and exhalation. After sufficient practice, this exercise can be lengthened in time and repeated multiple times over the course of the day.

## PROGRESSIVE MUSCLE RELAXATION

In addition to shallow breathing, another symptom of stress is muscle tension. Edmund Jacobson began his work on reducing muscle tension through progressive muscle relaxation in 1908. Jacobson believed that

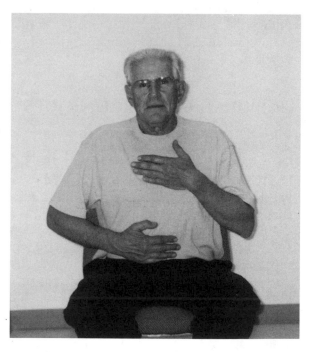

FIGURE 8.1   Belly breath.

tension can manifest itself in any muscle in the body, and in order to relax you must learn to differentiate between muscle tension and relaxation. Scientific inquiry has produced little evidence in support or refutation of this technique.

This may not be the ideal relaxation technique for people with painful arthritis or a heart condition. Clients with these conditions need to consult with their physician and may choose to eliminate or just to imagine the tension phase of the technique, or clients can focus exclusively on visualization, which tends to follow this technique.

One way to determine which sequence of muscle groups to tense and relax is to start from either your head or your feet, and continue in the opposite direction. For each part of your body, hold your breath and the tension for 3 or 4 seconds, and then relax. When relaxing, exhale slowly and steadily. After exhalation, spend a few seconds paying attention to the way you feel, and then move on to the next part of your body.

1. Tense your forehead by raising your eyebrows.
2. Wrinkle your nose and purse your lips together.
3. Tense your whole face, squeeze in like a prune.
4. Shrug your shoulders.
5. Tense your left arm, then tense your right arm.
6. Tense your left fist, then tense your right fist.
7. Tense your shoulders toward the back, slightly arch back, lift head up.
8. Squeeze your abdomen tight.
9. Squeeze your buttocks together.
10. Tense your left leg, then tense your right leg.
11. Bend your left toes, cock left ankle, then bend your right toes, cock right ankle.

After some practice at this technique you may begin to recognize and locate tension in specific parts of your body. You can then use a mini-version of this procedure to let go of tension in a specific area of your body at any time of the day.

## VISUALIZATION

Relaxation can be further facilitated by following progressive muscle relaxation with 10 minutes of visualization or imagery. One popular image is to recall the warmth of the sun, the sensation of a gentle breeze, the sound and smell of the ocean, and the sight of a swaying palm tree. Just visualize and relax.

Or, if you like wellness guru Donald Ardell's offbeat sense of humor (which I do), try the imagery that he suggests. "Picture yourself near a stream. Birds are singing in the crisp, cool mountain air. Nothing can bother you here. No one knows this secret place. You are in total seclusion. There is the soothing sound of a gentle waterfall, and the cool water is fresh and clear. And, without any effort, you can make out the face of the person whose head you are holding under the water."

Interactive guided imagery is a counterpart to visualization, but a technique that is guided by a therapist. The therapist may focus on visualization and relaxation or may direct your attention to an ailing part of your body (including internal organs) and ask you to enter into a dialogue with it. There is no research to date on the effectiveness of this technique. An organization that provides training for health professionals and laypersons, or that may be able to refer you to a local qualified therapist, is the Academy for Guided Imagery, P.O. Box 2070, Mill Valley, CA 94942; 800-26-2070.

## RELAXATION RESPONSE AND MEDITATION

The relaxation response is based on the technique of meditation, but without the Eastern spiritual overtones. It operates on the premise that the repetition of a sound or word (like *one* or *peace*) is equivalent to the repetition of a mantra (a one-or two-syllable sound) that is part of a meditation technique. (For more information on relaxation-response techniques and theory, see Benson, 1984).

Researchers at the Maharishi University in Fairfield, Iowa, have reported in academic journals that the technique of transcendental meditation—first brought to the United States in the 1950s by Indian guru Maharishi Mahesh Yogi and later popularized by the Beatles—is an effective option for lowering high blood pressure. Through randomized and controlled, single-blinded trials, the researchers report that meditation lowers blood pressure as effectively as hypertension drugs but without the side effects (Alexander et al., 1996; Castillo-Richmond et al., 2000; R. Schneider et al., 1995).

Both the relaxation response and meditation are based on the technique of letting all thoughts drift away from one's mind as they arise. This generally is referred to as emptying one's mind, but in actuality the technique is better described as thoughts that are allowed to pass through the mind as they arise, while the participant keeps returning to the chosen repetitive sound. The meditation may be performed in the following way:

1. Find a comfortable position. Most people prefer to be seated, though some choose to lie down. (Some people complain that they are likely to nap when they lie down; it is unclear if, or by how much, a short nap is less effective at revitalizing the body and mind).
2. Sit quietly with eyes closed; then run through a quick version of progressive muscle relaxation.
3. Begin to repeat to yourself, softly, your word or sound (choose one that is pleasing to you and that you are not likely to forget).
4. Continue for 20 minutes, opening an eye to check the time if you like, or set a timer in another room so you hear it as a soft auditory reminder.
5. Practice twice a day, preferably before a meal when digestive processes are not too distracting, and at a consistent time of the day (e.g., before breakfast and dinner) in order to establish a habit.
6. Most important, do not evaluate each session, even if you believe (and undoubtedly you will) that your thoughts have dominated your attention and prevented you from repeating your word or sound very often. Instead, choose a trial period (perhaps 3 weeks) and determine whether the sessions as a whole are having a favorable impact.

Although repeating a sound or word is the most popular meditative device, some people prefer to visually focus on the center of a yantra (a geometric form), or imagine a peaceful scene (such as the beach or the woods), or pay attention to their inhalation and exhalation pattern.

Stress management techniques like meditation are deceptively simple. As a past meditator for more than 20 years (I have preferred deep breathing techniques for the past several years), this technique is easy to learn but difficult to sustain. To help form a stress management habit, it is important to establish a consistent routine and it may be helpful to have a partner to encourage you and sometimes to remind you of your commitment.

## ACUPUNCTURE

One major source of stress is coping with chronic physical pain. In November 1997, a committee of independent physicians and scientists at the National Institutes of Health (NIH) reviewed a wide range of research findings and reported that acupuncture treatment—the 2,500-year-old Chinese needle therapy that has been on the fringe of American medicine for years—is effective for pain control and nausea, and has the promise to be beneficial in other areas as well.

The NIH committee encouraged insurers, both public and private, to cover acupuncture services for nausea caused by anesthesia, chemotherapy, and pregnancy, as well as for postoperative dental pain (NIH Consensus Development Panel on Acupuncture, 1998). Only 10% of health plans provide acupuncture benefits, however, and Medicare is not one of them.

The Chinese theory behind acupuncture—that the body is made up of channels of energy flow called Qi (pronounced chee) and that inserting needles into specific points on the body relieves energy blockages along these channels—has not received support from Western science. Research does support the idea, though, that acupuncture needles inserted into specific nerve junction points on the body and rotated or electrically stimulated will increase the production of the body's own natural painkilling chemicals.

In 1997, 34 states licensed or regulated the practice of acupuncture by nonphysicians and provided training standards for certification. In addition, the Food and Drug Administration regulates the needles as part of its medical device authority. The number of acupuncturists in the United States has grown to 10,000, including almost 3,000 physicians who are members of the American Academy of Medical Acupuncture. To find a licensed or certified specialist, contact the National Certification Commission for Acupuncture and Oriental Medicine (www.nccaom.org) or the American Academy of Medical Acupuncturists (www.med-icalacupuncture.org).

Research on the effects of acupuncture on cocaine addiction, rheumatoid arthritis, low back pain, asthma, emesis, and myocardial disease has been mixed at best (Chao et al., 1999; Margolin et al., 2002; Peterson, 1996; Shen et al., 2000). One study reported that therapeutic massage was more effective for persistent low back pain than acupuncture (Cherkin et al., 2001).

## THERAPEUTIC MASSAGE

Chances are you will feel better after a good massage. In addition, there are preliminary studies to suggest that it has a positive effect on lower back pain and migraine relief (Cherkin et al., 2001; Hernandez-Reif, 2001a, 2001b). For listings of licensed professionals in your area contact the American Massage Therapy Association (www.amtamassage.org).

## CHIROPRACTIC

Chiropractors focus on spinal and extremity manipulation, physical medicine modalities, rehabilitation, and nutrition. They are licensed in all

50 states and can become board certified in such subspecialties as orthopedics, sports medicine, and nutrition. Patients seek chiropractic doctors for musculoskeletal disorders, with low back pain being the most likely referral. Several studies report that manipulation by chiropractors provided as much or more pain relief, increased activity levels, and greater patient satisfaction than medical treatment for low back pain (Kaptchuk et al., 1998; Hurwitz et al., 2002; Sierpina, 2001).

One study reported that chiropractors spent more time with their patients than physicians explaining their treatment for low back pain, and advising them about self-care once they get home (Hertzman-Miller et al., 2002). Consequently, chiropractic patients were more satisfied with their care. Differences in satisfaction disappeared, however, when equal time was spent on explanations and advice about self-care.

It should also be noted that chiropractic manipulation is not without risk. If you want additional information on this practice or referral information, contact the American Chiropractic Association, 1701 Clarendon Boulevard., Arlington, VA 22209; 703-276-8800; www.acatoday.com.

## HYPNOSIS

The committee of independent physicians and scientists at the National Institutes of Health also reported that hypnosis may be effective for treating some types of pain. Hypnosis is a deep state of relaxation, accompanied by inertia, passivity, and a narrowing of consciousness. Guides are available to help clients learn self-hypnosis (M. Davis et al., 1995), and there is a professional society that focuses on hypnosis research (Society for Clinical and Experimental Hypnosis, www.sunsite.utk.edu/IJCEH).

## BIOFEEDBACK

The NIH committee recommended biofeedback for tension headaches. Biofeedback uses a machine to make you aware of bodily processes that you do not ordinarily notice (muscle tension, skin surface temperature, brain wave activity, skin conductivity or moisture, blood pressure, and heart rate), so that you can bring them under voluntary control. A directory of certified biofeedback practitioners in local areas is published by the Biofeedback Certification Institute of America, 10200 W. 44th Avenue, Suite 310, Wheatridge, CO 80033-2840; 303-420-2902; bcia@resourcecenter.com.

## MAGNET THERAPY

A few poorly controlled studies, associated with great publicity on their positive results, led to $200 million in sales in 1999 for magnets manufactured for healing purposes. When studies began to use control groups and participants could not be sure who was wearing real or sham magnets (Collacott et al., 2000; "Attracted to magnets," 2000) or ionized or placebo bracelets (Bratton et al., 2002), no differences in pain relief were found.

One recent magnet study utilizing a treatment and control group, however, was able to report differences in self-rated pain and physical function. But the claim of using a blinded sample was probably offset by the fact that the magnet pad attracted metal objects (Hinman et al., 2002). Although only 10% of treatment participants admitted to this detection, others may have noticed an attraction and experienced a placebo effect from the discovery.

## AROMATHERAPY

Aromatherapy may have been in use since 3000 B.C. It is based on the practice of treating patients with essential oils extracted from plants. There is speculation that beyond the effects of the treatment's pleasant smell, the oils may affect certain parts of the body when they are inhaled or absorbed by the skin.

One study found that 60% of severely demented patients who had lemon balm rubbed into their faces and arms twice a day for 4 weeks, reported a significant reduction in their symptoms of agitation, compared to only 14% of those treated with a placebo lotion (Ballard et al., 2002).

## LAUGHTER

There are laughter organizations that certify people as laughter leaders, there are laughter clubs, and there is an International Laughter Day (May 6—mark your calendar). There is even a study that reports an inverse relationship between laughter and heart disease (Clark et al, 2001). But does laughter ward off heart problems, or do people with heart disease lose their sense of humor? It doesn't matter. Go ahead and laugh. It can't hurt. For information on training and speakers, access the American Association for Applied and Therapeutic Humor at www.aath.org

# CAM AND MEDICAL EDUCATION

CAM has begun to establish a presence in medical schools and residency programs in the United States. Sixty-four percent of U.S. medical schools reported offering CAM courses, 68% as electives and 31% as part of required courses. Thirty-one percent of the courses were offered by departments of family practice and 11% by departments of internal medicine (Wetzel et al., 1998).

Similar results were found by another independently conducted study. Thirty percent of U.S. medical school family-medicine departments and nonuniversity-based family practice residency programs taught CAM in 1997, and an additional 6% were starting to teach it. The instruction was predominantly elective (72%) (Carlston et al., 1997).

This interest in CAM in medical education does not necessarily mean an endorsement of it. Many medical schools and residency programs are offering CAM courses and lectures in order to better inform physicians and students about what patients are doing ("Complementary curriculum," 2000). First-year medical students at one large midwestern medical school reported that most students (84%) were interested in learning about CAM because they perceive this knowledge will be important to them when they become physicians and their patients are using it (Greiner et al., 2000).

## NATUROPATHIC MEDICAL COLLEGES

Naturopathy emphasizes the healing power of nature, and practitioners attempt to support the body's own healing capacity with natural therapies. There are four naturopathic medical colleges in the United States, and 12 states in which licensed naturopaths can legally practice medicine as primary care physicians.

The state of Washington leads the country in naturopathic medicine. Seattle is the home to Bastyr University, the largest naturopathic school in the country, and in 1996 the state of Washington became the first to require insurance companies to cover complementary and alternative therapies in their benefit plans. The first publicly funded natural medicine clinic—staffed with naturopaths, other alternative therapists, and conventional health professionals—opened in the Seattle area in October 1996.

Naturopaths complete 4 years in a medical college and take national licensing exams. These physicians receive training that is similar in many ways to traditional physicians, plus they receive excellent training in the areas of nutrition (comparable to registered dietitians) and herbal medicine. These practitioners use herbal medicine, massage, and acupuncture; take X rays, blood, and urine tests; and in some states perform minor surgery and prescribe antibiotics.

Naturopaths are more inclined than medical doctors, however, to try treatments that have little or no credible scientific backing, such as homeopathy—prescribing infinitesimal doses of herbs and minerals that in larger amounts would produce an ailment's symptoms, in order to stimulate the body's curative powers; color therapy—wearing purple to lower blood pressure and yellow to prevent another stroke; and colonic irrigations—a powerful, machine-delivered enema. The Liaison Committee on Medical Education, the accrediting body for the 125 U.S. medical schools, does not recognize naturopathic medical colleges.

To acquire more information, contact the American Association of Naturopathic Physicians (www.naturopathic.org), or call 866-538-2267.

# MISCELLANEOUS

## CAM INSURANCE

Nearly two thirds of HMOs offer coverage for at least one form of CAM, usually chiropractic (65%) or acupuncture treatments (19%). About 8% offer coverage for massage therapy, biofeedback, or homeopathy ("Getting a boost," 1999). Coverage of chiropractic treatment is mandated by 42 states, acupuncture by 7 states, and massage therapy by 2 states. The state of Washington requires that insurers cover all categories of providers, including acupuncturists, massage therapists, and naturopaths.

Chiropractic coverage is endorsed by some insurers because there are studies that report this type of treatment is more successful at treating patients with chronic low-back pain and that it costs about 10% of allopathic care (Pelletier et al., 1999). CAM coverage is endorsed by other insurers in the hope of attracting higher-educated consumers with higher incomes and better health.

In general, however, CAM coverage is quite limited, with insurers waiting for research results on clinical efficacy and cost-effectiveness (Pelletier et al., 1999). When insurers do cover a CAM therapy, it is deemed for medically necessary reasons, visits are limited, and deductibles and copayments are high (D. Eisenberg et al., 1998).

Oxford Health Plans in Connecticut became the first major U.S. health care plan to offer comprehensive coverage for a wide range of CAM services. Its network of 2,000 alternative providers include licensed practitioners of acupuncture, chiropractic, naturopathy, massage therapy, nutrition, and other specialties like yoga and Tai Chi. These services are available for an additional premium (Lagnado, 1996).

Medicare began a demonstration program to evaluate Dean Ornish's Program for Reversing Heart Disease at selected sites for beneficiaries who meet clinical eligibility requirements. Ornish's program includes nutrition education, meditation, yoga, and other CAM therapies. Medicare is also evaluating the clinical efficacy and cost-effectiveness of biofeedback for the treatment of urinary incontinence, and acupuncture for specific medical conditions.

## WEIL AND CHOPRA

The two most popular purveyors of alternative medicine are physicians Andrew Weil and Deepak Chopra. Dr. Weil is on the medical school faculty at the University of Arizona in Tuscon where he has developed a 2-year residency program that integrates traditional medicine with other disciplines, such as meditation, nutrition, herbal medicine, acupuncture, and osteopathic manipulation. He has published best-sellers (*Spontaneous Healing* and *Eight Weeks to Optimum Health*) and reports receiving about 50,000 questions a week online (www.drweil.com).

Dr. Chopra is an entrepreneur who writes books and a monthly newsletter, recites lyrics and poetry on CDs, delivers lectures and seminars, sells tapes, herbs and aromatic oils, and has plans for breaking into movies and television, and establishing a chain of healing centers. The Chopra Center for Well Being in La Jolla, California, dispenses aromatherapy, massage, and spa food (for $3,000 a week, lodging not included), along with conventional medicine.

Charismatic health and spiritual gurus were on the rise at the turn of the new century, and included Tony Robbins, John Bradshaw, Robert Bly, Marianne Williamson, James Redfield, and many others. To the extent that they advocate critical thinking and do not denounce the medical mainstream, they can serve a useful purpose of expanding our strategies for improving our health. To the extent that they are interested in idolatry and the bottom line—Chopra enterprises brought in about $15 million in 1997—they may be expanding their wallets more than our health care options.

## CAM ORGANIZATIONS

The American Holistic Medical Association (AHMA) and the American Holistic Nurses Association (AHNA) are educational associations that focus on holistically oriented health care—health care that emphasizes the biological, psychological, social, and spiritual dimensions. These associations provide information on alternative healing therapies, as well as local referrals. Access AHMA (www.holisticmedicine,org); or contact AHNA at P.O. Box 2130, Flagstaff, AZ 86003: 800-278-2462.

The Center for Mind-Body Medicine provides information for health professionals and laypersons alike. Its projects include mind-body studies, community programs for the working poor and indigent, and support groups for people with chronic illness. For more information, contact The Center for Mind-Body Medicine, 5225 Connecticut Avenue, NW, Suite 414, Washington, DC 20015: 202-966-7338.

Commonweal is a support program for people with cancer who seek physical, mental, emotional, and spiritual healing, and a professional development program for health professionals who care for people with life-threatening illnesses. For more information, contact Commonweal, P.O. Box 316, Bolinas, CA 94924.

The National Wellness Institute is an organization for professionals and laypersons interested in promoting health and wellness. Its annual summer conference at Stevens Point, Wisconsin, attracts advocates who want to redress national health care policies that focus primarily on the treatment of sickness. For more information, contact the National Wellness Institute, P.O. Box 827, Stevens Point, WI 54481; 800-43-8694.

The Complementary & Alternative Medicine Program at Stanford is the only university-based research center focused on CAM and aging adults. The goal is to apply CAM therapies to enhance successful aging. To obtain additional information, contact the Stanford Center for Research in Disease Prevention (askCAMPS@med.stanford.edu; 650-723-8628).

## CAM JOURNALS AND NEWSLETTERS

- Alternative Therapies in Health and Medicine 800-899-1712
- Ardell Wellness Report Newsletter 813-251-4567
- Dr. Andrew Weil's Self Healing 800-523-3296
- Journal of Complementary and Alternative Therapy 212-289-2300

# DIETARY SUPPLEMENTS

For many years the conventional wisdom in the nutritional sciences has been that a balanced diet is sufficient to achieve all nutritional goals. Horwath (1991), for instance, reported that purchasing healthy foods within the context of a balanced diet is more effective and less costly than purchasing supplements. She also noted that the suspected value of any particular dietary supplement is subject to change with each new research finding. Horwath concluded that it is best to rely on the variety of good foods provided by nature.

Over the following decade, however, an increasing number of researchers have been finding evidence for the need for specific dietary supplements. For example, the research supporting folate as a supplement was so persuasive that the FDA required manufacturers of breads, cereals, pasta, and other grain products to fortify their products with it by January 1998. The American public, however, has gone one giant step further, finding the need to buy a wide range of dietary supplements. This need is so strong that one study reported that 71% of regular patrons of dietary supplements would continue to use them even if research proved them to be ineffective (Blendon et al., 2001).

## CAUTIONS

There are good reasons to be more cautious taking dietary supplements than the general public appears to be. It is not clear, for example, if dietary supplements are adequate substitutes for nutrients in foods. Most dietary supplements are narrowly targeted while the nutrients in foods work in synergy.

Phytochemicals are an example of this distinction. These are recently discovered chemical compounds found in abundance in fruits and vegetables, which seem to exert a powerful synergistic effect in cancer prevention (Hoeger & Hoeger, 1997). These compounds, however, are presently impossible to replicate in pill form. Adults who eat a poor diet and try to compensate with a variety of specific supplements will not derive the same benefits they would from healthy eating because of the inability to replicate synergistic chemical compounds in pill form.

Another caution with taking supplements is that they can be dangerous. An overdose of vitamin A can cause headaches, nausea, diarrhea, liver problems, and hip fracture (Feskanich et al., 2002). Too much vitamin D can cause appetite loss, fatigue, nausea, and constipation; can lead to abnormal calcium deposits in the body; and can adversely affect the kidneys. An overdose of bran can lead to seriously reduced calcium absorption. Excess vitamin $B_6$ can cause numbness; vitamin E, bleeding; and niacin, gastric problems and liver damage.

In addition, people on medication need to be careful with taking dietary supplements. For instance, a person taking coumadin, a blood-thinning medication, should avoid vitamin K, which can negate the effect of this medication; and also avoid several herbs like gingko biloba that can unsafely exacerbate the effects of blood-thinning medication.

Finally, people need to be cautious about the proclaimed benefits of dietary supplements, which are often exaggerated. If consumers acquire a false sense of security regarding supplements, it may contribute to a failure to pay sufficient attention to the nutritive value of the foods they eat.

## DIETARY SUPPLEMENT HEALTH AND EDUCATION ACT

Though researchers, health professionals, and the lay public are bullish on the prospects of dietary supplements, the Food and Drug Administration has logged more than 2,500 reports of side effects associated with dietary supplements, including 79 deaths (Neergaard, 1998). Because the federal government has decided to take a caveat emptor, or buyer beware, approach to regulating supplements, there has been insufficient consumer guidance about what works, what does not work, and what the potential side effects are.

Before 1994, the FDA regulated nutritional supplements through premarket safety evaluations, similar to the procedure required for food and drugs. Most herbs and all vitamins that were sold in dosages exceeding 150% of recommended daily allowance were considered to be prescription drugs in 1993.

In 1994, however, the federal government created the Dietary Supplement Health and Education Act, which eliminated premarket safety evaluations for a wide variety of dietary supplements, including many herbs, vitamins, minerals, and hormones. The FDA can now only intervene after consumers complain about illnesses from supplements, and even then the FDA can only restrict the product if it can be proven that the specific supplement caused the harm. This is difficult to accomplish because it is hard to separate out people who did not take the supplement as directed, or who exceeded the recommended dose, or who took different types of supplements simultaneously, or who engaged in some other confounding practice.

The 1994 legislation also allows advertisers to make unproven claims—for instance, that their product supports the immune system, improves memory, or arouses sexual desire. Even false claims on product labels, which are illegal, are not being punished because government agencies lack the resources for enforcement. Moreover, the unprotected consumer has to contend with the lack of regulation over product purity, that is, the amount of active ingredient in a supplement. Two packages of the same product may have vastly dissimilar amounts of active ingredients.

Without safeguards against grandiose advertisement claims, it is not surprising that dietary supplements became a booming business beginning in 1995. Dietary supplement sales went from $9 billion in the United States in 1995, to $16 billion in 2000 (or $31 billion if you add functional foods, i.e., foods "enhanced" by supplements). In 2000, 52% of Americans used dietary supplements on a sometime (32%) or regular (20%) basis (Blendon et al., 2001). A survey of Americans aged 50 and older reported that 59% used dietary supplements at least once a month, with 52% taking them daily (Eskin, 2001).

Utilizing herbs, vitamins, minerals, hormones, enzymes, and many other "natural" products, Americans have attempted to prevent cancer and heart disease, improve mood, increase sleep, ease achy joints, enhance memory, strengthen immune function, increase intelligence, or reverse the aging process.

Given the widespread public use and limited government regulation, it is important to examine the research on dietary supplements. Unfortunately, research studies in the United States have been limited because many dietary supplements are naturally occurring substances that cannot be patented, thereby reducing the incentive for manufacturers to invest money in research. Research on dietary supplements has been more common outside the United States, but the methodologies have been less rigorously designed.

# VITAMIN AND MINERAL SUPPLEMENTS

## MULTIVITAMIN

In an essay in the *Journal of the American Medical Association,* Ranjit Chandra (1997)—a physician twice nominated for a Nobel Prize in medicine—reported that deficiencies in vitamins and trace elements have been observed in almost one third of sampled older adults. However, it is expensive and impractical to analyze the blood levels of various nutrients in individuals on a periodic basis, so Chandra encourages all older adults to take a multivitamin containing modest amounts of vitamins and minerals as good preventive medicine practice.

A review of studies that were published between 1966 and 2002 also reported that all adults, but especially older adults, should take a daily multivitamin (R. Fletcher & Fairfield, 2002). Moreover, a review of nutritional interventions involving older adults in clinical trials concluded that nutritional supplements boost immunity among older adults (High, 2001).

A placebo-controlled, double-blind study resulted in the recommendation that older adults take a low-to-moderate dose of a daily multivitamin in order to make a significant difference in immune response (Bogden et al., 1995). Dr. Chandra conducted another placebo-controlled, double-blind study with 86 older adults and concluded that those who took the supplement showed significant improvement in short-term memory, problem-solving ability, abstract thinking, and attention, and a decline in infection-related illnesses. No improvement in cognition or immune response was found in those who took the placebo (Chandra, 2001).

Robert Butler, MD, Pulitzer Prize-winning author and former chair of the Department of Geriatrics and Adult Development at New York's Mount Sinai Medical Center, agrees with the practice of routinely taking a multivitamin. Butler once considered vitamin and mineral supplements a rip-off, but his concern about the methods of food production and processing led to the recommendation that older adults consume an inexpensive multiple-vitamin supplement on a daily basis (unpublished communication).

Although a significant percentage of older adults are deficient on several nutrients, it is unclear when these deficiencies begin. There is less evidence, for instance, on the benefits of dietary supplements for baby boomers in their 50s, than after age 65. Chandra recommends that middle-aged people take a good multivitamin once a week and slowly increase the frequency until they are taking it daily by their late 60s ("Building Immunity," 1997).

## CALCIUM AND VITAMIN D

In 1997, the Food and Nutrition Board of the National Academy of Sciences increased the recommended intake of calcium for adults over age 50 by 50%, to 1,200 mg of calcium daily. There is widespread recognition based on research findings and a recommendation by a National Institutes of Health panel, that even this amount may not be sufficient for postmenopausal women, and that 1,500 mg/d is recommended ("Calcium and Vitamin D," 1996).

The current average calcium intake for women is only 600 mg a day, and for women over 70 even less. To supplement this amount, most people cannot drink three or four glasses of milk every day or eat other calcium-rich foods like broccoli on such a repetitive basis. Moreover, calcium can be a difficult mineral to absorb; it clings tightly to wheat bran, for instance, making the calcium in the cereal milk go largely unabsorbed. Other foods that inhibit calcium absorption are spinach, green beans, peanuts, and summer squash. Also, high levels of protein, sodium, or caffeine in the diet have each been associated with high levels of excretion of calcium in the urine (Atkinson, 1998).

Thus, a calcium supplement is recommended by geriatricians for most postmenopausal women. Several cautions do apply. It is important not to take the supplement in one dose because the body absorbs best when smaller amounts—doses of 500 mg or less are ideal—are ingested throughout the day. Also, not all pills contain the same amount of calcium. Calcium carbonate (Tums, for example) is 40% calcium versus the 21% in calcium citrate, thereby requiring fewer tablets and less cost. Calcium citrate, on the other hand, is better absorbed than calcium carbonate (Heller et al., 2000) and does not have to be taken in conjunction with food.

Vitamin D enhances the absorption of calcium, and its recommended intake doubled several years back to 400 IU daily for people aged 51 to 70, and tripled to 600 IU daily for those 71 and older. This is the first time that the Food and Nutrition Board of the National Academy of Sciences has made recommended daily allowances for adults over age 70, making it official that the nutritional needs of younger adults, baby boomers, and older adults are different.

Most older adults are deficient in vitamin D for a variety of reasons. They are unable to absorb the vitamin from foods as efficiently as when they were younger. They also tend to be outside less where vitamin D can be produced from exposure to the sun. And while 15 minutes a day outside is sufficient for younger persons, the skin becomes less effective at absorbing vitamin D as we age.

During the colder months in northern climates it is almost impossible to receive the ultraviolet light needed for vitamin D production (Sharp, 1997). It is even more important at that time to eat fish, eggs, liver, and meat, which naturally contain vitamin D, or to drink milk fortified with vitamin D. Perhaps the best idea is to take a multivitamin or calcium supplement with sufficient amounts of additional vitamin D.

A randomized, double blind, controlled trial reported that supplements of high-dose vitamin D *without* calcium taken every four months for five years lowered the fracture rate by 22% among persons aged 65 and older living in the community (Trivedi et al., 2003). The cost of the supplementation was $1.58 a year per person.

For the first time, the Food and Nutrition Board has set upper limits for some vitamins and minerals. The upper intake level for calcium is 2,500 mg/d and for vitamin D, 2,000 IU/d. Too much calcium can contribute to kidney stones; too much vitamin D can actually cause bone loss.

If calcium and vitamin D supplements are discontinued by older adults, the positive effects are reversed (Dawson-Hughes et al., 2000)). The supplements offer only temporary benefit and, by themselves, are insufficient protection for bones. It is essential to engage in regular weight-bearing exercise like walking, which stresses the bone in a way that allows it to retain calcium.

## VITAMIN B$_{12}$

Vitamin B$_{12}$ (cobalamin) helps maintain red blood cells and nerve cells and is needed to make DNA. It is found naturally in animal foods such as meat, poultry, fish, eggs, and dairy products. A deficiency in B$_{12}$ can lead to fatigue, memory loss, balance problems, constipation, and depression.

The National Academy of Sciences, which advises the federal government on nutrition, urged people over age 50 to take a vitamin B$_{12}$ supplement or to eat cereals fortified with B$_{12}$ ("Take Vitamin B-12," 1998). The academy reviewed several research studies and concluded that up to 30% of persons over age 50 cannot absorb B$_{12}$ in foods, primarily due to the onset of atrophic gastritis—a reduction in the ability to secrete stomach acid that allows us to separate vitamin B$_{12}$ from the protein in food and thereby utilize it.

The Framingham Offspring Study reported that 39% of their national sample had low B$_{12}$ levels. Some participants had primarily a vegetarian diet and failed to get enough in their diets. Others did get sufficient amounts of meat, poultry, and fish but had difficulty with absorption. The authors speculated that an increased use of antacids may contribute to the absorption problem (Tucker et al., 2000).

Researchers are beginning to report, therefore, that persons over age 50 should consider increasing the recommended daily allowance for vitamin B$_{12}$ in their diet from 6 mcg to 25 mcg ("Vitamin B-12," 1998). Though most multivitamin supplements have only 6 mcg, Centrum Silver and other supplements designed for older adults typically have 25 mcg. An option to dietary supplementation that is nearly as effective is to eat B$_{12}$-fortified cereals and dairy products five or more times a week (Tucker et al., 2000).

# VITAMIN E

As is true of many areas of nutritional research, there seems to be a pendulum effect, and the new millennium brought in a pendulum that may be swinging away from recommending vitamin E supplementation.

At first there were a number of promising observational studies that associated high intakes of vitamin E with protection against cancer and heart disease. Studies of older adults taking vitamin E supplements of 200 IU/d (significantly higher than the 30 currently recommended) reported improved T-cell function and other immune function tests (Chandra, 1997, 1992; Meydani et al., 1997). As we age we produce fewer T-cells and antibodies that help us attack viruses and cancers and fight infection.

Vitamin E also appeared to be important in the reduction of risk for heart disease. It seemed to be a potent antioxidant that attaches directly to LDL cholesterol to prevent damage from free radicals. A study in the *New England Journal of Medicine* (Kushi et al., 1996) reported that older women who eat more food rich in vitamin E reduce their chance of heart disease by almost two thirds. A study in *Lancet* (Stephens et al., 1996) reported that adults who were given 400 or 800 IU of vitamin E a day for 18 months had a 77% lower risk of heart attack.

Vitamin E supplementation also appeared to reduce prostate cancer incidence and mortality in male smokers in Finland and provided some protection against colorectal and lung cancer among persons of this ethnic background (Heinonen et al., 1998). Yet another study reported that 1,000 IU of vitamin E twice a day slowed the progression of Alzheimer's disease, though it did not stop or reverse it (Sano et al., 1997).

The next generation of research studies was not quite as sanguine. A study of 9,500 patients at high risk for cardiovascular events reported that treatment with vitamin E for 4.5 years had no apparent effect on cardiovascular outcome in comparison to a randomly assigned control group (Heart Outcomes Prevention Evaluation Study Investigators, 2000). Another study reported that vitamin E supplements did not reduce the risk of cardiovascular disease over a 3-year period (Hodis et al., 2002). An additional study reported that 2 months of vitamin E supplementation had no significant effect on protecting fat molecules in cell membranes from oxidative damage (Meagher et al., 2001).

One interesting study reported that vitamin E intake in food (green, leafy vegetables and corn, whole grains, nuts, olives, and vegetable oils) may slow a decline in mental function among older adults, whereas a vitamin E supplement may not (M. Morris et al., 2002). Another study conducted with 5,395 residents in the Netherlands who were age 55 and older, reported a similar conclusion. Vitamin E intake from food sources may reduce the risk of developing Alzheimer's disease, while vitamin E from supplements may not (Engelhart et al., 2002).

Because most of the studies that supported vitamin E supplementation were observational rather than more rigorous clinical trials (for an examination of potential problems, see hormone replacement therapy section in chapter 3), two additional explanations emerge: a) persons taking vitamin E supplements may have also had a diet richer in vitamin E and this may have accounted for the positive results. b) persons taking vitamin E supplements may have also been more likely to include healthier lifestyle practices in their daily routines and this may have accounted for the positive results.

So what do the experts think? It depends on whom you ask. *Consumer Reports on Health* (2001) polled 16 experts on heart health and 13 experts on cancer prevention. Among the heart experts, three recommended vitamin E supplementation, seven believed the jury is still out, and six said no. Among the cancer experts, three recommended supplementation, one said the jury was still out, and nine said no.

For those who choose to supplement with vitamin E while the research continues to accumulate (several major clinical trials are underway as this book goes to press), it is not clear what the recommended amount should be. Researchers have been testing primarily between 200 and 400 IU of vitamin E a day, compared to the 60 IU that is currently recommended. Researchers also believe that though the body cannot tell the difference between natural and synthetic vitamins, this is not the case with vitamin E. Natural vitamin E (d-alpha tocopherol) is absorbed into the bloodstream about twice as well as the synthetic form (dl-alpha tocopherol) ("Is there a difference," 2000).

One final caution. Vitamin E supplementation is not recommended for individuals on anticoagulant therapy as vitamin E is an anticoagulant in itself.

## VITAMIN C

For almost 30 years, millions of people followed the lead of Nobel laureate Linus Pauling and consumed vitamin C pills to fight the common cold and cancer. The late Pauling earned his laurels for work in molecular structure, however, not vitamin C, and most scientists rejected his theory that vitamin C is an antioxidant that fights disease-causing free radicals.

Nonetheless, studies on the positive effects of vitamin C appear from time to time. The most promising of these studies suggest that vitamin C supplementation may prevent cataracts. Cataracts are thought to result from the oxidation of lens protein, and vitamin C may prevent this oxidation. One study of long-term vitamin C supplement use among 492 nondiabetic women over a 15-year period was associated with a 60% reduction in the risk of cataracts, when compared to no supplement use (R. Taylor et al., 2002).

This study corroborated an earlier report that linked 10-plus years of vitamin C supplements with far fewer cataract surgeries (Jacques et al., 1997). Another study associated the regular use of vitamin C, vitamin E, or multivitamin supplementation for longer than 10 years with a significantly lower risk for developing cataracts (Mares-Perlman et al, 2000).

Based on studies like this, the National Institutes of Health and the National Cancer Institute proposed raising the current RDA for vitamin C from 60 mg/d, to up to 200 mg/d (M. Levine et al., 1999). The advisory board of the UC Berkeley Wellness Letter recommends a daily supplement of 250 to 500 mg of vitamin C per day.

Most nutritionists argue that the recommended 5 daily servings of vitamin C-rich fruits and vegetables would easily meet the minimum recommendation for daily vitamin C. Unfortunately, only 9% of Americans eat the recommended minimum of five daily servings of fruits and vegetables ("Vitamin Report," 1994).

## ANTIOXIDANT COCKTAIL

The antioxidants vitamins are vitamin E, vitamin C, and beta-carotene. Many advocates of antioxidant vitamins recommend a cocktail of all three.

Antioxidants stabilize free radicals, which are unstable forms of oxygen. Oxygen is utilized during metabolism to change carbohydrates and fats into energy. During this process oxygen is converted into stable forms of water and carbon dioxide, but some oxygen (i.e., free radicals) ends up in an unstable form with a normal proton nucleus but a single unpaired electron. The unpaired electron seeks to steal a second electron from a stable molecule, and in so doing it damages proteins and lipids that likely contribute to heart disease, cancer, and other diseases. This chain reaction among unpaired electrons continues until antioxidants help stabilize the free radicals so they will not be as reactive.

Antioxidants are found in food, especially fruits and vegetables. As mentioned, though, few Americans get adequate servings of fruits and vegetables in their daily diet. Thus, there are nutritionists who recommend the *antioxidant cocktail* (Cooper, 1994; UC Berkeley Wellness

Letter, 1995). The typical cocktail guidelines range from 250 to 1,000 mg of vitamin C (no more than 500 mg at one time); 200 to 800 IU of vitamin E; and 10,000 to 25,000 IU of beta-carotene.

Based on more recent research the editorial board of the UC Berkeley Wellness Letter modified their earlier cocktail recommendation and suggested that the beta-carotene be obtained from natural food sources rather than through dietary supplements. This can be accomplished through the consumption of one medium raw carrot, which contains 20,000 IU of beta-carotene. Several well-designed studies have found that beta-carotene supplements offer no protection against cardiovascular disease and two studies even found an increased risk of lung cancer in smokers who took the supplements ("Beta Carotene Pills," 1997).

However, a modified version of the original cocktail—400 mg of vitamin E, 500 mg of vitamin C, but only 15 mg of beta-carotene—plus 80 mg of zinc (and 2 mg of copper to compensate for depletion caused by zinc) provided the first effective treatment for the leading cause of vision loss among older adults—macular degeneration. Among persons with macular degeneration who have not yet lost the central portion of their vision from the disease, the cocktail reduced their risk of vision loss by 20% (Jampol et al., 2001).

## HERBS

The medicinal benefits of plants are undeniable. Herbs are the basis for aspirin, morphine, digitalis, and many other medicines. Most of the millions of dollars that consumers spend on herbal remedies do not produce effective outcomes, however, and a not-insignificant number create health risks. Even among those products that appear to be helpful, the consistency of ingredients is unregulated and uncertain.

The regulation of herbs in Europe, where they are treated almost like drugs, sharply contrasts with America. In Europe, herbal labels warn people with diseases or conditions that might leave them susceptible to bad outcomes. Germany's Commission E of the Federal Department of Health has tested hundreds of herbs, approving those with absolute proof of safety and some proof of efficacy (though nowhere near the FDA's standard for efficacy in the United States). These clearly labeled herbal medicines outsell prescription drugs in most European countries.

In contrast, Americans can access herbs over the counter, but they must rely on books for safety and efficacy information—a good one is *Tyler's Honest Herbal* (Tyler, 1999)—or they need to contact the nonprofit educational and research organization, the American Botanical Council at www.herbalgram.org (or telephone 512-926-4900).

## GINKGO BILOBA

Ginkgo biloba is the best-studied and most popular herb in Europe. It is also the most popular herb used by older adults in the United States ("Herbal Hype," 2000) and is believed to be a memory enhancer. Numerous well-controlled studies show that an extract from the leaves of the ginkgo biloba tree dilates blood vessels and can improve blood flow in the brain and the extremities.

A placebo-controlled, double-blind randomized trial in the United States reported that ginkgo biloba is safe and appears capable of stabilizing, and in some cases improving, the cognitive performance and the social functioning of demented patients for 6 months to a year (Le Bars et al., 1997). This study, however, was limited by a high dropout rate and small differences between treatment and control groups. A team of Dutch researchers employed the same ginkgo preparation as did the U.S. study and did not find significant differences between gingko recipients and placebo recipients (van Dongen et al., 2000). Although both trials appeared to be methodologically sound, the Dutch trials had a lower dropout rate.

Another randomized controlled trial with 230 people over age 60 with no signs of memory impairment found that the gingko biloba supplement worked no better than a placebo on learning, memory, attention, concentration, naming, and verbal fluency outcomes (Solomon et al., 2002). Despite the absence of well-controlled studies to support the manufacturer's claim that gingko biloba improves memory and related cognitive function, sales reached $240 million in the United States in 1997.

## THE OTHER GS

In addition to gingko biloba, there are other popular herbs that begin with the letter g—ginseng, garlic, and ginger—that are anticoagulants and can increase the risk of bleeding problems, especially when taken with aspirin, warfarin (Coumadin), and other over-the-counter and prescription blood-thinning medications

Ginseng products are used for energy boosters and to cure a wide range of ills. The few well-designed studies of ginseng do not bear out the claims that it boosts energy (Engels & Wirth, 1997) or enhances psychological well-being (Cardinal & Engels, 2001) when compared with a placebo control group. Another problem is that authentic ginseng in standardized doses is difficult to find. *Consumer Reports* tested ten ginseng products and found that one contained almost none of the active ingredient and the remainder varied by 1,000%.

The typical claim for garlic is that it lowers cholesterol level and improves cardiovascular health. A panel of experts reviewed 1,800 studies on the potential health benefits of garlic and found little evidence that it lowers cholesterol, blood pressure, or blood sugar, or that it prevents heart attacks, cancer, or blood clots ("Garlic: Case Unclosed," 2000). Commission E, the agency that advises the German public and health professionals on herbal medicines, no longer recommends garlic for cholesterol reduction. The small reductions in cholesterol in some of the short-term studies were no longer evident at 6 months or longer.

Ginger is typically taken to relieve nausea associated with seasickness, motion sickness, and anesthesia. Studies of ginger extract and its effect on the lowering of cholesterol have been promising, but have focused on mice (Fuhrman et al., 2000). Ginger, like the other "G" herbs, can exacerbate internal bleeding.

## ST. JOHN'S WORT

St. John's wort (botanical name *hypericum perforatum*) is a weed native to the western United States and parts of Europe. This weed is named for St. John the Baptist whose birthday is celebrated on June 24th , about the time the plant puts forth its yellow blooms.

St. John's wort is the second most popular herb (after ginkgo biloba) in the United States, but is the most popular antidepressant in Germany where 66 million daily doses of the herb were prescribed in 1994, and where it outsold Prozac four to one.

St. John's wort was not effective in the treatment of moderate or severe depression in two separate studies (Hypericum Depression Trial Study Group, 2002; Shelton et al., 2001), but there was evidence that it was effective with milder depression in comparison to a prescription antidepressant (Philipp et al., 1999; Woelk et al., 2000). The studies of milder depression, however, have been criticized for the lack of rigor in their study design (Kupfer & Frank, 2002; Spira, 2001).

Prozac costs on average $80 a month, and a regimen of St. John's wort costs about $10 a month. Researchers warn, however, that the German studies supporting the efficacy of St. John's wort involved small numbers of patients, the trials were brief, the diagnosis of depression was not standardized, and the potency and dosages were varied.

St. John's wort can interfere with drugs for depression, cancer, heart disease, asthma, and AIDS, as well as with antibiotics. Clinicians warn about the adverse effects from stopping prescribed antidepressants on one's own or taking St. John's wort while taking prescription antidepressants like Prozac. Older adults are particularly susceptible to combining the herb with prescription antidepressants and are likely to experience dizziness, confusion, headaches, and anxiety.

Finally, several organizations have analyzed dozens of brands of St. John's wort and found serious deficiencies in a majority of the products ("St. John's worts and all," 2000).

## SAW PALMETTO

Saw palmetto is an herb that may improve urinary flow in men with non-cancerous enlarged prostate, or benign prostatic hypertrophy (BPH). A review of 18 randomized controlled trials examining saw palmetto extracts for the treatment of BPH was generally positive (Wilt et al., 1998). The United States Pharmacopeia, a quasi-governmental agency that sets manufacturing standards for drugs and advises health professionals, reported in April 2000 that there is moderate evidence of effectiveness for saw palmetto in men with BPH (Schardt, 2000b).

The potential market for saw palmetto extracts is huge, with half of all men over the age of 50 having enlarged prostates. Moreover, prescription prostate drugs have substantial side effects. Saw palmetto is definitely not a substitute for conventional medical treatment. In fact, it does not actually shrink the prostate, but may relieve the symptoms of enlargement such as the frequent urge to urinate. Saw palmetto is not effective when the dried berry or extract is made into a tea.

## ECHINACEA

Extracts of the plant echinacea are widely used in the United States and some European countries for the treatment or prevention of common colds (upper respiratory tract infections). A review of 16 randomized and quasi-randomized trials with 3,396 participants suggested that some echinacea preparations may be better than placebo (Melchart et al., 2000). A more recent study reported that compared with placebo, echinacea provided no detectable benefit or harm (Barrett et al., 2002).

Although the overall evidence is promising, there is insufficient evidence to recommend specific preparations or products containing echinacea.

## EPHEDRA

Ephedrine-containing compounds, sold under such names as ephedra and ma huang, stimulate the heart and central nervous system and are sometimes used for weight control. The efficacy of these drugs is not only unproved, but they can also cause heart palpitations, seizures, hypertension, heart attacks, and stroke. Given that products containing ephedra may supply doses varying from 1 to 110 mg of ephedrine, it is not surprising that they have been linked to 36 deaths ("Ephedrine's Deadly Edge," 1997). Products containing ephedra accounted for 64% of all adverse reactions to herbs in the United States, yet these products represented less than 1% of herbal product sales (Bent et al., 2003). The American Medical Association and consumer groups have called for it to be banned.

# HORMONE SUPPLEMENTS

## GROWTH HORMONE

Growth hormone is a synthetic version of a hormone produced by the pituitary gland. Growth hormone levels begin declining by age 30 along with the body's muscle mass. By age 70, hormone levels are only 25% of the peak reached by most people between the ages of 18 and 30. Injecting growth hormone appears to boost lean body mass.

This hormone has been promoted as an anti-aging remedy that improves strength, energy, and immunity, and as a treatment for heart disease, cancer, impotence, and Alzheimer's disease. Although these claims remain unproven, there is more evidence that the supplement can lead to carpal tunnel syndrome, edema, joint and muscle pain, high blood pressure, congestive heart failure, tumor growth, and worsen the effects of arthritis and diabetes. Two studies have associated growth hormone with increased mortality rates (Demling, 1999; Maison et al., 1998).

Growth hormone intervention does not yet translate into improved function for older adults, and the risk of adverse effects is substantial (Cassel, 2002). Researchers conclude that older person participation in this therapy should be confined to controlled studies (Blackman et al., 2002). Moreover, buying pills or getting shots that can cost up to $15,000 a year and is not covered by insurance is a poor financial investment (Boling, 2000).

On a related note, testosterone therapy to restore vitality in aging has also been disappointing. Testosterone therapy appears to be beneficial only to those with an original deficit in the hormone, regardless of age (Snyder, 2001). The National Institute on Aging formed a task force in 2003 to evaluate the benefits and risks of testosterone therapy (for more information, go to www.nia.hih.gov). There have been concerns that this therapy increases the risk for stroke and prostate cancer. And as we discussed in chapter 3, recent research on estrogen therapy for women has belatedly reported on increased risks.

### MELATONIN

Melatonin is a hormone produced in the brain by the pineal gland, and it is believed to set the body's sleep cycle. It became the first best-selling hormone supplement with 20 million new melatonin users in 1995 in the United States. Adults also use melatonin to reduce the effects of jet lag.

These uses of melatonin have not generated much research support. Scientists are not convinced that there is an age-related decline in melatonin levels, nor that sleep problems typical of older people occur because of this hormone (J. Duffy et al., 2002). Melatonin might not be an effective jet-lag antidote either. Traveling physicians randomly assigned to a melatonin treatment group or a placebo control group did not report differences in jet-lag symptoms after a trip from Norway to New York (Spitzer et al., 1999).

For free fact sheets on melatonin, DHEA, human growth hormone, estrogen, and testosterone, call the National Institute on Aging at 800-222-2225.

## OTHER DIETARY SUPPLEMENTS

### GLUCOSAMINE AND CHONDROITIN

Glucosamine and chondroitin in the human body are used to make cartilage and were touted as a way to reverse the effects of arthritis in the best-selling book *The Arthritis Cure* (Theodosakis, 1997). In supplement form, these compounds come from crab shells, cow tracheae, and shark cartilage, and appear to ease arthritic aches and slow the loss of cartilage.

In one study, persons with mild-to-moderate knee arthritis who took 1,500 mg of purified, standardized glucosamine once a day for 3 years had 20% to 25% less pain and disability than those taking a placebo pill.

Also, X-ray examinations showed that arthritis progressed slowly or not at all in the treatment group, while the placebo group continued to lose cartilage at the expected rate (Reginster et al., 2001).

There is also evidence to suggest that chondroitin is effective in the treatment of osteoarthritis (Leeb et al., 2000; Mazieres et al., 2001). In fact, a meta-analysis of 15 clinical trials of glucoasmine and chontroitin found a moderate treatment effect for glucosamine and a large effect for chondroitin (McAlindon et al., 2000).

Chondroitin, however, is a more expensive supplement, and it is difficult to make. Twelve of 14 glucosamine samples had at least 90% of the ingredient listed on the label, but only 5 of 32 chondroitin samples contained that amount (Schardt, 2000a).

It should be noted that the risk of long-term use of these supplements is uncertain, the ideal doses have not been determined, the quality of the ingredients varies tremendously, and it is unclear whether a combination of the two works best or if either would be more effective on its own. A study is underway by the National Center for Complementary and Alternative Medicine and the National Institute of Arthritis and Musculoskeletal and Skin Diseases to answer these questions, and results are expected in 2005.

## NUTRITIONAL DRINKS

Ensure, Sustacal, Nutra Start, and Boost are liquid meal supplements touted to increase energy. The supplements were originally designed for elderly persons who have debilitating health conditions that make it difficult for them to eat or keep their food down. Advertisers, however, are also promoting the products to baby boomers and the young-old who are still in good health but are seeking more vitality, for whom these supplements may be expensive and ineffective. Sometimes the nutrients in these supplements are not fully absorbed by the body and provide only a third of the calories (about 240 versus 750) of a meal if used as a substitute.

There are also many protein drinks on the market, some advertised as energy boosters and others as meal replacements. These drinks are two-thirds protein and are useful for the few adults who have a protein deficiency. But they lack some of the vitamins, minerals, fiber, phytonutrients, fat, and carbohydrates found in whole foods. Protein bars are likely to be less healthy than the drinks, as they tend to be high in saturated fat. And, based on tests by ConsumerLab.com, 60% of 30 protein bar products tested failed to meet their labeling claims.

he UC Berkeley Wellness Letter (2000): "Not since the early 1900s, vhen unregulated patent medicines were sold from circus wagons, has here been such a free-for-all."

# NUTRACEUTICALS OR FUNCTIONAL FOODS AND DRINKS

Americans have been eating fortified foods since 1924, when manufacurers added iodine to salt to prevent goiters. Since then, we have had vitmin D-fortified milk, calcium-fortified orange juice, flour enriched with vitamins and iron, and other useful products.

Nutraceuticals represent a new pathway in the field of functional oods: exploiting nutritionally weak foods and marketing them as health roducts. Waffles with refined flour and orange drinks with sugar and vater are now calcium-fortified. Corn chips have kava kava to promote elaxation. Donuts are vitamin-fortified and portrayed as healthy. A hocolate-chip cookie is laced with 500 mg of calcium and called Calcipokie. Tortilla chips contain St. John's wort to boost your mood. And otato rings have gingko biloba to increase memory and alertness. The inction of most functional foods and drinks is to make a profit for the aanufacturer. Sales reached $16 billion in 2000 and may triple by 2010.

Not all fortified products are soft drinks, breakfast cereals, and snack hips. Two margarines, Benecol and Take Control, are functional foods ith probable benefit. These products, as part of a low-fat diet, can educe the LDL cholesterol level up to 10%. The FDA allows the manfacturers of these products to claim that these margarines may reduce ie risk of heart disease. It is unclear, however, whether there is an nhealthy effect on the body from the unprocessed oils that are also in iese products.

Some foods are merely getting image makeovers. Ketchup is now ore than a mere condiment. Kethcup is the richest dietary source of copene, and lycopene may ward off prostate cancer (though the evince is still tentative). So squirt a little ketchup on a super-sized order ' french fries and ward off cancer. Milk (calcium), tea (flavonoids), grapes henols), carrots (beta-carotene), broccoli (sulforaphane), and beef noleic acid) are also undergoing image makeovers (Haney, 1999).

Some products may turn out to be useful, but manufacturers are willing to wait for the research to be completed. Glucosamine is a etary supplement that has much promise in the area of reducing pain om arthritis, so Coca Cola formed a partnership with Procter & Gamble

## CONSUMERLAB.COM AND DIETARY
## SUPPLEMENT VERIFICATION PROGRA

Unlike drugs, dietary supplements are not required to underg
ket safety testing, which means a brand may not contain the i
it claims on the label. In response to this situation, Consume
subjects different brands of dietary supplements to laborator
and posts the results on the Internet. Results appear every 4 t
and it is not uncommon when 25% or more of products fail
the labeled ingredients in the amounts described, or fail relat
disintegration and impurity levels. Recent results, for example
that 25% of gingko biloba product labels were inaccurate, as
of saw palmetto products.

Typically, when a product fails to contain the designated (
labeled ingredients, the amount of ingredients is inadequate–
times even nonexistent. However, a recent review of B vitam
ments (complexes and single B vitamins) found that 9 of 2
exceeded the established Tolerable Upper Intake Levels for ad
which there is increased risk of side effects with regular use.

The ConsumerLab.com Web site has its detractors. It does
the names of failing products. It samples only one batch of a p
herbal products are notorious for being inconsistent from bat
because of the nature of the plants and the processing technic
not test for bioavailability, that is, whether the substance will t
and actually utilized by the body. And finally, even if the label
does the product have any benefit?

The U.S. Pharmacopeia's (USP) launched a Dietary
Verification Program in 2002. The USP mark, which state
Supplement Verified," refers to the presence, quantity, and
supplement's ingredient. If a bottle of ginseng pills bears the
means that the product contains the amount of ginseng listed
and that the ingredient is free from contamination.

The USP seal does not verify safety or possible benefits. T
ginseng pills that bears the USP seal, therefore, does not veri
seng provides additional energy or that it is safe. Neither tl
nor the accompanying explanation makes that distinction cle

These steps are at least in the right direction. And other or
like Consumers Union are joining in. Unfortunately, the ov
to regulate dietary supplements remain woefully inadequate
emptor—buyer beware—is an inadequate descriptor of
events in dietary supplements. Perhaps the situation is best

and is testing a drink called Elations that has 1,500 mg of glucosamine added to it. Rather than wait for the National Institutes of Health study on glucosamine to be completed, the manufacturers decided to get an edge on the competition. If the test marketing goes well, the product will go nationwide, along with its motto: the drink that brings "Joy for Joints."

The good news is that the herbal supplements added to most functional foods is so miniscule that they are quite safe. The bad news is that you are wasting your money. The additional bad news is that junk foods and drinks with a supplement added are still junk. And the bad news on top of that is that manufacturers could start adding unsafe dosages of herbs without premarket safety testing. Then it will be up to a sufficient number of sick consumers to demonstrate that it was the functional food and not some other factor that caused their problem.

## QUESTIONS FOR DISCUSSION

1. Do you think CAM usage is more complementary or alternative? Why?
2. What category of CAM intrigues you the most? Why?
3. Read the descriptions of diaphragmatic breathing, progressive muscle relaxation, visualization, and meditation or relaxation response at the beginning of this chapter. Supplement your reading on one of these techniques. Then, try leading one other person or a small group if it is available to you. How did it go?
4. Can you imagine any medical problems that you might acquire in the future for which you would consider paying for the services of a licensed naturopath? Why?
5. An older client asks you what dietary supplements you are taking and whether you recommend taking vitamin E. As a health professional, how do you respond to these two requests for information?
6. St. John's wort, gingko biloba, and ginseng are among the most widely used herbs. What cautions would you recommend with these supplements?
7. If you are taking a dietary supplement, are you convinced of its efficacy? Or are you taking it "just in case"? If you are not taking a dietary supplement, have you given thought to trying one?
8. If you are doing a CAM activity, are you convinced of its efficacy? Or are you doing it for other reasons? If you are not doing a CAM activity, have you thought about trying one?

9. What CAM services or dietary supplements would you like to see generally covered by health insurance? Why?
10. How would you change the Dietary Supplement Health and Education Act so that it maintains as much consumer freedom as possible, while protecting the safety of the public?
11. Because many dietary supplements are naturally occurring substances and cannot be patented, how do you provide incentives to individual manufacturers in the United States to conduct more research?
12. Do you find the author of this book too skeptical about CAM, or not skeptical enough?

# 9

# Other Health Education Topics

**H**ealth professionals and older adults need to be informed about a great many health education topics. In this chapter, we will explore a few of these topics: smoking, alcohol, medication usage, injury prevention (fall prevention, and motor vehicle and pedestrian safety), and sleep.

## SMOKING

### PREVALENCE

Although most health educators proclaim the three leading causes of death to be heart disease, cancer, and stroke, others view these diseases as pathological diagnoses rather than as causes (McGinnis, 1992). The latter group cites the three leading causes of death as smoking, diet and activity patterns, and alcohol. From the perspective of these analysts, therefore, the number one cause of death is smoking tobacco. And the Americans who are most likely to die as a result of smoking are over the age of 60.

The prevalence of smoking in the United States declined between 1965 and 1990. In the mid-1960s, 44% of American adults smoked; in 1987, 29% smoked; and in 1990, 25.5% smoked (Fiore, 1992). By 2000, however, smoking had leveled off in the United States to about 25% of the population.

Tobacco is a worldwide problem and, unlike in the United States, it has been steadily increasing not only over the past half century, but the past decade as well. It is a leading cause of premature death in all developed countries (Peto et al., 1992). Each year, 20% of the more than 1.25 billion deaths worldwide can be attributed to tobacco.

## ASSOCIATED DISEASES

Cigarette smoke irritates and inflames lungs and air passages and produces excess mucus. Over time, these effects lead to or exacerbate a variety of lung diseases, including cancer and chronic obstructive pulmonary
disease (COPD). More deaths occur from lung cancer than from any other
type of cancer; yet lung cancer is rare among those who have never smoked
(Office on Smoking and Health, 1989). Smokers with a habit of two packs
or more per day have lung cancer rates about 20 times greater than those
who have never smoked (American Cancer Society [ACS], 1990).

Cigarette smoking accounts for more than 60,000 of the 80,000 deaths
each year that are due to COPD (Office on Smoking and Health, 1989).
Moreover, death from COPD usually is preceded by an extended period
of disability due, in most cases, to chronic bronchitis or emphysema
(NCHS, 1988). In addition, smokers are about 3 times more vulnerable
than nonsmokers to the incidence of coronary heart disease and to the
risk of sudden death (USPSTF, 1996). Smoking is a strong contributor to
stroke mortality and may also be a contributor to osteoporosis (Institute
of Medicine, 1990). Smoking is associated with cognitive decline in
midlife (Richards et al., 2003).

## QUIT RATIO

*I phoned my dad to tell him I had stopped smoking. He called me a quitter.*
                                                              —*Steven Pearl*

*It's not that difficult to quit. I did it a thousand times.*
                                                              —*Mark Twain*

The United States has approximately 48 million smokers, and 48 million
people have quit since 1976. In 1991, 34 million people wanted to quit, 17
million attempted to quit, but only 1.3 million did quit (Fiore et al.,
1992). However, the quit ratio (the ratio of former smokers to those who
have ever smoked) for the United States population increased from just
under 30% in 1965 to 45% in 1985 (Kottke et al., 1988) and to 49% in
1990 (CDC, 1992).

Age, race, and gender may have a small relationship to the quit ratio,
but it is formal educational level that is the most important factor. People
without a high school diploma, for example, are more than twice as likely to smoke than those with a college degree (38% vs. 16%), and those
without a college degree are less likely to quit than are those with a college degree (40% vs. 61%) (Fiore, 1992).

In general, the percentage of older adults who smoke is about half that
of younger adults. The lower rate may be attributable to a higher quit

rate (either self-initiated or in response to advice from a health care professional), but is more likely to be linked to a higher mortality rate. Smokers risk shortening their lives between 7 and 13 years.

## AGE-BASED OBSTACLES TO QUITTING

Older smokers are likely to be pessimistic about their ability to quit as a consequence of a longer history of unsuccessful quit attempts. Nonetheless, the number of failed attempts in the past appears to be unrelated to success in quitting (S. Cohen et al., 1990).

Older smokers do contend with: a longer smoking history; the tendency to be thoroughly addicted due to a heavy smoking habit; the likelihood of not being exposed to the nonsmoking norms and influences in the workplace; being less knowledgeable than younger adults about the physical effects of smoking; being more likely to have a fatalistic attitude regarding the benefits of quitting at their age; and being less likely than younger smokers to be told by their physician to quit (Rimer, 1988).

Two stereotypical attitudes about smokers who survive into old age are a) they must be resistant to the health hazards of smoking, and b) because of their advanced age, they no longer have time to benefit from a reduction in risk by quitting. In fact, smokers who continue to smoke as older adults continue to increase their risk of morbidity and mortality. Conversely, even 65-year-old men who quit smoking gained 2 additional years of life, and 65-year-old women gained almost 4 years (Taylor et al., 2002).

A factor that could motivate older adults to quit smoking is to provide them better education on the prospects of improving the quality of their life after they stop. Continued smoking in late life is associated with the development and progression of several major chronic conditions and declining physical function. Former smokers, even late in life, can improve their physical function and overall health in comparison to those who continue smoking (LaCroix & Omenn, 1992).

It appears that older adults are becoming more inclined to quit smoking. Quit attempts by older adults was less than 30% in 1987, but 15 years later was above 40% (Arday et al., 2002).

## GENDER

The prevalence of smoking among adults in general has declined over the past two decades. This decline, however, has been considerably lower among females; in fact, there has been a slight rise among female smokers who are age 65 and over. By 2000, the prevalence of older women smokers equaled that of men. The American Cancer Society predicts that as a consequence, women's deaths from smoking-related disease will exceed men in about a decade.

Lung cancer death rates are estimated to climb rapidly about 20 to 30 years after a large increase in the incidence of smoking. Men began smoking in large numbers after the turn of the century, and their death rate from smoking peaked during the first half of the century. Women's rapid rise in smoking began in the 1950s, and by 1986 lung cancer had surpassed breast cancer as the leading cause of cancer death among women (Brown & Kessler, 1988).

In 1991, 45% of women who had ever smoked had quit, versus 52% of men. Researchers believe that it is more difficult for women to quit smoking because they depend on cigarettes to control their weight. In fact, a nationwide survey of adults over age 35 revealed that women who gave up smoking gained an average of 11 pounds, and men 10 pounds (Flegal et al., 1995). Although from a health perspective a modest weight gain is much more desirable than continued cigarette smoking, it is a difficult trade-off for many female American smokers to make because of the perceived stigma associated with additional weight.

One study, though, reported that women who exercise while trying to quit smoking are twice as likely to quit—and only gain half as much weight—as those who did not exercise (Marcus et al., 1999).

## PHYSICIAN, NURSE, AND TELEPHONE INTERVENTIONS

About 70% of all adult smokers visit a physician each year, with almost 80% of the heavy smokers claiming that they would stop smoking if their doctors urged them to do so (ACS, 1994). Only half of all smokers, however, report having heard an antitobacco admonition from their physician (Morain, 1994). One problem is with the training of physicians. A majority of U.S. medical school graduates are not adequately trained to treat tobacco dependence (Ferry et al., 1999).

When client readiness is combined with the authority of the physician, even brief smoking cessation counseling by primary care physicians— especially when reinforced by follow-up visits or telephone calls during the first four to eight weeks—is effective in getting clients to quit (Davis, 1988; Kottke et al., 1988). An attempt to quit is "twice as likely to occur among smokers who receive nonsmoking advice from their physicians compared with those who are not advised to quit" (Glynn, 1990).

Physicians either overestimate the percentage of smoking patients that they counsel to stop smoking on a regular basis, or their patients do not hear them (NCHS, 1988). In one study, only 40% of smokers reported that they received counseling from a physician, although the great majority of physicians reported that they counsel smokers on a regular basis (Horton, 1986). Other studies show that most physicians report that they routinely inquire about patients' smoking habits, but only 25% (Taylor et al., 1982) to 50% (Marcus & Crane, 1987) of smokers say their physicians have told them to quit.

Physicians are more likely to communicate effectively with smoking clients if they are well prepared for the task (S. Cohen et al., 1989). One simple but effective smoking-cessation intervention consists of asking whether patients smoke, motivating them to quit, setting a date, providing a written reminder or prescription, and using either a nicotine patch or gum as a supplement. These principles have been incorporated into the Doctors Helping Smokers (DHS) system, which was developed in 1989 by Minnesota physicians Thomas Kottke, MD, a cardiologist, and Leif Solberg, MD, a family physician. The system was implemented in 31 Minnesota clinics and reimbursed through Blue Plus, a health maintenance organization.

DHS is based on the four As: *A*sk if patients smoke; *A*dvise them that smoking is harmful; *A*ssist them by providing self-help guides, education, and counseling; and *A*rrange for a follow-up visit, mailing, or telephone call as the proposed quit date nears. Nurses and receptionists assist the physician in counseling and follow-up duties. In addition, follow-up audits allow the team to devise ways to improve the system (American Medical News, 1992b).

Nursing interventions for smoking cessation appear to be effective, based on a meta-analysis of 16 studies. There were significant increases in patients' quitting rates due to nursing intervention, when compared to a control group or usual care (Rice & Stead, 2002). Moreover, there was no evidence that interventions classified as intensive had a larger effect on patients than less intensive ones, such as the offering of brief advice. If the latter finding even partially holds up, it could make it less challenging to incorporate smoking cessation interventions by nurses as part of the standard practice in hospitals, clinics and other settings.

Telephone services that offer smoking cessation counseling (quitlines) appear to be effective. More than 3,000 smokers were given self-help materials and then were randomized to a treatment group that received up to seven telephone counseling sessions or to a control group that did not. Abstinence rates were doubled over a 1-year period for those who received the counseling (Zhu et al., 2002). Thirty-three states have established quitlines for smokers, including 10 state quitlines that the American Cancer Society coordinates from Austin, Texas.

It should be noted that more than 90% of successful quitters do not participate in organized smoking-cessation programs. Nevertheless, some evidence suggests that those who smoke more heavily and more addicted smokers may be the best candidates for formal smoking cessation programs (Fiore et al., 1990). If every primary care provider offered a smoking cessation intervention to smokers, it is estimated that an additional 1 million would quit each year (Hypertension Detection and Follow-Up Program Cooperative Group, 1988).

## THE PATCH

It is estimated that more than 80% of smokers relapse after their first attempt to quit (Zajac, 1992). Withdrawal symptoms, such as irritability, anxiety, restlessness, and a craving for nicotine, are the major cause of relapse. Nicotine is the psychoactive drug that is primarily responsible for the addictive nature of tobacco use.

The nicotine transdermal delivery system, commonly referred to as the nicotine patch, was developed to combat withdrawal symptoms. In late 1991, the Food and Drug Administration approved 3 nicotine patches, Nicoderm, Habitrol, and ProStep. Nicoderm has been the best-selling patch and employs a weaning process that releases 21 mg of nicotine a day, then drops to 14 mg, followed by 7 mg over an 8- or 10-week period.

In 1996, Nicoderm became available over the counter as NicoDerm CQ, and soon thereafter increased its sales to about one half of the smoking-cessation aids market. Nicorette gum controlled 40% of the market, followed by Nicotrol, another patch, at 10%. Sales for a nicotine-containing lozenge, recently approved by the FDA, have been increasing.

Both the patch and the gum manufacturers highly recommend that their aids be used as a component of a behavior modification and support group program. These educational programs typically include self-monitoring of daily living habits to determine which habits need to be changed to support a lifestyle without cigarette use. Other program components usually include a combination of breathing and other stress management exercises, nutrition education, assertiveness training, exercise, peer support, and tips for relapse prevention.

After reviewing all placebo-controlled, double-blind nicotine patch studies with at least 6 months follow-up, Fiore and colleagues (1992) concluded that nicotine patches produced 6-month abstinence rates of

22% to 42%—higher percentages representing patches combined with education and support—while placebo patches produced quit rates of 5% to 28% (Fiore et al., 1992). Thus, education and support, in addition to the nicotine patches, appear to be significant factors in the long-term success of those who stop smoking.

## COMBINING INTERVENTIONS

The most effective behavior management strategy for smoking cessation employs a combination of approaches (USPSTF, 1996). One study reported that a patch followed by a nasal spray was more effective than a patch alone (Blondal et al., 1999), and the antidepressant Zyban combined with a patch was more effective than a patch alone (Jorenby et al., 1999). Given the risk of nicotine overdosing, the combined strategies require a physician's supervision and careful monitoring of blood pressure.

More frequently, combining interventions means combining a nicotine replacement aid with a behavioral strategy for enhanced results. The Medicare Stop Smoking Program, sponsored by the Centers for Medicare and Medicaid Services is a demonstration project that compares reimbursement for provider counseling alone, versus provider counseling and nicotine replacement therapy. Results of the study are expected to be available in 2005.

A health contract is another example of a strategy that can incorporate several behavioral techniques such as social support, contingency reinforcement, record keeping, problem-solving skills, and the involvement of a physician who prescribes a patch and signs the health contract.

Another popular behavioral strategy is to have clients prepare ahead for smoking cessation. Clients dispose of extra cigarettes and paraphernalia (ashtrays, lighters); self-monitor how much they smoke, when, and in which mood states, and eliminate some cigarettes that are easy to omit; switch to a lower-nicotine brand of cigarettes; announce a quit date to their physician, family members, and friends; stock up on cigarette substitutes (celery and carrot sticks); spend less time with smokers; and avoid smoking situations.

Other behavioral strategies include the following: 1. Solicit a wide range of social support among your physician, spouse, friends, and support group. 2. Employ response substitution. Instead of smoking after dinner, quickly clean your mouth by brushing your teeth, take a shower (where smoking will be difficult at best), or substitute a celery stalk or carrot stick for a cigarette. 3. Activate a stress management routine. Perhaps implement a daily-deep breathing regimen or progressive muscle relaxation.

Regardless of the combination of techniques utilized, it is wise to acknowledge the likelihood of relapses and not to exaggerate or overgeneralize the implications of a failure or associate it with future attempts. Estimates of relapses within a year after stopping vary from 50% to 80% (Brownell et al., 1986). Techniques that were successful in initially helping an individual quit should be reapplied following a relapse. Because it is unusual for smokers to achieve success the first time they attempt to quit, they should be urged to consider their failed attempts as learning experiences and be encouraged to try again. Clients who are not ready to quit smoking can be moved toward greater readiness (Glynn, 1990).

## TAXES

In 1988, a California state referendum increasing cigarette taxes by 25 cents per pack, required that 20% of the tax money be used for smoking cessation programs, especially for an antismoking television campaign. The state of Nevada also adopted a 25 cents per pack cigarette tax, but did not institute a smoking cessation campaign. The result? The reduction rate in cigarette smoking almost quadrupled in California but was not significantly affected in Nevada (*American Medical News,* 1993). The decision to quit smoking, at least in Nevada, is not made on economic grounds alone.

Smokers will do what it takes to minimize economic disincentives. A study of the effects of taxes on cigarette consumption from 1955 through 1994 reported that state taxes are less effective than federal taxes because smokers will bootleg cigarettes across state lines to avoid state taxes (Meier & Licari, 1997). Children, however, have had fewer options in this regard. California raised its excise tax on cigarettes by 50 cents on January 1, 1999, and sales went down 29% over the next 6 months—particularly among children—compared with the previous year ("California cigarette sales," 1999).

In 2002, many states struggling with budget deficits raised their cigarette taxes substantially, mostly for the purpose of raising revenue. In New York, for instance, additional taxes raised the price of a pack of cigarettes to $7.50. As a consequence of the steep price increases, smokers became a lot more creative at dodging them. Popular strategies include buying over the Internet, on American Indian reservations, in low-tax states like Virginia and Kentucky, and from illegal sources. The black market in contraband cigarettes in 2003 appeared to be a lot more robust than it was in 1999 after the 50 cent cigarette tax increase in California resulted in only 5% of cigarette buyers turning to low-tax or no-tax sources.

Since the California Tobacco Control Program was initiated in 1988, the Centers for Disease Control and Prevention reported a 14% decrease in lung cancer in that state over the following decade, compared to only 2.7% in the rest of the country ("Tough anti-tobacco," 2000). The tobacco control program was also associated with lower rates of death from heart disease during this same time period (Fichtenberg & Glantz, 2000).

## Secondhand Smoke and Attacking the Tobacco Industry

In January 1993, an Environmental Protection Agency (EPA) report that was widely publicized in the media declared that passive tobacco smoke is a human carcinogen responsible for 3,000 lung cancer deaths annually among U.S. nonsmokers and that there is an increased risk of cancer, lower respiratory tract infection, and severe asthma symptoms among children. Subsequent research has also documented the link between secondhand smoke and lung cancer (Bennett et al., 1999; Kreuzer et al., 2000), heart disease (Kawachi et al., 1997), stroke (Bonita et al., 1999), and respiratory symptoms (Janson et al., 2001).

With the accompanying media attention, the 1993 report contributed to the implementation of smoking restrictions in the community. Restaurants and other public places imposed restrictions in response to the fear of legal action by patrons and employees. Excise taxes on tobacco were raised to fund educational programs for the public, especially ones targeted to nonsmoking children and the spouses of smokers about the dangers of secondhand tobacco smoke.

About the same time, Michael T. Lewis, a personal injury lawyer from Clarksdale, Mississippi, developed a strategy for attacking the tobacco industry on the basis of secondhand tobacco smoke and tobacco-related illnesses. Realizing that smokers as plaintiffs had had little success winning conventional lawsuits, this small-town lawyer convinced the Mississippi attorney general to sue the tobacco companies to recover money the state spent in Medicaid bills for cigarette-related illness. By April 1997, 25 states had filed copycat suits against the tobacco industry.

Also during the 1990s, FDA commissioner David Kessler, MD, became convinced that the smoking industry deliberately relied on nicotine to hook smokers and also that they intentionally marketed to minors. In 1996, in fact, daily smoking among 12th graders had reached its highest level (21.6%) since 1979. Dr. Kessler unveiled a proposal to restrict the sale and marketing of cigarettes to minors and, in 1996, President Clinton, realizing that smoking curbs on young persons would be politically viable, allowed the FDA to enforce it.

In 1998, California became the first state to extend a smoking ban to bars, casinos, and even private clubs. The main motivator was not a clamor from the public, but the state's legal liability to waitstaff and bartenders who were forced to inhale secondhand smoke during the workday. After the ban took place, the respiratory health of bartenders improved dramatically with the establishment of a smoke-free environment. Respiratory irritations to eyes, nose, and throat decreased from 77% to 19% among bartenders, and coughing, wheezing, shortness of breath, and phlegm symptoms decreased from 74% to 32% (Eisner et al., 1998).

Attacked on economic, legal, and political fronts, the tobacco industry in 1998 paid a $206 *billion* legal settlement for the Medicaid expenses associated with smoking-related illnesses. Other features of the settlement included FDA regulation of nicotine content, advertising and labeling restrictions especially as they related to minors, and tobacco company financial penalties if youth smoking rates did not decrease. In exchange, the tobacco industry received immunity from lawsuits for punitive damage that their products cause and a cap on other damages.

In turn, the tobacco companies raised the price of cigarettes 44% over the next 2 years and increased their marketing budget by 33% in 2000. They also shifted more attention to exporting tobacco products to overseas markets. In addition, only 5% of tobacco settlement money has been spent by state governments on smoking control (with North Carolina spending some of its settlement money to fund a tobacco auction house and to create a video history of tobacco cultivation). Given these trends, it is not surprising that the World Health Organization reported that cigarette consumption did not decline in the United States in 2000 and had significantly increased in developing nations.

## BLOODY MOUTHS

When it comes to truth in advertising, American tobacco companies thought they had it bad in the mid-1960s when they had to make space on cigarette packs for a warning that cigarette smoking is a health hazard. In 2001, the Canadian government went one giant step further: Over 50% of each cigarette pack had to be adorned by a graphic warning of what those health hazards look like. Among the 16 designs they may choose from are bloody mouths in acute periodontal distress, cancerous lungs, stroke-clotted brains, and damaged hearts. It remains to be seen if this strategy will be more effective than the United States' warning on cigarette packs, which appears to have slipped out of the consciousness of most Americans.

## ADDITIONAL PROGRAMS AND MATERIALS

Fresh Start is a group smoking-cessation program that is offered by many local chapters of the American Cancer Society. To locate your local chapter or to obtain free publications on smoking cessation, contact the American Cancer Society, 1599 Clifton Road, Atlanta, GA 30329; or call 800-227-2345 (information service).

Two booklets, *Clearing the Air—A Guide to Quitting Smoking and Guide to Quit Smoking for Your Health and Your Family* (the latter available in Spanish as well), offer strategies and suggestions for quitting and staying a nonsmoker. These booklets (up to 200 copies free) are available from the Office of Cancer Communications, National Cancer Institute, Building 31, Room 10A24, Bethesda, MD 20892; 800-422-6237.

*Freedom From Smoking* is offered by local affiliates of the American Lung Association. To locate your local chapter or to obtain manuals, audiotapes, videotapes, films, posters, and buttons, contact the American Lung Association, 1720 Broadway, New York, NY 10019-4374; 212-315-8700; 800-586-4872.

The *Smoking and Health Bulletin;* a free guide entitled *Out of the Ashes: Choosing a Method to Quit Smoking;* a free bibliography on smoking and health, and materials on smoking cessation techniques are available from the Office on Smoking and Health, Park Building, Room 1-16, 5600 Fishers Lane, Rockville, MD 20857; 301-443-5287. Smoking cessation kits are available from the American Academy of Family Physicians at 800-944-0000.

Interested in quitting? Try one of these online resources: www.cdc.gov/tobacco/quit/canquit; www.cdc.gov/tobacco/quit/quittip; www.lungusa.org; www.quitnet.org; or the toll-free New York Smokers' Quitline 888-609-6292.

# ALCOHOL

## DEFINITION

No consensus exists among alcohol researchers and other experts regarding what constitutes moderate drinking and what constitutes alcoholism (Dufour et al., 1992). The Department of Agriculture (1990) somewhat arbitrarily defined moderate drinking as no more than 2 drinks a day for men and 1 drink a day for women, with a drink defined as approximately 12 ounces of beer, 5 ounces of wine, or 1.5 ounces of spirits.

Dufour and colleagues (1992) conclude, however, that "given the dramatic increase in the proportion of body fat with aging and the concomitant decrease in volume of total body water," a maximum of one drink a day is advised for older men.

It may be best when attempting to define alcoholism to avoid associating it with a specific number of drinks. One definition states that alcoholism is "impaired control over drinking, preoccupation with the drug alcohol, use of alcohol despite adverse consequences, and distortions in thinking, most notably denial" (Morse & Flavin, 1992).

The diagnostic criteria for alcohol dependence used in the *Diagnostic and Statistical Manual of Mental Disorders* [DSM-IV, 1994] is the persistence for a month or more, of 3 or more of the following 9 criteria:

1. Drinking more or over a longer period than previously
2. Persistent desire or unsuccessful efforts to cut down or control use
3. Considerable time spent in obtaining, drinking, or recovering from the effects of alcohol
4. Intoxication or withdrawal when expected to fulfill major obligations
5. Important activities given up or reduced because of drinking
6. Continued use despite knowledge of having persistent or recurrent psychological or physical problems related to alcohol
7. Marked tolerance
8. Withdrawal symptoms
9. Drinking to relieve or avoid withdrawal symptoms

## TYPES

About one third of elderly alcoholics are late-onset, reactive problem drinkers. Late-onset alcoholics are likely to be the product of a life-cycle crisis, such as the death of a spouse or the loss of a physical function. Once the precipitating event is identified and therapy is pursued, the condition may be reversible. A return to moderate drinking may be viable for late-onset alcoholics. Early-onset drinkers have had a drinking problem for many years and have either avoided, or have undergone unsuccessful, treatment. While the prognosis for successful treatment of chronic, lifelong problem drinkers is poor, it is not impossible to treat.

## ASSESSMENT

During the early stages of alcoholism, no physical signs nor symptoms signal the shift from health to disease. Often, though, behavioral problems, such as repetitive accidents or injuries or ongoing family or work problems, accompany alcohol misuse.

It may be especially difficult to detect alcohol problems among retired persons, who have few opportunities to experience problems in the work or community setting. It appears to be particularly difficult for physicians to detect. When presented with early symptoms of alcoholism, only 6% of 462 physicians mentioned substance abuse as a possible diagnosis (Schmid, 2000). It is estimated that physicians make the correct diagnosis of alcoholism in older adults in only 22% to 37% of actual cases seen in emergency departments or during hospitalizations ("AMA Reports," 1995).

Even when alcoholism is recognized, the physician is less likely to initiate or recommend treatment for older clients than for younger clients (Curtis et al., 1989). Some physicians believe it is too late in their older patients' lives to do anything about the problems of alcoholism (Butler et al., 1998). Other physicians believe it is too difficult and time-consuming to accurately assess.

One of the most popular assessment tools for busy health professionals and one that has been tested with older clients is the CAGE questionnaire. It has good sensitivity and specificity for alcohol abuse in general, though is less sensitive to early problem or heavy drinking (USPSTF, 1996). The four questions in this instrument ask:

Have you ever

| Thought about | *Cutting down?* |
| Felt | *Annoyed when others criticize your drinking?* |
| Felt | *Guilty about drinking?* |
| Used alcohol as an | *Eye opener?* |

Two or more affirmative responses to the above questions suggest an alcohol problem.

Although the CAGE instrument is practical for the busy health care professional, more sensitivity and specificity can be obtained with longer questionnaires, especially the 25-item Michigan Alcohol Screening Test (MAST) that has been tested with older adults (Schonfeld, 1993). The MAST, however, is too lengthy for routine screening.

There is a brief version of the MAST, but it and the CAGE lose sensitivity when used in a community where the base rate of alcoholism is low (Crowe et al., 1997). Moreover, a study comparing the short version of the MAST and the CAGE concluded that they were capturing different aspects of unsafe drinking, and perhaps both instruments need to be used (Moore et al., 2002).

A third commonly used assessment tool is the Alcohol Use Disorders Identification Test (AUDIT). The value of the AUDIT is that it also incorporates questions about quantity, frequency, and binge behavior

(USPSTF, 1996). Conversely, the AUDIT focuses on drinking during the previous year and is less sensitive for past drinking problems that can help the clinician distinguish between late-onset versus long-term drinking problems.

Another assessment option is a biochemical test for diagnosing alcohol abuse. The carbohydrate-deficient transferrin test was approved by the Food and Drug Administration in 2000. It improved upon the specificity and sensitivity of previous biochemical tests and may help break through the denial and rationalization of a patient.

## PREVALENCE

Estimates of the percentage of older Americans who are problem drinkers vary widely, from 2% to more than 10% (Butler et al., 1998). The National Health and Nutrition Examination Survey reports that 7% of older adults are heavy drinkers of alcohol (Moore et al., 1999). About 10% of patients who go to an emergency room with an alcohol-related problem are over age 60 ("Measuring Alcohol's Effect," 1996), though the prevalence of alcohol-related hospitalizations declines with age for both men and women (Adams et al., 1993).

It is not easy to estimate the scope of problem drinking in late life because much of it may take place out of the glare of work and community life. It is easier to predict that alcohol abuse and dependence are likely to increase in the coming decades, due to baby boomers having a history of greater alcohol consumption than current cohorts of older adults (Reid & Anderson, 1997).

## ASSOCIATED DISEASES AND PROBLEMS

Although problem drinking in late life is less than for younger adults, the risks of alcohol abuse for older drinkers are elevated in terms of falls and accidents, dementias, medical problems, reaction time, memory, and interactions with prescription and over-the-counter drugs (Butler et al., 1998; Schonfeld, 1993). Nutritional deficiencies, particularly vitamin and protein deficiencies, are more common among older alcohol drinkers as well because of the increased inhibition of the absorption of many nutrients.

With age, the body absorbs a higher percentage of the alcohol consumed. This occurs because alcohol is soluble in water and not in fat; and as we age, lean body mass that is high in water content decreases, and body fat that is low in water content increases. Thus, alcohol reaches a higher concentration in the blood of an older person. Also, as we age there is a decline in the stomach enzyme—alcohol dhydrogenase—that can break down alcohol before it reaches the bloodstream. This further increases the blood alcohol level and places an extra burden on the liver where most alcohol metabolism takes place.

Moreover, as we age, blood flow through the liver declines, as does kidney function, which means that alcohol is eliminated more slowly from the blood. Consuming the same amount of alcohol as a younger person, the older person will have a blood alcohol level that is 30% to 40% higher.

Although alcohol adds calories to the diet, it adds almost no nutrients; therefore, malnutrition becomes a problem as well. Other problems of excess alcohol consumption are an increased risk of injury or accident, especially when driving, and (along with excess caffeine and medications) an adverse affect on sleep.

At least 100 of the most commonly prescribed medications interact negatively with alcohol. This interaction effect, along with the increased vulnerability of older adults to alcohol abuse, accounts for the fact that older adults are hospitalized as often for alcohol-related problems as for heart attacks (Adams et al., 1993).

## INTERVENTION AND REFERRAL

Most patients with suspected drinking problems receive no counseling from primary care physicians. One study cited that about a third of physicians report having counseled patients on alcohol abuse (Rosen et al., 1984). However, the percentage is likely to appear much lower when patient records are examined. One study of patient records, in fact, revealed that only 18% of patients were counseled by physicians (Hayward et al., 1987). When physicians do offer problem drinkers advice and additional workbook materials, problem drinking may be reduced and maintained for at least a year (Fleming et al., 2000).

Older adults often drink in response to depression and loneliness, whereas younger adults are likely to use multiple substances to assuage their anger, frustration, tension, interpersonal conflicts, and social pressure (Schonfeld et al., 1992). If interventions are to be effective, most older adults with alcohol abuse problems will need to be referred by their health professionals to groups or specialists who recognize the different needs of older versus younger persons.

Some evidence indicates that persons referred to age-specific support groups remain in treatment longer and complete treatment more often than those in age-mixed groups (Kofoed et al., 1987). Problems such as widowhood and retirement, which are not of universal concern, may be particularly difficult for older people to share in support groups of mixed ages (Schonfeld, 1993). Borkman (1982) reports that older adults might also be reluctant to air their problems in Alcoholics Anonymous (AA) groups with predominantly younger memberships.

About a third of those who attend AA meetings are over age 50, and many communities operate programs specifically for older adults. The geriatrician Robert Butler, MD, suggests: "Because of the magnitude of drinking problems among older people, it would be useful to have AA programs set up especially for them—perhaps called Ala-elder" (Butler et al., 1998, p. 178).

## TREATMENT ALTERNATIVES

Detoxification programs focus on the drying-out process, providing medical supervision to addicted persons who are going through periods of withdrawal. Because withdrawal symptoms can be severe, most but not all detoxification programs are affiliated with hospitals and under the supervision of a physician.

Alcoholics Anonymous (AA) employs a strategy that encourages public confession, intense social support, contrition, and a spiritual or philosophical awakening (N. Robertson, 1988). Founded in the 1930s, AA today has about 89,000 groups around the world, and about 1.8 million members (Butler et al., 1998). Companion organizations have been set up for the spouses (Al-Anon), teen-age children of alcoholics (Alateen), and adult children of alcoholics.

The anonymous nature of membership in AA makes it difficult to evaluate this type of intervention. Older alcoholics may be unprepared for the openness that characterizes these types of support groups, or they may not have access to a support group with other older alcoholics to whom they can relate. Professionally led programs, therefore, should be viewed as complementary to peer support groups, rather than as being in competition with them.

Professionally run treatment programs may be more effective than Alcoholics Anonymous groups for some individuals, but they have their disadvantages as well. They are typically costly and time-bound, in comparison to support groups that can and do meet frequently (sometimes, several times a week) and that continue on an ongoing basis.

The self-management strategies outlined under smoking cessation and the vulnerability to relapse are applicable to alcohol addiction as well. Behavior management techniques may need to be reapplied on multiple occasions.

## POSITIVE EFFECTS

Two studies found that individuals who consume moderate amounts of alcohol reduce their risk of heart failure; and if a heart attack occurs, these individuals are more likely to survive it in comparison to teetotalers or heavy drinkers (Abramson et al., 2001; Mukamal et al., 2001). Moderate alcohol consumption also appears to have a protective effect on ischemic stroke (Sacco et al., 1999). People who drank only 1 or 2 drinks daily had a 45% lower risk of stroke caused by insufficient blood flow to the brain. It is not clear why moderate drinking appears to have a positive effect on health, but it may act to lower blood pressure, raise protective HDL cholesterol, or reduce the likelihood of blood clots.

A survey of 490,000 adults, ranging in age from 30 to 104, concluded that taking 1 alcoholic drink a day provides a slight edge in longevity compared to nondrinkers (Thun et al., 1997). People who drank a small amount of alcohol on a daily basis reduced their incidence of heart disease and stroke, which modestly outweighed the increased risks associated with regular drinking, that is, death from cancer (especially breast cancer) and accidents. The study authors were not touting alcohol as the preventive therapy of choice because limiting oneself to one drink of alcohol daily is not the drinking pattern of many Americans.

"Reasonably small and controlled alcohol intake may be of benefit to the elderly, as it may stimulate appetite, increase socialization, and may play a 'protective' role against coronary artery disease" (Lamy, 1988). Nursing homes may be one type of facility where the introduction of controlled alcohol intake can be an effective preventive therapy. Research findings indicate that moderate alcohol drinking in nursing home institutions improves mental health and physical functioning, although the effects of an increased opportunity for socialization and increased personal control may be contributing to the positive outcomes as well.

## RESOURCES

For written material and other resources on alcohol abuse, contact:

- Alcoholics Anonymous, 475 Riverside Drive, 11th floor, New York, NY 10115, or the Web site, www.aa.org; or the local chapter of Alcoholics Anonymous, Al-Anon, and Adult Children of Alcoholics, listed in area phone books, or the Web sites, www.al-anon-alateen.org or www.health.org/nacoa.
- National Clearinghouse for Alcohol and Drug Abuse Information, P.O. Box 2345, Rockville, MD 20852; 800-729-6686.

- Hazelden's brochure "How to Talk to an Older Person Who Has a Problem With Alcohol or Medications" and other materials, call 800-I-DO-CARE, or go to the Web site, www.hazelden.org.
- Smart Recovery (provides online and other types of support groups for abstaining from alcohol addictive behavior) at 7537 Mentor Avenue, #306, Mentor, Ohio 44060, www.smartrecovery.org.
- National Institute on Alcohol Abuse and Alcoholism, at www.niaaa.nih.gov.

# MEDICATION USAGE

More than 10,000 prescription drugs are currently available to Americans, and over a billion prescriptions are dispensed per year. There are also countless over-the-counter medications consumed, including 600 that would have required a prescription just a few years ago. It is not unreasonable to suggest that most Americans consider taking medications a normal part of life.

Because vulnerability to chronic disease increases over time, medication usage becomes more typical with age. Although adults aged 65 and over comprised 12.4% of the population, they accounted for over 34% of outpatient prescription medications and nearly half of those purchased over-the-counter ("Protecting Yourself," 1996). Older persons rely on drugs to alleviate pain and discomfort and to give them a sense of security and control in sometimes frightening health situations. Drugs, however, can make matters worse as well as better. The potential for serious adverse drug reactions is great.

## MISUSE

About 50% of prescriptions are not taken properly, and according to the National Council on Patient Information and Education, an estimated 125,000 Americans die each year from prescription drug misuse. In fact, you are more likely to die from prescription medication than from an accident, pneumonia, or diabetes (Lazarou et al., 1998).

On an outpatient basis about 5% of Medicare patients are made ill by their medications during the course of a year, leading to as many as 1.9 million drug-related injuries (Gurwitz et al., 2003). More than half of these adverse drug events are preventable, ranging from monitoring mistakes made by physicians to failure of patients to adhere to medication instructions.

About 15% to 20% of hospital and nursing home admissions are the result of adverse drug reactions ("Protecting Yourself," 1996), and about 11% of emergency department visits by older adults are due to adverse drug reactions (Hohl et al, 2001). These percentages are probably under-estimated because medical personnel are not enthusiastic about filing the additional reports required by the FDA (Lazarou et al., 1998). Adverse drug reactions probably affect older adults three times as often as the general population (Sloan, 1986).

To avoid adverse drug reactions, patients need to comply with their medication regimen, report unexpected side effects, and show caution with over-the-counter medications. They also need to know more about their medications. Only 15% of elderly patients who visited an emergency department were able to accurately report on their medications, dosages, frequencies, and indications (Chung & Barfield, 2002), despite the fact that patients who were disoriented or medically unstable were excluded from the study.

Conversely, physicians need to take a good drug history, carefully assess the dosage, communicate the rationale for the drug treatment and the expected response and common side effects, and monitor patient reactions. The aging process complicates this course of action because it affects the absorption, distribution, metabolism, and excretion of medications (Pollock & Mulsant, 1995).

Physicians also need to know which medications are inappropriate for older persons. About 1 million older patients were prescribed 1 of 11 medicines that a panel of geriatric medicine and pharmacy experts had agreed should always be avoided by older adults (Zhan et al., 2001). A slightly higher percentage of Finnish older patients may also be taking at least one inappropriate medication (Pitkala et al., 2002).

Overprescribing is common as well. "Even when non-pharmacological treatments are suitable for a given condition, physicians often prescribe medications. Predictably, the greater the number of drugs prescribed, the greater the risk of inadvertent or intentional misuse of drugs by the patient or caregiver" (Montamat & Cusack, 1992).

Polypharmacy is the use of more medications than are clinically indicated. Older adults are particularly vulnerable to polypharmacy because most of the chronic conditions associated with aging are potentially responsive to medications. This leads to the increased risk of multiple drug use among older adults, complicated by the fact that many older patients see more than one health care provider. With more than one provider, prescription and over-the-counter drug usage may not be coordinated, and older clients are vulnerable to potential interactions (drug-drug, drug-allergy, drug-food, drug-drink, and drug-disease), and therapeutic duplication.

This challenge has been met, to some extent, by the fact that almost all pharmacies in this country are using computers. Nonetheless, many pharmacies do not have complete computer records of all the medication usage of their clients.

Based on an article by Montamat and Cusack (1992), I have developed 10 patient-related and physician-related factors that contribute to polypharmacy and other types of drug misuse:

Patient-Related Drug Misuse Factors

1. Expectation of physician to prescribe medication
2. Inadequate reporting of current medications being taken
3. Failure to complain about medication-related symptoms
4. Use of multiple, automatic refills without visiting a physician
5. Hoarding and using prior medications
6. Use of multiple pharmacies or multiple physicians
7. Borrowing medications from family members or friends
8. Self-medication with over-the-counter drugs
9. Impaired cognition or vision
10. Underuse of medications due to side effects and cost considerations

Physician-Related Drug Misuse Factors

1. Presuming that patients expect a prescription
2. Treatment of symptoms with drugs without sufficient clinical evaluation
3. Treating conditions without setting therapy goals
4. Communicating instructions in an unclear, complex, or incomplete manner
5. Failure to review medications and their possible adverse effects at regular intervals
6. Use of automatic refills without adequate follow-up
7. Lack of knowledge of geriatric clinical pharmacology, leading to inappropriate prescribing practices
8. Inadequate supervision of medications in long-term care
9. Failure to simplify drug regimens as often as possible
10. Failure to identify and adequately communicate the equivalency of cost-effective generics

## PREVENTION

One of the most effective prevention strategies against drug abuse is to avoid unnecessary medication. Many Americans unthinkingly take pills to alleviate constipation, insomnia, indigestion, headache, and other types of pain or discomfort. Diet, exercise, and stress management, however, may be effective alternatives that avoid the danger of medication side effects.

Elderly clients with high blood pressure are susceptible to severe adverse drug reactions (Potter & Haigh, 1990). Treating some patients with modestly high blood pressure with nonpharmacological alternatives, therefore, may be appropriate. Older adults can be responsive to a reduction in sodium intake (Horwath, 1991), and exercise can reduce the risk of elevating blood pressure levels (W. Evans et al., 1991).

"Physician and patient must have an understanding of the . . . degree to which [the other] favors chemical or psychological coping devices" (Taylor et al., 1982, p. 299). Many patients, and some physicians, believe that a productive medical encounter requires the writing of a prescription. In support of this assertion, about 75% of all physician visits result in the prescription of a drug (Kemper et al., 1985). Along with unnecessary prescriptions, older clients are more likely to be inadequately knowledgeable about the drugs prescribed for them (American Board of Family Practice, 1987).

If prescriptions become the treatment of choice, more patients may be willing to participate actively in choosing among medication alternatives (type, dosage, and schedules) than the physician feels comfortable with (American Board of Family Practice, 1987). Yet active participation in choosing drugs is likely to lead to better compliance (R. Taylor et al., 1982).

## ADVICE FROM PHARMACISTS

Since January 1993, pharmacists have been required to give Medicaid patients advice about their prescription drugs. When the federal Health Care Financing Administration implemented these rules, some state boards of pharmacies expanded them to cover all patients.

In addition to informing patients verbally and in writing, pharmacies must maintain files of patient information (including a list of the medicines and health care devices being used by the patient). The pharmacist must provide specific information about each medication, its common side effects, potential interactions, and contraindications, and must instruct patients on monitoring their responses, explaining what to do if a dose is missed, and how to store the medicine. Since 1995 pharmacies have been required to provide an area suitable for confidential patient counseling. It is not uncommon for these laws to be ignored.

The consumer who is most disadvantaged, especially in monitoring potential interaction effects, is the one who pharmacy-hops for either financial purposes or convenience. It is not unusual for a patient to obtain prescription drugs from multiple sources, such as a community pharmacy, a hospital pharmacy, a mail-order pharmacy, and directly from the physician. To offset this diversity, a credit card system could be implemented to enable patients to carry prescription records with them wherever they go.

## A PHYSICIAN'S EXPERIENCE

"Recently, I spoke to a group of older people. I told them that as a young doctor I had spent most of my time putting patients on drugs. But now that I'm an old doctor, I spend a lot of my time taking patients off drugs. I thought the remark might elicit a few smiles or chuckles. Instead, they rose as a body, cheering and clapping (Morgan, 1993)."

## ADVERTISING

Only the United States and New Zealand permit advertising of prescription medicines to consumers. As the number of advertisements continue to rise, along with spending on advertised prescription medications, this practice becomes more controversial. The 50 most advertised prescription medicines in 2000 probably contributed to an additional $10 billion in spending on medications.

Merck & Company spent $161 million on Vioxx, an arthritis drug, in 2000, and sales of that one drug alone increased more than 1 billion dollars. The amount of advertising for Vioxx that year was more than PepsiCo spent to advertise Pepsi or Budweiser spent to advertise beer. Besides prescription arthritis drugs, the most heavily advertised medications were cholesterol-lowering drugs, antidepressants, allergy medicine, and heartburn medicine (Petersen, 2001).

As geriatrician John Morley, MD (2002) noted, "Nancy Reagan's 'Just say no to drugs' campaign may have been more effective if it had been aimed at adults rather than teenagers."

## RESOURCES

Many readily available booklets on medication provide a good consumer safety tool for today's cohort of older adults. These booklets remind consumers of important questions to ask their physicians and pharmacists about their medications, offer several ideas to improve daily compliance in taking medications, provide a listing of generic equivalencies, note commonly reported side effects of particular medications, and offer blank charts for listing all prescriptions and over-the-counter medications prior to visiting a physician.

Consumers who are vulnerable to psychological and emotional factors that may affect their use of medications, can obtain free copies of a booklet entitled *So Many Pills and I Still Don't Feel Good: Suggestions for Preventing Problems with Medications.* The booklet helps individuals recognize times when they may be at risk for misuse of medications, suggests ways to manage medications, lists questions to ask the doctor or pharmacist about medications, and suggests things to do if there is a problem with medication usage. Up to 50 free copies are available from AARP Fulfillment, 601 E Street, NW, Washington, DC 20049; order #PF 4767 (1091) D14581 (no telephone orders).

Two other booklets that I recommend from having utilized them in community health education classes are provided free by AARP: *The Smart Consumer's Guide to Prescription Drugs* (PF 4297(389)-Dl3579) and *Using Your Medicines Wisely: A Guide for the Elderly* (PF l436(ll85)-D3l7). Contact AARP Publications, Program Resources, 601 E Street, NW Washington, DC 20049.

To get answers about the drug approval process, drug reactions, and new and approved medications, contact the Food and Drug Administration, Center for Drug Evaluation and Research, CDER Executive Secretariat (HFD-8), 5600 Fishers Lane, Rockville, MD 29857, 301-295-8012; or go to the Food and Drug Administration Web site at www.fda.gov and click on 'Information for Consumers,' and then on 'D' for Drug Interactions.

To learn about AARP's Check Up on Your Prescriptions campaign and to find links to other useful sites, go to www.aarp.org/wiseuse. AARP's mail-order pharmacy is for members of AARP (who are aged 50 and older and pay a small annual membership fee). This network of regional pharmacies provides information on common prescription drugs, their side effects, and cost differences between brand names and generic drugs: AARP Pharmacy Services, 500 Montgomery Street, Alexandria, VA 22314, 703-684-0244 or 800-456-2277.

Three sources of free information on older persons and medications are: The Elder Health Program, School of Pharmacy, University of Maryland at Baltimore, 20 N. Pine Street, Baltimore, MD 21201, 410-706-3011; the National Institutes on Aging, P.O Box 8057, Gaithersburg, MD 20898-8057 (800) 222-2225; and for taking prescriptions safely, go to www.prescriptionforsafety.com.

Finally, contact the National Council on Patient Information and Education for free booklets and other information on prescriptions. For the free booklet "Prescription Medicines and You," call 800-358-9295. For additional information, go to www.talkaboutrx.org. To find out about nonprescription products, go to www.bemedwise.org.

# INJURY PREVENTION

Unintentional injuries were the fifth leading cause of death in the United States in 1998, accounting for 97,000 deaths. And while the percentage of deaths from unintentional injuries was lower among persons aged 65 and older, the mortality rate from injuries for older adults was more than twice that of other age groups.

Among older adults, some injury problems appear to be getting worse. During the decade of the 1990s, the *Healthy People 2000 Final Review* reports that among people 65 years of age and older, the hospitalization rate for hip fractures increased from 714 to 863 hospitalizations per 100,000 persons.

Two of the main antecedents of injuries are falls and motor vehicles. A number of physical and environmental factors associated with age contribute to the greater frequencies and seriousness of injuries due to both falls and motor vehicles. Diminished vision and hearing, poor coordination and balance, slower reaction time, arthritis, and neurological disease all are intrinsic to the increased vulnerability to falls and motor vehicle accidents of older adults. In addition, medication use, which increases with age, can produce drowsiness, confusion, and depression, and increase the probability of accidents (Spirduso, 1995).

Other factors are extrinsic to the increased incidence of accidents among older people. Homes age along with people; uneven floor surfaces and the absence of safety equipment (such as grab bars for bathtubs and showers) in older homes contribute to accidents. Other environmental culprits are throw rugs, inadequate lighting, steep stairs, and lack of railings on stairs.

Accidents can also increase as road repairs and improvements and law enforcement fail to keep pace with the increased demands of automobile traffic. Transportation systems and cars are not designed with older people's capacities in mind. And few cities acknowledge the need to lengthen the duration of walk signals at crosswalks to accommodate older pedestrians.

## FALL PREVENTION

Approximately 60% of persons who die from falls are age 65 or older, and about half of the older adults who are hospitalized from a fall do not live more than 1 year (Rivara et al., 1997; Spirduso, 1995). People age 75 and older account for 59% of all fall deaths, even though they are only 5% of the population ("Accidents Don't Just Happen," 1995). Also, falls account for 87% of all fractures in older adults, and a majority of older adults who have serious hip fractures never regain their previous function (Rivara et al., 1997; Spirduso, 1995).

Falls result not only in decreased physical functioning, but also in decreased confidence and the fear of falling. The fear of falling can then lead to a cycle of social isolation, further functional decline, and depression (Rubenstein et al., 1994; Tinetti et al., 1994).

The primary risk factors for falling are balance abnormalities, muscular weakness, visual disorders, gait abnormalities, cardiovascular disease, cognitive impairment, medication usage, and environmental hazards (Spirduso, 1995). Many of these risks are preventable. Tai chi, for instance, improves balance and reduces falls (Wolf et al., 1996; Wolfson et al., 1996). Weight-bearing and other types of exercise reduce the risk of hip fracture and falls (Campbell et. al., 1997; M. Robertson et al., 2001; Rubenstein et al., 2000; Tinetti et. al., 1993).

Persons with osteoporosis—which can lead to falls—can be helped by treatment with alendronate and other medications that increase bone density (Morley, 2001). Environmental changes (e.g., night-lights, placement of objects and furniture, removal of tripping hazards, use of nonslip floor mats, and installation of grab bars in the bathroom) recommended by nurses, physical therapists, and occupational therapists, can also lead to a reduction in the incidence of falls by older adults (Turkoski et al., 1997).

Regarding environmental hazards, up to 40% of older adults living in the community fall each year, and 75% of these falls occur within the home (Kiernat, 1991). It behooves the health professional, therefore, to recommend a home assessment to identify conditions that increase the risk for falling, to suggest environmental changes, and to educate their clients to reduce the risks. An environmental assessment of the homes of 1,000 persons aged 72 and older was conducted in Connecticut, and the prevalence of environmental hazards was high. Two or more hazards were found in 59% of the bathrooms, and in 23% to 42% of the remaining rooms (Gill et al., 1999).

Two thirds of all deaths due to falls in the home are preventable (Ferrini & Ferrini, 1989). The following is a list of 10 simple precautions that can reduce the risk of falls within the home:

1. Provide proper illumination and convenient light switches—by the bed, at the end of the hall, and at the top and bottom of stairs. Older persons generally need two to three times as much illumination as younger persons do.
2. Install handrails and place nonslip treads in strategic locations.
3. Tack down or remove loose throw rugs and repair torn carpet.
4. Install grab bars and use adhesive strips in shower and bath. Only about 6% of the dwelling units of older persons have grab bars in their bathrooms.
5. Eliminate such hazards as trailing electrical cords, sharp corners, slippery floors, and household items that require a step stool to reach.
6. Lower bed height for ease in getting in and out.
7. Wear footwear that provides adequate traction, such as supportive, rubber-soled, low-heeled shoes.
8. Exercise to improve balance, flexibility, strength, and coordination.
9. Avoid the misuse of medications and alcohol.
10. Limit fluids after dinner, which can reduce nighttime trips to the bathroom.

Several health conditions place older individuals at risk for falling. Some of these conditions are dizzy spells, osteoporosis, arthritis, alcoholism, structural diseases of the feet, stroke, visual or hearing impairments, gait and balance disorders, physical weakness, and the use of medications that impair coordination and balance or result in frequent trips to the bathroom at night. A multidisciplinary geriatric assessment can identify those at risk and thereby help to prevent serious injuries from falls.

An increasing number of departments of internal medicine and family medicine at university medical schools, as well as private practitioners, provide multidisciplinary geriatric assessments. Teams invariably include a physician and nurse; and those with enhanced benefit to consumers include several of the following health professionals: occupational therapist, physical therapist, counselor, social worker, health educator, pharmacist, and dentist.

There are several innovations to protect older adults at risk of falls. A telephone emergency alert system, for instance, has a signaling device that is worn around the neck or on the belt of older adults who have a tendency to fall. Anatomically designed external hip protectors can reduce the risk of hip fracture among frail elderly adults (Kannus et al., 2000). And universal design is an architectural philosophy that is being applied to both new homes and to the modification of existing ones, to make them safer for older persons and those with disabilities.

Universally designed homes may include grab bars that look like towel racks, counters with stripes around the edge to create definition for people with poor vision, showers with pull-down seats, entrances with no steps, doorways that are wider to accommodate wheelchairs, and bedrooms and bathrooms on the same level as the main entrance so that stairs will never bar access. For more ideas on applying universal design to a home, contact the AARP Web site at www.aarp.org/universalhome.

A guide that includes summaries of innovative programs to prevent falls, short descriptions of research findings on the topic, a home safety/fall prevention assessment tool, and educational strategies is provided by the AARP. For a copy of *The Perfect Fit: Creative Ideas for a Safe and Livable Home or Fall Prevention Guide,* contact AARP/Program Resources, 601 E Street, NW, Washington, DC 20049.

## MOTOR VEHICLE AND PEDESTRIAN SAFETY

On July 16, 2003 an 86-year-old driver killed 10 people and injured 45 more when he drove into a crowded farmer's market in Santa Monica, California. Despite widely publicized tragedies like this one, older drivers kill fewer motorists and pedestrians than any other age group and have the lowest crash rates per licensed driver (Swoboda, 2001).

As older drivers increase, however—there were 18 million registered drivers over age 70 in 2001, and 40 million are expected by the year 2020—they will account for an increasing share of the motor vehicle accidents each year. And once having been in an accident, older adults are more prone to serious injury and death.

A number of physiological changes affect the driving of older adults. Arthritis makes it difficult to turn the head and directly observe cars coming up from behind. Slower reflexes make emergencies more dangerous to contend with. Susceptibility to glare, poor adaptation to dark, and the need for additional light make night driving riskier. Cognitive impairment rises with age and has been linked to higher motor vehicle crash rates in elderly individuals (Retchin & Anapolle, 1993). Medical conditions, and comorbidity in particular, are correlated with decreased driving amount and driving cessation (Forrest et al., 1997).

Driving in late life is not necessarily an all-or-nothing proposition. Older adults who find driving an automobile increasingly difficult can restrict their driving to areas with little traffic, avoid rush hours, and abstain from driving at night. In addition, older adults may need to be vigilant about restricting their driving to those periods of time when their medications are not slowing their reaction time or compromising their vision.

Measures to Prevent Motor Vehicle Accidents

1. Enroll in a driver safety class designed for midlife and older motorists, such as a course through AARP 55-Alive or the state motor vehicle department.
2. Adjust to hearing and vision losses, that is, keep radio, air conditioner, and heater noise low; crack windows open to hear warning signals; wear good-quality sunglasses; and keep windows clean inside and out.
3. Time trips to minimize the effects of medications.
4. Stop frequently to stretch muscles and rest eyes.
5. Limit driving to the safest times of day and to familiar areas.
6. Use seat belts all the time, even on short trips and in cars with airbags in order to prevent injury from side collision.
7. Keep the car in good working condition.
8. Avoid drinking while driving.
9. Lobby for state policies that are more responsive to the functional abilities of older drivers.
10. Lobby for state policies that require physicians to report motorists who have health problems that could affect their driving ability.

In regard to advocating for more responsive state policies (#9), selected states have begun to make the following traffic improvements: wider highway lanes, larger road signs with larger letters and numbers, more reflective pavement markers to better illuminate roads at night, and street names displayed well in advance of intersections.

In regard to advocating for more responsible physician reporting (#10), five states—California, Delaware, Nevada, North Dakota, and Texas—require physicians to report motorists who have health problems that could affect their driving ability. In one study using a convenience sample of older patients at a medical clinic in Hawaii, 24% of older adults with poor brain function said they currently drove. This poor cognitive performance, however, was often unrecognized by their physicians. Doctors identified mental problems in only 5% of the older adults with intermediate impairment and 11% of older adults with poor mental performance (Valcour et al., 2002).

The National Institute on Aging estimates that 600,000 people age 70 and older give up their driving each year. One interesting study reported that older adults will live up to 10 years after they stop driving, during which time they will need to rely on other forms of transportation (Foley et al., 2002). In the same way people prepare for retirement, older adults will need to plan ahead for the resources they will need after they stop driving. If attention is not paid to this challenge, social isolation and depression may result.

There is little guidance for older adults on when to stop driving. State bills to require drivers age 75 and older to take regular behind-the-wheel road tests have consistently failed. Among 16 states that considered road tests for those age 75 and older, only Illinois and New Hampshire passed such legislation. Charges of age discrimination, and the millions in additional costs to test older drivers have served as deterrents. A compromise bill in Missouri did pass, and allows family members, physicians, and others to report an "impaired driver," who is then required to take a road test.

Older adults are more likely than members of any other age group to be injured by motor vehicles while crossing a street, and experience the highest death rate from pedestrian accidents (USDHHS, 1985). A study of 1249 residents aged 72 or older from New Haven, Connecticut revealed that fewer than 1% of these pedestrians had a normal walking speed sufficient to cross the street in the time typically allotted at signalized intersections (Langlois et al., 1997). Crosswalk markings at sites with no traffic signal or stop sign are particularly hazardous to older pedestrians (Koepsell et al., 2002). Motor vehicles struck and killed 4,882 pedestrians in the United States in the year 2001, with older pedestrians at especially high risk. People aged 70 and older accounted for nearly 20% of all pedestrian deaths in 2001, nearly double what would have been expected on the basis of age-related pedestrian statistics.

Measures to Avoid Pedestrian Accidents

1. Wear highly visible clothing, preferably of light-colored or even fluorescent material.
2. Do not assume that drivers in moving vehicles see pedestrians.
3. Do not return to the curb if the Don't Walk sign begins to flash. Continue to walk at maximum comfortable speed, moving your arms to be more visible.
4. Lobby local officials to install properly timed pedestrian traffic signals.

AARP's 55 Alive/Mature Driving Program was launched in 1979 and is available around the country. It is an 8-hour, classroom-based (no actual driving), driver education refresher course for persons 50 and older, and is taught by instructors who are also 50 and older. Almost 600,000 older drivers enrolled in AARP's classes in 2000, an increase of 60% over the 1990 figure. In some states, drivers who complete the course are eligible for a discount on automobile insurance. For more information, contact the American Association of Retired Persons, either toll-free at 888-227-7669, or at the Web site www.aarp.org/55alive.

For tips on driving safety for older adults, the AAA Foundation launched a Traffic Safety Web site www.seniordrivers.org. Other useful Web sites are the National Highway Traffic Safety Administration at www.nhtsa.gov and the Insurance Institute for Highway Safety at www.highwaysafety.org.

# SLEEP

Although the diagnosis of chronic, primary insomnia in older adults is estimated at 5% to 10% (Ohayon et al., 1996), as many as 40% of older adults complain about sleep problems (Vitiello, 1997). Significant sleep disturbance is likely to impact on quality of life. Insomniacs are 2.5 times more likely to have accidents than other drivers, are more likely to be anxious, depressed or forgetful, and may recover more slowly from an illness (Mestel, 1997b).

A national survey conducted by the National Sleep Foundation reported that 56% of Americans experienced one or more symptoms of insomnia, including difficulty falling asleep, waking up during the night, waking up too early, and waking up feeling fatigued (D. Shelton, 1999). Forty percent of the adults in this survey were so sleepy during the day that they reported it interfered with their daily activities. Yet only 4% were seeing a health care provider for advice or treatment.

## INTERVENTIONS

Identifying the cause of sleeplessness can be rather complicated. Insomnia can result from arthritis, a hyperactive thyroid, sleep apnea, restless leg syndrome, too much caffeine, poor circulation, inadequate sleep hygiene, anxiety, and too little exercise. The first line of attack is lifestyle change, such as restricting caffeine, keeping a regular schedule of going to bed and waking up, using relaxation techniques, limiting or eliminating daytime napping, avoiding reading and watching television in the bedroom, limiting drinking—particularly alcohol—after dinner, avoiding heavy meals late in the evening, and getting more exercise.

Regarding exercise, older adults with moderate sleep complaints slept almost an hour longer and cut in half the amount of time it normally took to fall asleep as a consequence of participating in a low-impact aerobic program (King et al., 1997). Even a sample of healthy older adult caregivers who were without initially reported sleep complaints reported improvements in sleep quality after completing a moderate-intensity exercise program (King et al., 2002).

After 8 weeks of an insomnia study, it was reported that behavioral therapy was slightly more effective than drug therapy. Follow-up assessments up to 14 months, however, indicated that only behavioral therapy led to sustained benefits (Morin et al., 1999). Sleeping medication may be almost as effective as behavioral therapy in the short run, but in the long run individuals build up tolerance, the dosage must be raised, and the risk for memory impairment, hypertension, and more frequent accidents is increased.

Another study reported that two behavior programs significantly improved sleep patterns among older adults with chronic illnesses who had trouble sleeping. The cognitive behavioral program consisted of group education sessions. The home audio relaxation treatment consisted of audiotapes that instructed listeners in muscle, breathing, and cognitive relaxation techniques. The audiotapes included techniques similar to the ones taught in the cognitive behavioral program.

Fifty-four percent of participants in the cognitive behavior program, 39% of persons in the home audio relaxation treatment, and 6% of the members in the control group significantly improved their sleep efficiency, the time awake after sleep onset, and total time in bed (Rybarczyk et al., 2002). The authors concluded that older adults with chronic illness are able to make substantial improvements in their sleep patterns without resorting to medication. This is particularly important among older persons who already take other drugs for existing chronic medical conditions.

Seventy-five patients (mean age 55) with persistent primary sleep disorder for an average of 13 years were randomly assigned to cognitive behavioral therapy (attitude and bedtime habits), relaxation techniques, or a placebo. After 6 weeks, the cognitive behavioral group reduced wake time once asleep by 54%, the relaxation group by 16%, and the placebo group by 12% (Edinger et al., 2001). These improvements persisted 6 months later.

One controversial study reported that 8 hours of sleep or more led to *shorter* life expectancy (Kripke et al., 2002). This study contradicted all preceding studies that reported that many Americans suffered from too little sleep, not too much. The study received a substantial amount of public media attention, but little note was made of the fact that it was based on a questionnaire that was not designed to analyze sleep issues. The study also did not examine morbidity and other qualities of life that may be affected by sleep deprivation—depression, memory problems, relationship difficulties, and increased accident risk.

Although data on the United States is not available, the median amount of time spent on sleep related issues in medical training in the United Kingdom is 5 minutes (Stores & Crawford, 1998). Not surprisingly, the typical treatment for chronic insomnia by physicians is to prescribe benzodiazepines, which have known side effects, rather than cognitive behavioral interventions (Montgomery, 2002).

Finally, many herbs are reputed to act as sedatives, such as chamomile, exotic passionflower, and valerian extract (Mestel, 1997b), but their effectiveness is not supported by randomized, controlled research studies. The same holds true for the popular hormone, melatonin, which is found in most health food stores and drugstores. There has been little controlled research on its utility as a sleeping aid, and prolonged use may be unsafe.

## RESOURCES

If conventional solutions for older adults do not work, it may be necessary to contact an accredited sleep clinic, by writing to the American Sleep Disorders Association, 1610 14th Street, #300, Rochester, MN 55901.

A toll-free 24-hour hotline that provides information on sleep is called the Shuteye Sleepline, at 1-800-*shuteye.*

The National Sleep Foundation posts research and lists sleep treatment centers at www.sleepfoundation.org.

For a course syllabus on sleep education, contact Gregg Jacobs, PhD, an instructor in medicine at Harvard Medical School at 110 Francis Street, Suite 1A, Boston, MA 02215, 617-632-7369.

# QUESTIONS FOR DISCUSSION

1. An alcohol abuse specialist and a smoking cessation specialist, both of whom have focused their practice exclusively on young adults, are being confronted for the first time with older clients. What advice would you give to help each of them become more responsive to the needs and interests of older clients?

2. Think about your classroom space, your neighborhood, and your home. What steps can you take to reduce the chances that an older person will have an accident in one of these three locations?

3. You are interested in reducing drug misuse and have applied for a grant that forces you to focus on only one population for your study, from among the following three options: older persons, physicians, or pharmacists. Which population would you choose, and why is it more preferable than the other two choices? What strategies would you recommend?
4. The author criticizes direct-to-consumer advertising of medications. Can you make the case that it is more useful than detrimental?
5. What do you think is the single best way to prevent older pedestrians from getting killed?
6. An older adult has voluntarily given up driving, and you want to reduce their chances of becoming isolated and depressed. What ideas can you suggest that might enhance the older adult's ability to continue to be connected to the world?
7. Prepare an outline for a presentation to older adults at a senior center on improving sleep hygiene. Make sure it is an interactive presentation. What kinds of questions will you ask them in order to generate discussion?

# 10

## Social Support

*You need an experience with at least one person who cares about you. It doesn't matter at what age this person appears. If you didn't have a close relationship when younger, and you now have one close person in your life, that makes up for the early deficiency. That person can appear at any time in the life cycle, even on the day of death. One does not need to make up for lost time.*

—*Weininger & Menkin, 1978*

I was struck by this quotation, even though it is not an evidence-based assertion. What it says to me is that at this moment in life—whether it is among our last moments or not—we need to believe that someone cares about us. The benefits that accrue from believing that we have the support of another person will be the subject of this chapter.

## DEFINITION OF SOCIAL SUPPORT

Social support can be defined as the perceived caring, esteem, and assistance that people receive from others. Support can come from spouses, family members, friends, neighbors, colleagues, health professionals, or pets. The literature is rife with elaborate taxonomies of social support (Eng & Young, 1992), yet it can be reduced to three basic types:

1. *Emotional support* provides people with a sense of love, reassurance, and belonging. When individuals feel they are being listened to, and valued, they develop a healthy sense of self-worth. Emotional support has a strong and consistent relationship to health status (Israel & Schurman, 1990).

2. *Instrumental support* refers to the provision of tangible aid and services that directly assist people who are in need. Examples are financial help and household maintenance. Good instrumental support has been correlated with a decrease in psychosomatic and emotional distress, and with greater life satisfaction (Revicki & Mitchell, 1990).
3. *Informational support* is the provision of advice, feedback, and suggestions to help a person address problems.

Social networks, unlike social support, are defined in terms of structural characteristics: the number of social linkages, the frequency of contacts, and so on. Although the characteristics of people's social networks do not correlate with the quality of their social support, they do correlate with positive health outcomes.

There is a tendency, however, for social networks to shrink with age—older adults have about half as many friends and associates as younger people—because older persons cease relating to people who are less close or less important to them. With older adults, though, the quantity of relationships may decrease over time, but the quality of social relationships may be better and lives may be more satisfying (Lang, 2001).

Social support appears to boost the immune system, reduce the likelihood of illness, speed up the recovery process, diminish the need for medication, reduce psychological strain and cognitive impairment, and lower the risk of death from heart disease (Bassuk et al., 1999; Eng et al., 2002; Fratiglioni et al., 2000; Koenig et.al., 1997; Larson, 1995; Sarafino, 1990). S. Cohen and colleagues (1997) gave nasal drops containing viruses to a large sample of participants and discovered that those with more diverse social networks had greater resistance to upper respiratory illness. A population study of social and productive activities that involved little or no physical activity among older Americans, reported that these non-physical social activities are as important as fitness activities when it comes to impacting on mortality (Glass et al., 1999).

Unfortunately, people who provide social support can also set bad examples and offer poor advice. The correlation of negative relationships, such as those characterized by hassles and mistrust, with poor mental health is stronger than the association of social support with good mental health (Israel & Schurman, 1990).

## FAMILY, FRIENDS, CHURCH, AND OTHERS

Large-scale epidemiological studies have shown that membership in a social network of family, friends, church, and other support structures is correlated with lower mortality risk. The classic research endeavor in this area, led by the epidemiologist Lisa Berkman, was a study of 7,000 residents of Alameda County, California. The research team found that residents who were married, had ample contact with extended family and friends, belonged to a church, and had other group affiliations were half as likely to die over the course of the 9-year study as those with less adequate social supports (Berkman, 1983).

The results of research on the relationship between social support and mortality have been replicated in other large studies of both healthy and sick adults (J. Goodwin et al., 1987; House et al., 1988; R. Williams et al., 1992), most of which have controlled for other factors that might affect mortality, such as lifestyle, socioeconomic status, age, race, and access to health care. House and colleagues (1988), in fact, have shown that social isolation has as strong an effect on mortality as does smoking or high cholesterol levels.

Studies report the importance of a spouse or supportive family in helping people adopt or sustain good health habits. One study, for instance, reported that lifestyle interventions targeted at men and women as couples rather than as individuals resulted in a greater reduction in cardiovascular risk factors like cigarette smoking, systolic blood pressure, and cholesterol level (Pyke et al., 1997). The authors report that targeting the couple may strengthen outcomes through the mutual reinforcement of lifestyle changes.

Another study reported that women on insulin treatment were found to be more likely to experience metabolic control (i.e., a good fasting blood glucose level) if they were part of a supportive family (Cardenas et al., 1987). Supportive families were also found to be important in reinforcing eating behaviors, sustaining regular exercise, and helping individuals sustain weight loss (J. Murphy et al., 1982; Stuart & Davis, 1972; Zimmerman & Connor, 1989). Men with supportive wives were twice as likely at those whose wives had neutral or negative attitudes to continue in a physical activity program (Heinzelmann & Bagley, 1970).

Spouses as a source of support, however, are increasingly less available with age, particularly among older women. Although 84% of males and 67% of females live with their spouses during late middle age, the percentages drop to 65% of males and 21%(!) of females at age 75 and over. Fortunately, older women living independently manage pretty well psychologically and may fare even better than women living with a spouse, provided they have supportive relationships from other relatives and from friends (Michael et al., 2001).

And though adult children are a major alternative source of social support for older adults, their support for parents has to compete for time and energy with their own needs and those of their children. Because of the limitations of spousal and child support, friendships take on increasing importance in late life (Wykle & Musil, 1993). In one sample, support from friends was found to be more important for preventing depression than support from children (Dean et al., 1990).

In 1995, Robert Putnam published an article entitled "Bowling Alone: American's Declining Social Capital," and then followed up subsequent criticism of his article with a book, *Bowling Alone: The Collapse and Revival of American Community* (Putnam, 2000). Putnam argued that both television and a generation that is less civically engaged than their parents has created more social isolation—to the detriment of themselves and society. His conclusion generated much discussion, including from those who argued that there has only been a change in *type* of social support (e.g., cyberspace, nontraditional small groups like book clubs and support groups, and prayer fellowship) in contemporary America, rather than the quantity or quality of social involvement.

The question of whether there is a trend toward less social support or to different types of social support in American society remains unanswered. But Putnam's writing has emphasized the importance of monitoring social activity in America, and it has stimulated discussion on what we should do to sustain or improve it.

## LAY SUPPORT

"Professionals do not take the time to first gauge the ways that ordinary people help one another and then try to strengthen the helping processes that work for them" (Gottlieb, 1985). Different terms and definitions are used to describe lay support, but the commonalties tend to crosscut these differences. One such definition is that of *lay health advisors,* referring to "people to whom others naturally turn for advice, emotional support, and tangible aid. They provide informal, spontaneous assistance, which is so much a part of everyday life that its value is often not recognized" (Israel, 1985). A concept similar to lay health advisors is *natural neighbor,* coined by Collins and Pancoast (1976), which refers to people who are prompted by empathy or a desire to help others. Many do volunteer work at churches or community organizations.

Some lay health advisors or natural neighbors may not be as "natural" or as skillful as others but are willing to participate in paraprofessional training programs to increase their skills and to better identify persons who are in need of support. Two such programs, sponsored by the federal government, are the Senior Companion Program, in which low-income persons, aged 60 and over, receive a small stipend (below minimum wage) to provide companionship to peers in need; and the Foster Grandparent Program, in which low-income persons, aged 60 and over, receive a small stipend to provide companionship and guidance to children with exceptional needs, especially in hospitals, centers for those with mental retardation, correctional facilities, and other institutions that serve children. Studies of these programs report that in addition to providing benefits to the young and the old in need, the older volunteers improve their own mental and physical health (ACTION, 1984, 1985).

## ONLINE SUPPORT

There are thousands of different self-help groups available online. The American Self-Help Clearinghouse's *Self-Help Sourcebook* (White & Madara, 2002) provides information on more than 1,000 national and international self-help support groups for addictions, bereavement, physical health, mental health, disabilities, caregiving, and other stressful life situations. Information on starting and sustaining a group is also provided. The sourcebook can be accessed at www.mentalhelp.net/selfhelp

One Internet support group that was utilized by nurses and other health professionals focused on support for caregivers of persons with Alzheimer's disease. A computer support network was implemented by nurses who provided information, communication, and decision-support functions for caregivers. During a 1-year study, access to this network enhanced caregivers' decision-making confidence (Brennan et al., 1995).

There is a downside to cyberspace support as well. On the Internet there is rarely a professional available to intervene when bad advice, faulty information, or inappropriate support is being given. Moreover, it is not uncommon to spend an excessive amount of time on the Internet to the exclusion of other responsibilities or people who are important to you. Ironic as it might seem, there are Internet addiction support groups on the Internet to help people with such afflictions.

## PET SUPPORT

It is estimated that between one third and one half of all households in the English-speaking world contain pets, yet there has been limited empirical research on the effects of animal companionship (Siegel, 1993). Though meager, however, the research results are also consistently positive. And most of the existing studies have focused on older persons, who are believed to have the greatest need for companionship.

Pet ownership, adjusting for other variables, was associated with less deterioration of physical function among older adults over a 1-year period (Raina et al., 1999). Pet therapy in long-term care facilities reduced loneliness in comparison to older residents in a control group (Banks & Banks, 2002). Medicare enrollees revealed that pet owners demonstrated lower levels of stress and less utilization of health services for non-serious medical problems than did those who were not pet owners ("Health and Fitness," 1991). Pet owners with heart disease had a significantly higher 1-year survival rate than did those who did not own pets (Friedmann et al., 1980).

The majority of the evaluations of pet intervention programs have not been rigorous, and few have included control groups. Also, the positive effects of pet companionship have not been separated out from participating in a novel or intriguing activity of any sort, as well as the involvement of children and young adults who are a part of many of these programs. Nonetheless, the evidence to date has been consistently positive and suggests that it would be desirable if more "community and volunteer organizations would play a constructive role in facilitating pet ownership among people who wish to own pets" (Siegel, 1993).

## THE EDEN ALTERNATIVE

Pet therapy and pet visitation programs with older adults in institutionalized settings appear to result in a variety of mental health benefits, though most of these programs were limited by temporary contact with pets, which restricts the bonding potential (Boldt & Dellmann-Jenkins, 1992). Unlike most previous pet therapy programs, however, dogs, cats, and other pets live *permanently* with residents in long-term care facilities through the Eden Alternative. The basic premise of the Eden Alternative is that nursing homes should treat residents as people who need attentive care in a homelike setting. To accomplish this goal, nursing homes need to contain not only pets, but also plants, children, and other amenities that make life worth living (see Figure 10.1).

The Eden Alternative was initiated by William Thomas, MD, in 1991 when he was medical director at a nursing home in New York. Since then, it has been replicated at least partially by about 300 nursing homes nationwide. Studies that support the benefits of the program—lower

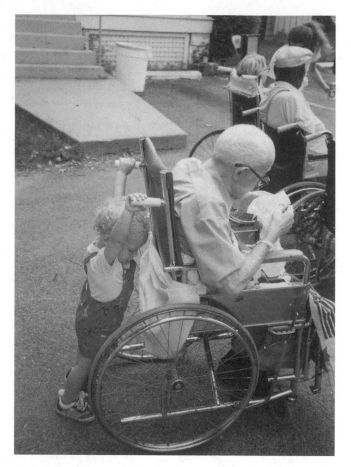

FIGURE 10.1  The author's son visiting a resident in a nursing home (1984).

mortality rates, urinary tract infections, respiratory infections, staff turn-over, resident depression, and medication costs—are reported in Thomas's book *The Eden Alternative* (1995).

Beginning in 2003, the first of 12 small (10-person) "green houses" was erected to serve persons with skilled nursing needs who desired an alter-native to the larger nursing home institution. The brainchild of William Thomas, the Green House Project (web site http://thegreenhousepro-ject.com) refers to houses that will be "filled with the laughter of children, the growth of green plants, and the presence of animals." With support from the Robert Wood Johnson and other foundations, green houses will be built in Mississippi, New York, Michigan, and Nebraska.

An Eden Alternative Train the Trainer Program was launched in 1996. The 3-day program demonstrates how to create a long-term care environment that supports residents emotionally and spiritually as well as physically. To find out about the training or where there are Eden Alternative sites in your state, go to the Web site www.edenalternative.com.

## OTHER PET SUPPORT OPTIONS

In contrast to the Eden Alternative is the uniquely bad idea (based on this author's personal opinion) that was implemented by two researchers from the veterinary school at Purdue University. They pilot-tested robotic dogs with older adults in retirement homes and reported that they observed positive psychological effects on the older residents. The researchers noted that the older adults not only responded well to the robot dogs, but also they did not have to worry about remembering to feed them or about being fit enough to walk them (A. Eisenberg, 2002). The downside of this experiment might be the novelty of the situation producing immediate results that do not survive more than a few encounters, and the less-than-ideal tactile sensation that the robot dog provides.

Although much less common than nursing home and retirement home programs, pet therapy programs based in hospital units under the leadership of nurses have been implemented as well. One nurse manager evaluated a hospital-based pet therapy program by reporting that the staff appeared to be smiling more and laughing more with the patients, and everyone seemed to work much more as a team while the pets were on the unit (Willis, 1997).

There are organizations that promote pet ownership and visitation on a national basis. Some of them—like Jeff's Companion Animal Shelter, which provided isolated older adults with companion dogs—survive less than a decade. The Delta Society, however, is an exception. It is an international, not-for-profit organization that provides training for volunteers and animals in visiting and therapy programs. Its program, Pet Partners, brings volunteers and their pets to nursing homes, hospitals, and schools. The society sponsors an annual conference and publishes a bimonthly magazine. For more information, contact the Delta Society, 289 Perimeter Road East, Renton, WA 98055, 425-226-7357; www.deltasociety.org.

To observe the effects of one visiting dog, see Figure 10.2.

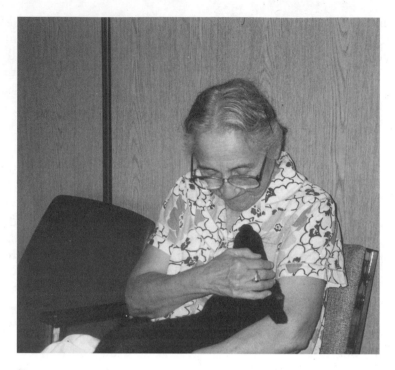

FIGURE 10.2   Dog from a pet companion program visiting an older adult in the author's community health education class.

## RELIGIOUS OR SPIRITUAL SUPPORT

During the 1990s there was considerable research supporting the idea that people who engage in religious or spiritual activity are more likely to live longer or in better health. *Religious* and *spiritual* activity are often used as interchangeable terms, and most research linking spirituality to longevity or health has, in fact, been measured by way of religious beliefs or practices (Koenig, 2000). When a distinction is made, religious activity is more likely to be organizationally based and more traditional in its manifestation.

Religious people not only live longer, but they also have stronger immune systems, are physically healthier, and are less depressed than those who are not (Koenig et al., 1999, 1997; Larson, 1995). The relationship between religious activities and good health remains even when researchers control for potentially confounding variables, such as chronic illnesses, functional abilities, age, race, and other health and social factors.

Explanations for the positive relationship between religion and health range from the impact of religion on healthy lifestyles (e.g., less addiction to smoking and drinking); positive and supportive social relationships; positive ideologies and prayer which lower harmful stress hormones; and more stable marriages (Idler, 1994; Strawbridge et al., 1997; "Studies Suggest", 1996).

Although church attendance decreases with age, a shift to such personal practices like Bible reading and listening to religious radio programs increases. Reduced attendance at religious services is due primarily to decreased mobility and transportation problems rather than declining interest.

One interesting study on the effect of religious involvement on health status reported that Christians and Jews tended to die less frequently in the month before their own group's religious holidays (Idler & Kasl, 1992). Another remarkable—and considerably more controversial—study reported that intercessory prayer (praying long distance for others) was an effective adjunct to standard medical care, when analyzed as part of a randomized, controlled, double-blind, prospective, parallel-group trial (in other words, as part of an allegedly rigorous study) (W. Harris et al., 1999). Patients in the coronary care unit treatment group had lower overall adverse outcomes than control group patients. Even more startling, the patients in this study were unaware that they were being prayed for, and those who did the praying did not know and never met the patients for whom they were praying.

A less controversial study on prayer reported that people who engage in private prayer before surgery are more optimistic on the day before surgery than those who do not; and people who are optimistic before surgery for coronary heart disease recover from surgery more effectively than those who are not (Ai et al., 2002). Conversely, sick patients who are pessimistic about their religious faith had a higher risk of mortality within 2 years (Pargament et al., 2001).

As might be expected, 94% of one sample of outpatients agreed with the statement that in times of medical crisis physicians should ask them whether they have beliefs in prayer and other religious and spiritual practices (Ehman et al., 1999). A bit more surprising is that about 70 medical schools offer instruction in how to address patients' religious beliefs (Duenwald, 2002).

Harold Koenig, a physician and leading researcher on religion, spirituality, and medicine, reviewed 350 studies on the impact of religious involvement on physical health and reported that the majority of the studies support the finding that religious people are physically healthier and require fewer health services. Moreover, an additional 850 studies examined the relationship between religion, spirituality, and mental health, and about 70% of these studies reported that people experience better mental health and adapt more successfully to stress if they are religious (Koenig, 2000).

## AND NOW FOR THE REST OF THE STORY

Led by two psychologists from Columbia University, there are researchers who state that there is no compelling evidence of a relationship between religious or spiritual activity and health and longevity. The psychologists reviewed all 266 articles published during the year 2000 on religion and medicine, and reported that only a few demonstrated the beneficial effects of religious involvement on health (Sloan & Bagiella, 2002).

One of the common mistakes made by the researchers in the studies they reviewed—including the one on intercessory prayer (W. Harris et al., 1999)—is the failure to control for multiple comparisons, commonly referred to in research as a fishing expedition. In other words, if you examine enough variables you will find some of them significant on the basis of chance alone. When the studies with multiple dependent variables are statistically corrected for—a standard practice in statistical analysis when examining multiple comparisons—the significance levels of these variables disappear (Sloan & Bagiella, 2002).

The psychologists also noted that many studies were correlational rather than causal, and that religious behavior can be the product of good health, rather than its cause; and the lack of religious behavior can be the product of poor health, rather than its cause. In other studies that were examined, the analysts reported that improved physical and mental health functioning was based solely on self-report with no independent assessment; that researchers were not blinded to the data collection process, which can compromise objectivity; and that an analysis of covariates that might explain the relationship between religion and health was omitted (Sloan & Bagiella, 2002).

One study that supported these contentions was a 14-year longitudinal study that carefully controlled for potentially confounding covariates and found that religious activity no longer had predictive value in terms of physical health or psychological well-being (Atchley, 1998).

The research battles wage on, and there is no declared winner as yet on whether religious and spiritual activities improve physical health or extend longevity. In the meantime, perhaps it is reasonable to endorse the idea that health professionals who work with older clients should be sensitive to their religious and spiritual needs and provide the time to listen to, and empathize with, their concerns. In addition, health professionals can strengthen the belief systems of their clients by finding out whether they have access to a pastor, rabbi, or religious study group or, if primarily homebound, they are receiving visits from volunteers at their previously attended church or synagogue.

Also, it should be noted that religious activity may not affect all older adults equally. It may, for instance, be especially important as a source of social support for Black elders. Holding strong religious or spiritual beliefs seems to protect elderly African Americans from contemplating or committing suicide (Cook et al., 2002). Involvement in religious activity correlated with greater self-esteem and personal control in a sample of older Blacks (Krause & Van Tran, 1989). Black caregivers were found to be more likely than White caregivers to use religion as a means of coping (Wykle & Segal, 1991). And the effects of religious consolation or religious comfort are stronger among African Americans than White church members who are faced with adversity (Ferraro & Koch, 1994).

Finally, a national sample of 1,500 older adults, equally divided between Blacks and Whites concluded that "older Black people are more likely than older white people to reap the health-related benefits of religion" (Krause, 2002).

## AGING AND SPIRITUALITY RESOURCES

Health professionals seeking innovative ideas or wanting to identify model programs in the area of spiritual health and the older adult should access *Aging and Spirituality*, published by the American Society on Aging's Forum on Religion, Spirituality, and Aging. To receive a copy, contact the American Society on Aging, 833 Market Street, Suite 512, San Francisco, CA 94103. Another useful publication is the *Journal of Religious Gerontology*, a quarterly publication of the National Interfaith Coalition on Aging, which is affiliated with the National Council on the Aging. Contact NCOA/NICA at the National Council on the Aging, 409 Third Street, SW, Washington, DC 20024-3204.

An argument can be made that Boulder, Colorado, is currently the home base of spirituality and aging. Two organizations in Boulder that focus on this topic are Naropa University and the Spiritual Eldering Institute. Naropa University houses a master's degree program in gerontology that is headed by the well-known gerontologist Robert Atchley. This unique program focuses on infusing administrators (and future administrators) of elder programs and long-term care facilities with the capacity for compassionate care. This gerontology program not only pays attention to the knowledge and skills required to be an effective professional, but also to the student's inner development and their attitude of service toward older adults.

Alongside coursework, gerontology students at Naropa University engage in contemplative practices like meditation and yoga, so that they can be more aware and fully present to the spiritual development of themselves and their older clients. For more information, contact Naropa University in Boulder, Colorado, at 1-800-772-6951, or visit the Web site, www.naropa.edu.

Another innovative organization in Boulder is the Spiritual Eldering Institute. This multifaith organization is focused on the spiritual dimensions of aging and provides a variety of workshops and other educational opportunities on this topic. There is also a training program to produce leadership in spiritual eldering. The founder and president, Rabbi Zalman Schachter-Shalomi, has written a book about his philosophy entitled *From Age-ing to Sage-ing: A Profound New Vision on Growing Older* (Schachter-Salomi, 1995). He also serves on the board of Naropa University's gerontology program, while Robert Atchley serves on the board of the Spiritual Eldering Institute. For more information, contact the Institute at 303-449-SAGE, or www.spiritualeldering.org.

One final comment for the reader about the spiritual aspects of aging: consider reading *Still Here: Aging, Changing and Dying* by Ram Dass (2000). Ram Dass, well-known spiritual leader and former Harvard professor, suffered a crippling stroke while writing this book, and the septuagenarian managed eloquently to include this experience in his writing. As he notes in his book: "These days I'm the advance scout for the experiences of aging, and I've come . . . to bring good news. The good news is that the spirit is more powerful than the vicissitudes of aging" (Ram Dass, 2000, p. 204).

## CAREGIVING, SEXUALITY, AND OTHER TYPES OF INTIMATE SUPPORT

Caregiving for an older adult often has a negative impact on health, personal freedom, employment, privacy, finances, and social relationships (Hooyman & Kiyak, 1999). And yet even this onerous task has its intimate qualities. One study of older caregivers reported that more than 70% of the caregivers had positive feelings towards at least one aspect of caregiving for an older adult (C. Cohen et al., 2002). Some of the positive aspects included companionship, fulfillment, enjoyment, and the satisfaction of meeting an obligation. In addition, caregivers are typically not isolated in their role. One study reported that 88% of caregivers had social support from others who helped them with their caregiving role (Penrod et al., 1995).

Older adults can share intimate support in many ways other than caregiving. Some older adults, for instance, cherish playing with grandchildren, watching a sunset, feeding ducks by a pond, walking in the woods, and enjoying sexual intimacy. Playing, watching, feeding, and walking, however, are not problematic for most older adults, but sexual intimacy may present a problem.

According to studies by the Duke University Center for the Study of Aging and Human Development, the majority of older couples remain sexually active between the ages of 65 and 75. Sexuality, however, increasingly focuses on warmth, sharing, touching, and intimate communication. As consumers of research, we might find it useful to pay more attention to the studies that report on individual perceptions and experiences, than to those that emphasize physiological parameters and statistical frequencies (Starr, 1985).

In one study of 800 people between the ages of 60 and 91, 36% reported that sex grew better over time, whereas only 25% said it was worse (Starr & Weiner, 1981). The sexuality of some aging Americans, however, can get waylaid by psychological factors, such as depression, guilt, monotony, performance anxiety, and anger. Young and old alike can be hampered by negative cohort attitudes that reveal hostility toward the expression of sexuality in late life.

Physical limitations are yet another cause of sexual dysfunction. Arthritic pains, cardiovascular disorders, respiratory conditions, hormonal imbalances, and neurological disorders can interfere with sexual performance. In addition, various medications can lead to sexual dysfunction (Ebersole & Hess, 1990).

But the most significant cause of sexual inactivity, particularly after age 75, is widowhood or lack of opportunity. This problem is exacerbated in older adults who are not accepting of alternative intimacy practices. Family members might try to expand the options of an older adult by arranging to have a respected health professional prescribe the reading of *The Joy of Sex* (Comfort, 1972), in which the physician-author, Dr. Alex Comfort, presents a wide variety of ideas on sex and intimacy for the open-minded.

A survey conducted by the AARP reported that women aged 45 through 59 are more tolerant about their attitudes toward sex, which should hold them in good stead as they age. These women are much more likely to approve of sex between unmarried partners and to engage in oral sex and masturbation (S. Jacoby, 1999).

Intimacy for older adults, however, is often as simple as touching. The importance of touching was clearly demonstrated to me when a yoga class, which had been enthusiastically received by older adults at senior centers and congregate living facilities (Haber, 1983a; 1986), was presented at 10 nursing homes (Haber, 1988a). After unsuccessful attempts to engage these nursing home residents were made during the first three classes, we decided to begin each class with massage—mostly instructor-to-resident massage (with help from student assistants), but also resident-to-resident and self-massage (see Figure 10.3).

As a consequence of this innovation we witnessed a dramatic increase in—there are no other words that come to mind—*fun and intimacy*. The nursing home residents enthusiastically awaited the remaining classes.

This demonstration of the need for touch and intimacy brought to mind a passage from a book by Ebersole and Hess (1990): "When a group of Boy Scouts completed their performance for (a group of nursing home) residents, (an old woman) beckoned to the scout leader and said, 'Do you suppose I could hug one of those little boys?'"

# TERMINALLY ILL

Initial research efforts reported that not only did peer social support improve quality of life among seriously ill persons in comparison with persons in control groups, but also that survival rates improved as well (Fawzy et al., 1995; Spiegel et al., 1989). Subsequent research has not in general supported these findings (Spiegel, 2001). Peer support groups, for instance, did not prolong survival in women with metastatic breast cancer, but it did improve mood and the perception of pain (P. Goodwin et al., 2001).

David Spiegel is the physician whose initial research on peer support had caused the stir about prolonging survival rates (Spiegel et al., 1989). In response to the current wave of research studies that are less supportive of a survival extension benefit, he reminds us that in addition to the research question not being definitely answered, there is consistent evidence of a mental health benefit. As he aptly states, "Curing cancer may not be a question of mind over matter, but mind does matter" (Spiegel, 2001, page 1768).

## HOSPICE SUPPORT

The philosopher Woody Allen once said, "I don't mind dying. I just don't want to be there when it happens." This sentiment may be shared

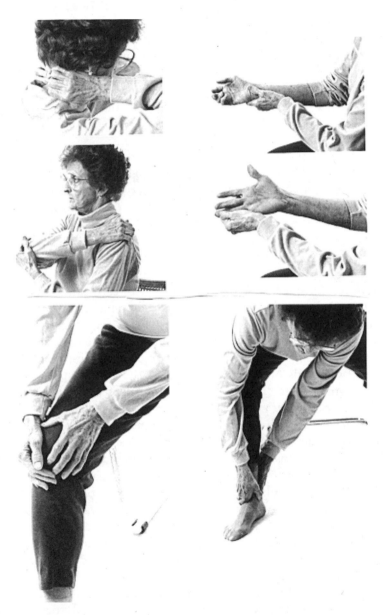

FIGURE 10.3  Massage *(Easy Does It Yoga)*.

by many Americans. For those who *are* willing to be there and who want an open acknowledgement of the experience surrounded by family, friends, and compassionate caregivers, there is hospice.

St. Christopher's Hospice, near London, was established in 1967 by the physician Cicely Saunders, who wrote about her experiences launching a hospice (Saunders, 1977). The St. Christopher's Hospice prototype was an independent institution that provided inpatient care for dying patients. The first American hospice, Connecticut Hospice in New Haven, was founded a few years later in 1974 and modeled after the London exemplar.

The growth of the hospice movement since then has been tremendous. By 1990 the number of hospice programs in America had increased to 1,800; the number of terminally ill persons served, to 210,000. Six years later, in 1996, the number of hospice programs increased to 3,000, and the number of clients served almost doubled—to 400,000. In 1999, more than 500,000 patients used hospice care, most of them older people on Medicare.

Hospice programs have also expanded their service sites, providing not only inpatient care but care in private homes, nursing homes, and other settings. Hospice has evolved into a type of care, rather than the site of care. Its distinguishing characteristic is the emphasis on psychosocial and spiritual support over medical procedures. By focusing on psychosocial and spiritual support, hospice attempts to improve the mental health and quality of life of clients, even as their physical bodies deteriorate.

About two thirds of America's dying, or 1.3 million persons, die in hospitals compared to the 15% who die in hospice settings. There are several barriers to why more persons do not receive hospice care. First, many physicians are still reluctant to refer patients to hospice, seeing it as an admission of defeat. Many family members also see it in the same negative way. Second, most insurance companies including Medicare require that the physician certify that the patient has less than 6 months to live. The problem is that only late-stage cancer tends to be that predictable. Emphysema, congestive heart failure, Parkinson's disease, and other conditions are not that predictable. Third, minority older adults are less likely to use hospice services due to fewer minority staff and volunteers, less trust of the health care system, and cultural beliefs that discourage the use of hospice care (Haber, 1999).

Finally, a major difficulty facing hospice clients and their families in the future may be the lack of a sufficient number of social support providers, especially for clients who choose to stay at home. Seventy-three percent of hospice clients are over the age of 65 and 83% are living in a private residence (Haupt, 1997). Their spouses and their adult children are often elderly themselves and physically unable to bear the exhausting burden of supporting the terminally ill in conjunction with hospice support. It is problematic whether we will be able to find sufficient numbers of volunteers to help meet the additional support needs of the terminally ill elderly that hospice does not provide.

Inadequate social support not only prevents some older adults from participating in hospice, but it may also characterize those who die in a hospital setting. Dying in a hospital largely means dying by oneself. According to one hospital study that used video cameras taped to patient doorways, seriously ill hospital patients were spending 75% of their day alone. Patients received an average of only 321 minutes a day of visits from hospital staff and family members combined (Sulmasy & Rahn, 2001).

Since 1983, Medicare has covered hospice care provided by Medicare-approved agencies or facilities for terminally ill older persons who elect it in lieu of standard hospital treatment. Most private health insurance plans and some state Medicaid programs also pay for hospice care. For more information on hospice, including where to locate the one closest to you, contact the National Hospice Organization, 1700 Diagonal Road, Suite 625, Alexandria, VA 22314, 800-658-8898. Other good sources of hospice information are the National Hospice Foundation (www.hospiceinfo.org) and the Hospice Foundation of America (www.hospicefoundation.org).

# PEER SUPPORT

Growing older presents the challenge, for many people, of coping with chronic conditions—either their own or those of loved ones. A significant number of these people are discovering the rewards of belonging to a peer support group. Such groups unite people with common concerns so that they can share their ideas and feelings, exchange practical information, and benefit from knowing they are not alone. In short, they attempt to help members learn to live as fully as possible despite the limitations that accrue with age.

A peer support group can be organized around a health-promoting theme (e.g., weight reduction, exercise, alcohol restraint, or smoking cessation), or it can exist to cope with almost any chronic health condition—Alzheimer's, Parkinson's, cancer, arthritis, heart disease, lung disease, stroke, hearing or visual impairment, and others. It appears that support seeking is a higher priority for persons with stigmatizing illnesses such as alcoholism, breast cancer, and depression, than it is for less stigmatizing conditions like heart disease (Davison et al., 2000). Other peer support groups are organized around specific activities like caregiving, or life cycle events like widowhood.

Besides the obvious mental health focus of group activities, group members—even if organized around a specific disease—typically exchange health-promoting ideas on nutrition, exercise, stress management, smoking cessation, and moderating alcohol patterns.

Peer support groups have certain commonalties: most operate informally, meet regularly, and do not charge fees. Most distribute leadership responsibilities among their peer members, and many involve health professionals in a significant way. Peer support groups, however, can differ widely in the way they operate. Most Alzheimer's groups, for example, focus primarily on the emotional needs of caregiving members. Other groups may emphasize education, while others focus on health advocacy in the legislative arena. Some groups meet in an institutional setting with strong professional leadership that differs markedly from groups that meet in a home or church and do not include professional involvement.

Regardless of how they operate, research suggests that peer support groups benefit most members (Lieberman & Borman, 1979). This research focus may be selective, however, in that good groups may draw researchers to them. I have personally visited groups that appeared to me to be effective, but also those that appeared to be ineffective. An example of an ineffective group that I attended is when the peer leader made inappropriate comments regarding medical care and about what constitutes good coping practices.

By any standard, the self-help group movement is a phenomenon to be reckoned with. By 1979, there was an estimated 15 million participants in 500,000 different groups, and the growth has been steady since then. In 1983, based on a probability sample of over 3,000 households, self-help groups were the number one source of assistance to persons with mental health problems. More individuals participated in self-help groups (5.8%) than sought help from mental health professionals (5.6%) or consulted with clergy or pastoral sources (5%) (Mellinger & Balter, 1983).

Fitzhugh Mullan, former director of the Bureau of Health Professions and a physician, suggests to newly diagnosed patients "instead of simply going to that white-coated doctor and medical establishment (go) to people who have already 'been there' in some way . . . people who have already had the condition, or who are coping with it" (1992).

## EMPOWERMENT THEORIES

There are a wide variety of untested theories on how peer support empowers its participants. One way is through the "helper" principle: helping others brings mental health benefits upon oneself (Wheeler et al., 1998). Another way is through modeling behaviors: giving encouragement and advice to others may help us clarify our ideas and become increasingly conscientious about our own health behaviors. Yet another way that peer support groups may empower is through the exchange of information about community resources, assistance with transportation needs, and encouragement to be assertive with health care professionals and within the health care system.

Support group members may also empower each other by validating their feelings in a sympathetic environment and developing new behaviors, attitudes, and identities. Support group members with medical disabilities, for example, may view outsiders as "temporarily able-bodied" or as potential victims of future disabilities, thereby enhancing their personal capacity for accepting adversity.

The peer support group may also empower its members by providing them opportunities to participate voluntarily in group advocacy activities, to share leadership functions, and to work for causes that are larger than themselves. For example, one support group in New York City, Friends and Relatives of the Institutionalized Aged, blocked the New York State Health Department's attempt to relax standards for nursing home care, and pressured the New York State Department of Social Services into revising regulations to allow more residents access to nursing home beds following hospitalization.

Another example of advocacy in peer support groups was initiated by a member of the Self-Help Group for the Hard of Hearing in Omaha, Nebraska. One older man expressed frustration with a recalcitrant hearing aid provider who refused to stand behind his promise of "satisfaction guaranteed." The subsequent threat of picketing this provider's establishment by a dozen support group peers quickly led to the successful resolution of the hearing aid consumer's problem.

## AGE-RELATED PEER SUPPORT GROUPS

Evidence indicates that peer support groups may be especially appropriate for aging persons who need chronic care and their caregivers. Age-related peer support groups may prosper because of the declining ability to depend on younger family support persons. Declining birth rates beginning with the baby boom generation mean that fewer children and grandchildren are available to serve as support persons. Job mobility, retirement relocation, and neighborhood growth and renewal result in the dispersion of family, friends, and neighbors. And an increasing percentage of women—who constitute most of the 13 million caregivers in America—who enter the workforce reduces the number of caregiving hours available to frail older adults.

Butler and colleagues (1998) also noted that older persons tended to be reluctant to seek help from mental health professionals due to a perceived stigma and a distaste for large, impersonal, and highly bureaucratic organizational structures. Conversely, some mental health professionals perceive mental health problems as irreversible in old age, and are less enthusiastic about treating older adults.

In response to these societal factors, I have built a peer support group component into most of my research and demonstration grants that focus on health promotion, health education, and caregiving training programs for older adults. Some participants in these peer support groups continued to provide social support and practical assistance to each other for years after the funded project—and the participation of health professionals—was terminated (Haber, 1983b, 1984, 1986, 1989, 1992a; Haber & Lacy, 1993).

One health education class, for instance, continued to meet a decade later as a monthly peer support group. A member of the group sent me the letter that appears in Figure 10.4.

Peer support groups may be especially important for the mental health of widowed older persons. Studies have reported that widows in support groups adjust better to bereavement and undergo reductions in their depression, anxiety, social maladjustment, somatic symptoms, alcohol use, psychotropic medications, and time needed to recover former activities and develop new relationships (Constantino, 1988; M. Lieberman & Videka-Sherman, 1986; Vachon et al., 1980), compared to widows who do not utilize support groups. The impact of self-help groups is comparable to that of psychotherapy intervention with bereaved older adults (Marmar et al., 1988). Lieberman and Borman (1979) also noted that support groups for older widows may be underutilized. Although half the widows in the general population were over age 60, widows over age 60 represented only 20% of those who joined widowhood support groups nationwide.

Older adults, however, may prefer the comfort of one-to-one peer support to that of group support. AARP's Widowed Persons Service, for example, has served thousands of persons who were widowed, through

April 1

Dear David,

    You might already know - but the outgrowth of your classes is a continuation of socialization among nearly 20 persons. The "Prime Timers" are going strong - we meet once a month.
    We are never at a loss for agenda! April 24, we will meet at Kountz Memorial Church for Fred Aliano's famous spaghetti, and a relaxation tape to improve our mental health.
    Everyone sends love and we miss you. From your friends....

*Jackie Devaney,*
*secretary for the day*

**FIGURE 10.4**   Dear Dr. Haber letter.

this type of one-to-one peer support program. For more information, contact the Widowed Persons Service, American Association of Retired Persons, Program Department, 601 E Street, NW, Washington, DC 20049; or go to griefandloss@aarp.org.

## HEALTH PROFESSIONALS AND PEER SUPPORT

In its early years, the peer support movement met with resistance from many health professionals. The groups were labeled nonprofessional or antiprofessional and were accused of potentially causing harm by "practicing medicine without a license." Although these attitudes have subsided—indeed, many professionals now initiate or are actively involved in self-help groups—they have not disappeared altogether.

Peer support groups are best labeled as nonprofessional, as are most family members who comprise them. Although nonprofessional, peer support groups are rarely antiprofessional. The role of the groups is to complement the services of health professionals. A few self-helpers may rail against professionals, but the overwhelming majority do not. Self-help group members are just as likely as those who do not join self-help groups to seek, or to encourage other people to seek, professional assistance (Lieberman & Borman, 1979).

Peer support group members may help health professionals by meeting existing service gaps, uncovering new knowledge, providing the ongoing social and emotional support that health professionals cannot provide, and helping to identify individuals who need a referral to a health professional. Health professionals may aid peer support groups by improving their effectiveness through training in facilitation skills, providing current research knowledge or resource materials, providing feedback through evaluation studies, and making referrals to existing support groups or starting new groups or peer pairings (Haber, 1989).

Many health science students come into contact with mutual help groups during their educational process. Students who visit a single group, though, need to be concerned about whether they are adequately informed about groups in general. Groups differ in the unique personalities of their members, how they are run, where they are located, and so forth. What can health professionals do to educate themselves about peer support groups? 1. Visit different types of groups, especially those that represent problems that are typical of their clientele. Most groups welcome observers who want to educate themselves. 2. Volunteer to make presentations to some of these groups, allowing plenty of time for questions. 3. Refer clients to these groups, and get feedback from them on the groups' effectiveness. 4. Start a specific group if none exist currently, or arrange for peer support between two patients.

## PEER SUPPORT ORGANIZATIONS

If you cannot locate the nearest local Area Agency on Aging (because "area agency on aging" is typically not part of the name of a local organization) in order to identify peer support groups in your community, contact the National Association of Area Agencies on Aging, at 202-96-8130 to obtain the address of a local area agency on aging. Professional associations relating to cancer, arthritis, and a number of other medical conditions are another source of information on local peer support groups (see national professional associations in chapter 12 on Community).

One such professional association is the Arthritis Foundation, for people with arthritis and their family members who wish to meet with peers for mutual assistance in satisfying common needs and overcoming common problems. Knowledgeable professionals are readily available to assist lay leaders who have been trained to be positive role models. Generally, groups meet monthly with sessions that include films, lectures, panel presentations, or group discussions. For individuals who prefer one-to-one support over group support, PALS, or volunteers from local Arthritis Foundations, will call or visit. For additional information on support options, as well as other activities and location of local groups, contact the Arthritis Foundation, P.O. Box 19000, Atlanta, GA 30326, or call 800-283-7800.

Some older adults may be more willing to seek counseling support from their peers than with professional counselors. Peer counseling is affordable and can provide positive role models for older adults. Santa Monica's Senior Health and Peer Counseling program is a model training and service program that has been replicated at sites throughout California. Since its establishment in 1978, many volunteer counselors aged 55 and over have been trained to provide counseling service to their peers. For more information, contact Senior Health and Peer Counseling Center, Director of Community Relations, 2125 Arizona Avenue, Santa Monica CA 90404-1398; or call (310) 828-1243.

VIEWS (Volunteers Involved for the Emotional Well-being of Seniors), another model peer counseling program, provides training to older peers to prepare them to conduct home visits to elders in need and provide additional counseling by telephone. In addition to one-to-one counseling, there are a half dozen peer-led groups. For more information, contact Cascadia Behavioral Health Care, Mt. Hood Community Mental Health Center, 400 NE 7th Avenue, Gresham, OR 97030; or call Judy Strand at 503-661-5455.

## INTERGENERATIONAL SUPPORT

Though older adults and children are not age peers, they are peers in the sense of being mostly outside the full-time employment phase of the life cycle. The Foster Grandparent Program is a national program that trains volunteers aged 60 and over to serve 20 hours a week with children in hospitals, shelters, and special-care facilities. Low-income volunteers receive a small stipend. For more information, contact the Foster Grandparent Program, ACTION, 1100 Vermont Avenue, NW, Washington, DC 20525.

The Off Our Rockers program is a model program that I visited and was very impressed with. It trains volunteers aged 50 and over to visit for 1-hour with kindergarten through third-grade students in the Dallas area schools (see Figure 10.5). For more information, contact Suzanna Swanson, Senior Citizens of Greater Dallas, 1215 Skiles Street, Dallas, Texas 75204, 214-823-5700.

For information and ideas on intergenerational programs and projects, order a free copy of the Intergenerational Projects Idea Book from AARP Fulfillment, 601 E Street, NW, Washington, DC 20049, and request stock #D15087.

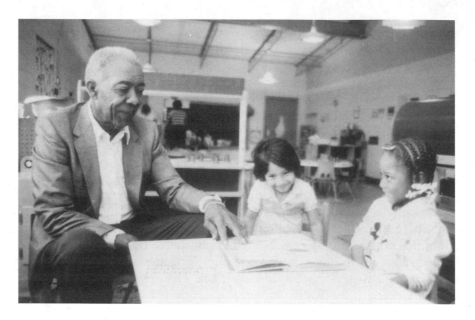

FIGURE 10.5   Off Our Rockers.

## PHYSICIAN SUPPORT

Nearly 80% of the American population visits their physician at least once a year. And older adults visit or consult with a physician more than any other age group—about 13 times during the preceding year (Federal Interagency Forum on Aging-Related Statistics, 2000). Because of their unusual degree of access to the older adult population, and the fact that 85% of adults say a doctor's recommendation would motivate them to get more involved in positive health practices (L. Harris et al. 1989), physicians are in a unique position to occupy a key role in promoting the health of older patients.

The physicians' potential for providing social support to older patients and helping them change their health behavior, however, is not being realized (Haber, 1993b; Maheux et al., 1989; Wechsler et al., 1996; F. Wheeler et al., 1989). A national survey of 2,250 primary care physicians revealed several barriers to counseling patients on health topics, including the lack of time, training, teaching materials, knowledge, and reimbursement (Kearney, 1998a; Kushner, 1995). With older patients, physicians are even less likely to discuss changing a health behavior habit than they are with younger patients (E. Callahan et al., 2000).

The Council of Scientific Affairs of the American Medical Association (*Journal of the American Medical Association*, 1990) has concluded that although physicians are well situated to play a leadership role in health promotion, they either do not act on these opportunities or are ineffectual in their daily practice. The council has suggested, therefore, that physician involvement with patient education should be embedded in a cost-effective framework "by using allied health personnel and providing advice in small-group settings to reduce per capita costs" (USPSTF, 1996). Two research projects supported the idea that physician counseling to change the health behaviors of older patients is likely to be more effective if supplemented by cost-effective health educators or other staff persons (Calfas et al., 1996; M. Goldstein et al., 1999).

Using physician health prescriptions or referral forms, I have involved physicians with my health science students and practitioners-in-training to perform this type of supportive health education role. The physician-health educator partnership has consistently led to positive health behavior change on the part of older patients (Haber, 2001b; Haber et al., 2000, 1997; Haber & Lacy, 1993).

## QUESTIONS FOR DISCUSSION

1. What is the difference between social support and social network? How are they similar?
2. Robert Putnam has argued that there is more social isolation in America today than in generations past. What is your opinion about this assertion, and on what is it based?
3. What are the major advantages and disadvantages of online social support for older adults?
4. If you have not already done so, visit two different peer support groups. Describe your experience in neutral terms to an older adult who has never attended a peer support group. What is the older adult's opinion of such a group and does it agree with your own?
5. Think about an older adult you know—a family member, friend, client—who could benefit from a strengthened social support network. What new sources of social support could be relevant to this person? How could you effectively communicate these suggestions to this person?
6. Do you think it is likely that in 10 or 15 years the majority of Americans will die with hospice support? What would it take for this to happen?

7. What are three reasons that a nursing home administrator might offer in resistance to the idea of converting his home into an Eden Alternative? How would you address each of these barriers and help change the mind of this administrator?

8. Do you believe that health professionals should concern themselves with the religious beliefs and practices of clients? If so, to what extent and how? If not, why?

9. Are you undecided on whether religious activity promotes physical health and extends longevity? Or do you think the research findings, as presented in this chapter, are persuasive in one direction or the other? Support your answer.

10. What is the single most significant barrier to sexual activity among older adults?

11. The anecdote on the importance of touch should probably have included a cautionary note: what would that be?

# 11

# Mental Health

*This life is only a test. If this were an actual life, you would have been given better instructions.*

—*Myrna Neims*

Of course, if it does turn out that this is our actual life, it is not surprising that, given the lack of instructions, maintaining mental health can be such a challenge.

## MENTAL HEALTH AND MENTAL ILLNESS

Mental health is a multifaceted concept and difficult to define. It may include such ideas and terms as life satisfaction, the statistically normal, the ability to cope, positive functioning, seeking meaning and purpose, self-actualization, and so forth. If mental health is defined as life satisfaction, researchers consistently report that the vast majority (about 85%) of older adults are satisfied with their lives, and that older adults are at least as satisfied with their lives as middle-aged and younger adults (George, 1986).

Moreover, neither the average 50% reduction in income at retirement, nor the increases in emotional losses, physical losses, and caregiving responsibilities in later life, result in the persistent reduction in life satisfaction among most older adults. As sociologist Linda George (1986) notes, "Older adults are apparently masters of the art of lowering aspirations to meet realities" (p. 7).

Although we need to acknowledge the mental health resiliency of older adults, we should also attach importance to the 15% to 20% of older adults who contend with mental disorders. A review of the mental health literature in the clinical and research arenas, in fact, leads one to believe that we pay a disproportionate amount of attention to mental disorders. In addition to the greater attention paid to mental illness than to mental health, there is greater scientific precision associated with it. Operational definitions of mental illnesses usually follow the specific criteria of the American Psychiatric Association's *Diagnostic and Statistical Manual of Mental Disorders* (DSM-IV, 1994). Clinicians and researchers refer to these guidelines or state how they are deviating from them.

This chapter reflects a combination of the two perspectives. As is true of most of the literature on mental health, I have organized chapter subheadings largely around mental illness terms. But I have also attempted to focus at least as much attention on mental health content as on mental illness. Thus, in addition to examining a topic like depression, I explore life reviews; and in addition to examining Alzheimer's disease, I explore cognitive fitness. Additional mental health content is provided in other chapters, like social support in chapter 10 and community involvement in chapter 12.

Finally, I want to note that a primary source of material on the mental disorders component of this chapter was obtained from chapter 5 in the Surgeon General's Report on Mental Health. The Surgeon General's report can be accessed through the Web site www.surgeongeneral.gov.

# DEPRESSION

The most likely causes of depression in later life are the emotional losses of a spouse or family support, chronic medical conditions and pain, loss of functional independence, and difficulty adapting to changing circumstances within the home, family, or living situation (Lantz, 2002). These emotional and physical losses not only can lead to depression, but depression in turn can lead to more physical decline (Penninx et al., 1998a).

Though the mechanism is not understood, depression increases the likelihood of mortality from cancer (Penninx et al., 1998b) and heart disease (Frasure-Smith et al., 1995). The mortality rate for depressed patients with cardiovascular disease is twice that of those without depression (Lantz, 2002). Even mild depression can weaken the immune system in older persons if it goes on long enough (McGuire et al., 2002).

Depression also plays a significant role in suicidal behaviors, and older persons have the highest suicide rate of any age group. Older adults account for 25% of all suicide deaths, though they make up only about 13% of the general population. This elevated suicide rate, however, is largely accounted for by White men aged 85 and older. The suicide rate of this age/gender category is 6 times higher than the overall national rate (CDC, 1999).

Depression in older adults often goes undetected until it is too late. Between 63% (Rabins, 1996) and 90% (Katon et al., 1992) of depressed older patients go untreated or receive inadequate treatment. One retrospective study of older adults who had committed suicide revealed that 51 of the 97 patients studied had seen their primary care physician within 1 month of their suicide date. Of these 51, only 19 were even offered treatment, and only 2 of the 51 patients studied were provided adequate treatment (Caine et al., 1996).

A substantial proportion of depressed older patients receive inadequate treatment from physicians in primary care settings. And yet, according to the Surgeon General's Report, up to 37% of older adults in the primary care setting (and between 8% and 20% in the community) suffer from depressive symptoms. These figures are higher than those reported elsewhere (see chapter 3 on Clinical Preventive Services), and some of this discrepancy may have to do with the definition of major depressive disorder versus depressive symptoms of lesser scope or intensity.

Older adults are *less* likely than younger adults to report feelings of dysphoria (sadness, unhappiness, or irritability), which is part of the standard criteria for depression (Gallo et al., 1994) by the *Diagnostic and Statistical Manual of Mental Disorders* (DSM-IV, 1994). Older adults are more likely to report some depressive symptoms—such as the loss of interest or pleasure in activities, weight change, sleep disturbance, agitation or fatigue, feelings of worthlessness, loss of concentration and recurrent thoughts of death or suicide—but not the scope or intensity of symptoms that qualifies them for a full-fledged major depression. And although these reported symptoms, also referred to as mild depression, are not yet recognized by DSM-IV, they nonetheless are a major clinical concern for older adults and interfere with their performance of social roles and quality of life (George, 1993).

Barry Lebowitz (1995) of the National Institute of Mental Health estimated that 15% of Americans aged 65 and over suffered from serious and persistent symptoms of depression, but only 3% were reported to be suffering from the clinical diagnosis of major depression as defined by the DSM-IV. In other words, though depressive disorders that fulfill rigorous diagnostic criteria are relatively rare, subthreshold disorders are considerably more common, infrequently diagnosed or treated with prescribed antidepressants, and because they usually go untreated, are likely to become chronic conditions (Beekman et al., 2002).

Detection of depression is hampered not only by the underreporting of symptoms by older patients, but by biases on the part of physicians and family members. In one study, 75% of physicians thought that depression was understandable in older persons, that is, a normal facet of old age (Gallo et al., 1999). Family members may also view the signs and symptoms of depression as "normal aging," when in fact the persistence of depressive symptoms is not normal.

## TREATMENTS FOR DEPRESSION

There are many modalities for the treatment of depression among older adults, including medication, cognitive-behavioral therapy, physical exercise, social support and pet therapy to reduce isolation, and bereavement and other forms of counseling.

The treatment of depression by medication is effective for up to 80% of older adults (NIH, 1992; L. Schneider, 1996), a rate that is comparable to younger adults. Older adults had more frequent and serious adverse reactions than younger adults did to the earlier generation of tricyclic antidepressants (Alexopoulos & Salzman, 1998). The newer generation of antidepressants, selective serotonin reuptake inhibitors (SSRIs), have produced fewer side effects among older adults (Small & Salzman, 1998). Moreover, combining SSRIs with cognitive-behavioral therapy appears to be superior to either treatment modality by itself (Keller et al., 2000).

Cognitive-behavioral therapy is designed to modify thoughts, improve skills, and alter emotional states that contribute to mental disorders. In a 2-year follow-up study of cognitive-behavioral therapy, 70% of formerly depressed older patients no longer met the criteria for major depression and maintained treatment gains (Gallagher-Thompson et al., 1990). A study of group cognitive therapy found this treatment to be more effective with older depressed patients than those who were randomly assigned to medication alone or to the placebo control group (Beutler et al., 1987).

Because depression is a relapsing disease and maintenance antidepressant medication often reduces the rate of relapse, it is of interest to find out if cognitive therapy can prevent relapse as well. One study applied cognitive therapy over a 2-year period, and depression relapse was significantly reduced (Jarrett et al., 2001).

Another technique, problem-solving social skills, was taught to depressed older persons and significantly reduced symptoms of major depression (Arean et al., 1993). One study employing problem-solving therapy reported that it was as effective as antidepressant medication, with over 50% of patients in both groups recovering from depression (Mynors-Wallis et al., 1995).

Interpersonal psychotherapy, which focuses on grief, role disputes, role transitions, and interpersonal failings, also has been effective in the treatment of depression of older adults (Pasternak et al., 1997; C. Reynolds et al., 1994; Schneider, 1995). Psychodynamic therapy, which focuses on the mourning of lost capacities, promoting acceptance of losses, and addressing fears of dependency, has been successful with older depressed patients as well (Gallagher-Thompson et al., 1990; L. Lazarus & Sadavoy, 1996).

As noted in chapter 5 on Exercise, physical activity, aerobics, and weight lifting can be effective treatments for depression, or reduce the risk of becoming depressed, among older adults (Blumenthal et al., 1999; Lawlor & Hopker, 2001; Singh et al., 2001; Strawbridge et al., 2002). And the most common form of physical activity in these studies—walking—reveals that neither high intensity exercise nor elaborate equipment is necessary for significant results.

Many of these interventions are nonmedical in nature, and a national survey reported that between 1957 and 1996, Americans increasingly relied on nonmedical mental health interventions for mental health problems. Individuals relied more on informal social supports (chapter 10), exercise (chapter 5), and psychosocial treatments rather than their primary care physicians for their mental health concerns (Swindle et al., 2000).

## THE LIFE REVIEW PROCESS

A life review refers to an autobiographical effort that can be preserved in print, by tape recording, or on videotape. The review can be stimulated by memories, a family album, a scrapbook, other memorabilia, a genealogy, or a trek back to an important place in one's past. It can be conducted by oneself, in a dyad, or as part of a group process. A life review is more likely to be conducted by or with an older adult who is relatively content with his or her life and not seeking therapy than it is to be used therapeutically with an older adult. Nonetheless, life reviews are believed to have therapeutic powers.

The psychiatrist Robert Butler first extolled the benefits of the life review process to his colleagues and the public as early as 1961, as a way of incorporating reminiscence in the aged as part of a normal aging process. Dr. Butler described the life review as more comprehensive than reminiscence, and perhaps more important in old age when there may be a need to put one's life in order and to come to an acceptance of present circumstances (Butler, 1995).

The review of, and reflection upon, positive and negative past life experiences by older adults has enabled them to overcome feelings of depression and despair (Butler et al., 1991; Butler, 1974). Another study of the life review process reported positive outcomes in terms of stronger life satisfaction, psychological well-being, self-esteem, and less depression (Haight et al., 1998).

Although life reviews are usually helpful for improving the mental health of most older adults who are seeking meaning, resolution, reconciliation, direction, and atonement, health professionals find it is too time-consuming to listen to the reminiscences of older clients in this era of managed care. Health professionals can, however, provide a key role in referring older clients to appropriate forums or helping them obtain relevant life review materials. One book by the psychologist James Birren and colleagues (1996) helps guide and provide structure for the life review process by suggesting a focus on several themes, such as love, money, work, and family. Birren also suggests supplementing life reviews with small-group discussion in order to help in the retrieval of memories as well as with the acceptance of memories (Birren & Cochran, 2001).

With careful monitoring, Birren noted that in his years of experience he has not had a group member report having become depressed as a result of a life review (Birren & Deutchman, 1991). He warned, however, that persons who are already depressed or otherwise needing therapy should be under the supervision of a qualified professional.

# ALZHEIMER'S DISEASE

There are no biological markers for Alzheimer's disease, except to examine by biopsy or autopsy the neurofibrillary tangles inside cells and the neuritic plaques deposited outside cells. Thus, it is a disease that is difficult to diagnose. One researcher reported that only 3% of patients with mild cognitive impairment were identified as early Alzheimer's disease by general practitioners, and only 24% of those with moderate dementia (D. Callahan et al., 1995). Identification of Alzheimer's disease becomes easier over time. The duration of this illness, from onset of symptoms to death, averages 8 to 10 years.

The most common symptom in early Alzheimer's disease and other types of dementia is diminished short-term memory. Word-finding becomes difficult and may be accompanied by personality changes, emotional lability, and poor judgment (Beers & Berkow, 2000). As persons progress to intermediate dementia, their ability to dress, bathe, toilet, and perform other activities of daily living becomes impaired. Persons with severe dementia are totally dependent on others, and the ability to recognize even close family members may be lost.

Alzheimer's disease is the most common form of dementia affecting older adults, accounting for two thirds of cases. Other types of dementia include vascular dementia, alcohol-associated dementia, infection-related dementia, and so forth. There are also reversible conditions that mimic dementia, such as hypothyroidism, depression, and vitamin $B_{12}$ deficiency.

About 8% to 15% of adults over the age of 65 have Alzheimer's disease (Ritchie & Kildea, 1995), and the prevalence appears to double every 5 years: 1% of persons aged 60–64; 2% of 65–69; 4% of 70–74; 8% of 75–79; 16% of 80–84; and 30% to 45% of those persons age 85 and above (D. Evans et al., 1989; Jorm et al., 1987). In addition to a strong correlation with age, Alzheimer's disease may be correlated with educational level: the higher the level, the lower the susceptibility (Fritsch et al., 2001).

## COGNITIVE FITNESS

K. Warner Schaie (1997) suggests that "use it or lose it" does not apply only to muscles, it applies to our brains as well. He reports that by 80 years of age, virtually everybody has some decline in mental function, but how much you slip in your 60s and 70s depends in part on mental stimulation. A higher level of education or greater engagement with cognitively stimulating activities over the life cycle may delay the onset of mental decline (Del Ser et al., 1999; Friedland et al., 2001; Fritsch et al., 2001; R. Wilson et al., 2002).

The research studies most widely publicized in the popular media on the factors that may delay the effects of Alzheimer's disease were conducted by Snowden and colleagues (2000) and referred to as the Nun Study. The Nun Study has been longitudinal in design and began with the analysis of handwritten autobiographies of 678 Catholic sisters from 7 Notre Dame convents across the country. From a research perspective, these types of religious groups provide the advantage of relatively uniform backgrounds to study and fewer variations in lifestyle to confound the data.

The participating sisters agreed not only to allow researchers access to their autobiographies that had been written before they took their religious vows, but to annual mental and physical examinations, as well as to brain donation after death. The researchers found that lower linguistic ability in terms of ideas and sentence structure (Snowdon et al., 2000) and greater negative emotional content (Danner et al., 2001) in early life writings had a strong association with dementia and premature death in late life.

Another study of 801 older Catholic nuns and priests without dementia at baseline rated their frequency of participation in cognitively stimulating activities. The study results reported that the higher the participation in cognitively stimulating activities, the lower the risk of contracting Alzheimer's disease (R. Wilson et al., 2002).

However, as noted in chapter 3 on Clinical Preventive Services, cause and effect are difficult to identify from population studies that are unable to employ random assignment to treatment and control groups. It is possible, for instance, that some of the persons studied were already in the earliest stage of Alzheimer's disease—before symptoms were detectable—and that this accounted for the association with reduced linguistic ability, the negative emotional content, and the lack of participation in cognitively stimulating activities, rather than the reverse.

In addition, these types of observational studies are still without a good biological explanation as to why increased mental activity may impede the development of Alzheimer's disease.

In addition to the possible association between mental fitness and Alzheimer's disease, there is evidence to support a potential relationship between physical fitness and dementia. Dr. Marilyn Albert of Harvard Medical School and her colleagues (1995) conducted interviews with 1,192 people aged 70 to 79 and concluded that not only mental stimulation—crossword puzzles, reading, and discussion versus passive television entertainment, idle chit-chat, and doing things from rote—may help stave off dementia and memory loss, but physical stimulation may as well. They reported that physical activities may affect the blood flow to the brain and help sustain mental faculties.

Other researchers also report a connection between physical and mental fitness. Psychologist Robert Dustman (1996) reported that after 4 months, sedentary people over age 55 who increased their aerobic capacity also increased their mental acuity. Also, people who have been physically active between the ages of 20 and 60 demonstrated a lower risk for Alzheimer's disease in later life (Friedland et al., 2001).

## COPING ABILITY

Due to the protracted period of decline with Alzheimer's disease, Alzheimer's patients are at risk for abuse by caregivers (Coyne et al.,

1993) and caregivers in turn are at risk for depression, anxiety, and somatic problems (Light & Lebowitz, 1991). Behavioral therapy, which helps caregivers identify, plan, and increase pleasant activities for the patient, improves the mood and depressive symptoms of Alzheimer's caregivers and care recipients alike (Teri et al., 1997; Teri & Gallagher-Thompson, 1991).

A meta-analysis of 18 studies reported that a variety of interventions reduced caregiver burden and dysphoria, including education, support, cognitive-behavioral therapy, and self-help (Knight et al., 1993). Adult day care provides respite for caregivers of persons with dementia and reduces caregiver stress and depression (Zarit et al., 1998). Support for caregivers can delay the institutionalization of patients with dementia by almost a year (Mittelman et al., 1996).

## OTHER MENTAL DISORDERS

Anxiety disorder is associated with at least three of the following symptoms: restlessness or edginess, fatigue, difficulty concentrating, irritability, muscle tension, and sleep disturbance. It is a difficult mental disorder to assess in those who are elderly, and psychological testing is rarely of benefit. The most common anxiety disorders, in order of prevalence, are generalized anxiety disorder, phobia, panic disorder, obsessive-compulsive disorder, and post-traumatic stress disorder (PTSD). PTSD is expected to increase in prevalence among future cohorts of older adults as Vietnam veterans age.

About 11% of adults aged 55 and older meet the criteria for an anxiety disorder (Flint, 1994; Pontillo et al., 2002), and an additional 8% of older adults may have anxiety symptoms that do not fulfill the criteria for a specific anxiety disorder (Himmelfarb & Murrell, 1984). It should be noted, however, that these types of prevalence rates for anxiety disorders vary greatly and have been the source of controversy (Smyer & Qualls, 1999).

Treatment with medications for anxiety disorders tends to be similar between older and younger patients. Benzodiazepines and other anxiety medications, however, are marginally effective in treating chronic anxiety in older patients. For anxiety associated with depression, an antidepressant is often effective. For anxiety associated with mild dementia, a more structured environment may alleviate symptoms. For anxiety associated with bereavement, cognitive behavioral therapy or an exercise program may be of benefit.

Schizophrenia, characterized by delusions, hallucinations, paranoia, disorganized speech, catatonic behavior and affective flattening, can extend into or first appear in later life. Prevalence of schizophrenia among older adults, however, is only 0.6%, about half the rate for the population aged 18 to 54. Pharmacological treatment of schizophrenia in late life is challenging, as the previous generation of antipsychotic medications have had a high risk of persistent and disabling side effects. The newer generation of antipsychotics, like clozapine and risperidone, may be more effective with older adults than the earlier neuroleptics.

Alcohol abuse and misuse of medications are also considered to be in the category of mental disorders, but these two topics are examined in chapter 9 on Other Health Education Topics. A related mental disorder, illicit drug abuse, rarely occurs among older adults, affecting less than 0.1% (Regier et al., 1988).

Finally, there are compulsive behaviors that are being labeled as mental disorders and treated with the new generation of antidepressants, selective serotonin reuptake inhibitors (SSRIs). These behaviors include such activities as gambling addiction, kleptomania, shopping addiction, and social phobia. Some argue that these are legitimate mental disorders that should be treated medically. Others contend that these behaviors are everyday maladies that are escalated into medical problems by drug-company marketing.

With the advent of Prozac, the most popular SSRI, the threshold has been lowered for what constitutes an emotional disorder that needs medication. Prescriptions for the new generation of antidepressants tripled during the 1990s, and sales for these types of drugs are expected to double between the years 2000 and 2005 (Szegedy-Masak, 2001). An increasing percentage of these drugs were directed toward compulsive behaviors.

# INSURANCE COVERAGE

Unequal Medicare coverage is provided for mental illness versus physical illness. Medicare patients pay 50% of Medicare-approved amounts for most outpatient mental health care, but only 20% for other medical services. Medicare also imposes a 190-day lifetime limit on inpatient psychiatric hospital care, but no cap on care in a general hospital. In addition, Medicare carriers automatically flag any claims for Alzheimer's disease as subject to the 50% out-of-pocket policy even when the care warrants 80% coverage. A September 2001 government memorandum to correct this bias against Alzheimer's disease did not seem to be working almost a year later, as noted by one analyst (Aston, 2002).

In addition, Medicare's lack of coverage for outpatient medication is especially troublesome for the treatment of mental illness, given the effectiveness of SSRI drugs and their significantly higher cost due to patent protection. At the same time that older patients are having difficulty affording these medications, the treatment of choice for mental illness has shifted to these outpatient medications. Between 1987 and 1997, for instance, the proportion of depressed individuals who were treated with antidepressant medications increased from 37% to 75%, whereas the proportion that received psychotherapy declined from 71% to 60% (Olfson et al., 2002).

Older Americans account for only 7% of all inpatient mental health services, 6% of community-based mental health services, and 9% of private psychiatric care (Persky, 1998). Clearly there are patient and provider barriers to this care, most notably the mistaken belief that mental health problems such as depression are natural or inevitable conditions of older age. Equally clear is that Medicare's lower reimbursement for mental health conditions is a barrier for older Americans in terms of access to mental health services.

Moreover, the disparity in Medicare reimbursement between physical and mental treatments serves to further the stigma surrounding mental illness in older adults, particularly among older men and minority groups (Unutzer et al., 2003). The disparity also fuels the misperception that mental illness cannot be treated as effectively as physical conditions in older adults. However, as noted by the surgeon general's report on mental health, when properly diagnosed and treated, 65% to 80% of depressed older adults improve with medication, psychotherapy, or a combination of both—a success rate higher than many current common medical treatments for nonpsychiatric illnesses.

# CHRONIC STRESS

Harvard physiologist Walter Cannon coined two terms, *homeostasis* and *fight or flight.* Homeostasis refers to the body's attempt to preserve the constancy of its internal environment. When cold, for instance, the body shivers to generate heat and when hot, sweats to reduce heat.

When a challenge produces fear, homeostasis is disrupted and the organism prepares for flight or fight. Adrenaline is released, and there is an increase in heart rate, respiratory rate, blood pressure, and blood flow to the brain and large muscles of the extremities.

Fight or flight, in response to a physical challenge, prepares the organism to move more quickly, see better, think better, and reduce blood loss. In modern times, however, stress is more likely to be emotional than the reaction to a physical threat. Fighting or running away is often inappropriate. For instance, if we are pressed for time and trapped in big-city traffic, there is nothing to fight and no way to flee. The fight or flight response can be harmful, both physically and emotionally.

Stress research began with Hans Selye. His General Adaptation Syndrome consisted of three stages: a) an alarm reaction, which mobilizes the body's resources, b) a stage of resistance, in which the body tries to adapt to the stressor, and c) a state of exhaustion. The trapped commuter, who can neither fight nor flee, is vulnerable to being in a prolonged state of resistance. This prolonged stress response, which is harmful to health, may produce pathologic changes, including hypertension, heart disease, arthritis, asthma, and peptic ulcers.

Chronic stress contributes to depression and anxiety disorders, and with aging will interfere with normal memory processing (Small, 2002). Several days of exposure to high levels of the stress hormone cortisol leads to memory and learning impairment (Newcomer et al., 1999). Similar results have been obtained with animal studies (Sapolsky, 1999).

## MEASUREMENT

Perhaps the most widely known stress measurement tool is the Social Readjustment Rating Scale (SRRS) developed by Thomas Holmes and Richard Rahe (1967) at the University of Washington School of Medicine. The SRRS ranked 43 life-change events according to a score derived from more than 5,000 interviews over two decades.

Men and women of different socioeconomic status, age, and marital status were asked to assign numeric values higher or lower than an arbitrary score of 50 for marriage. Ten of the top 15 scores related to the family, with death of a spouse receiving the top score of 100. Surprisingly, the ratings of events were consistent across ethnicities (African Americans and Mexican Americans) and countries (Europe and Japan).

Holmes and Rahe (1967) correlated the ratings of life-change events over a 12-month period with health risk. Thirty-seven percent of the individuals who scored under 200 underwent an appreciable change of health, compared to 79% of those who scored over 300.

An interesting facet of the SRRS scale is its validity despite its mechanistic approach to life events. The instrument does not, for instance, determine whether the individual's perception of a life event is stressful or not. Thus, the death of a cantankerous and burdensome spouse may be met with relief, while a codependent spouse may experience hysteria.

Researchers have been looking for ways to make stress-measuring instruments more precise and powerful by weighing individual perceptions of stressful events. Lazarus and colleagues have focused on daily hassles (e.g., weight gain, rising prices, losing things) and have found stronger statistical associations with health outcomes than those obtained by merely counting life events (Lazarus & Folkman, 1984).

Over the past decade it has also become clear that the Holmes and Rahe scale is not responsive to the life events of the later years and that many of the items included are unlikely to occur in late life. About a dozen age-specific scales have been developed since (Chiriboga, 1992).

## PERSPECTIVES

Stress can be viewed from three perspectives. The first perspective is external, focusing on threatening stimuli from the environment. Measuring stress from this perspective may consist of counting stressful events like divorce and widowhood (Holmes & Rahe, 1967), or calculating hassles, such as being stuck in traffic (Lazarus & Folkman, 1984), that have taken place within the previous year.

A second perspective on stress focuses on internal forces, such as our psychological response to stressors. Being stuck in traffic, for instance, can produce anger, anxiety, and frustration. Or we can perceive the traffic delay as an opportunity to converse with our companions or listen to a few additional audiotapes.

The fact that we do not all perceive events in the same way is illustrated by the well-known picture in Figure 11.1. Do you see a young woman or an old woman? Is it difficult to shift your perception between the two?

From the third perspective, stress is viewed as a transactional process, an interaction between forces in the environment and our perception. For example, because we are in a hurry, traffic triggers a stress response. Our anger and frustration then escalate our stress. In this transactional process, however, we can deliberately take a pause from our escalating stress level and choose to do a deep-breathing exercise. Thus, we can attempt neither to fight nor flee but to flow.

## PSYCHONEUROIMMUNOLOGY

Over the past two decades, researchers have found a number of physiological linkages between the nerve cells of the brain and the immune

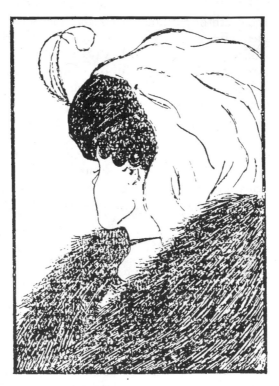

**FIGURE 11.1   What do you see?**

system (Goleman & Gurin, 1993). These nerve cells connect the brain with the spleen and other organs that produce immune system cells. When the brain perceives, for example, a stressful event, immunological changes result, such as a decline in the cells that fight tumors and viral infections.

Unfortunately for stress researchers, many other factors can also suppress immunity, for example, lifestyle habits (alcohol consumption, smoking, nutritional habits, etc.) and the overall status of the immune system. This latter variable is particularly relevant for older adults because the robustness of the immune system declines with age.

One study, which examined the relationship between lifestyle stress and the immune system of older adults, compared 69 older caregivers of spouses with Alzheimer's disease to a matched sample of older adults living in the community. During this 13-month study, the chronic stress of caring for a family member with dementia led to the reduced function of the immune system of the older caregivers, which in turn led to more frequent respiratory tract infections compared to the matched sample in the community (Kiecolt-Glaser et al. 1991).

Another study reported that the brain's perception of mental stress may be a better predictor of future heart problems than physical stress recorded through conventional treadmill testing with heart function measured on an electrocardiogram. Persons who responded adversely to mental stress testing (which included reactions to engaging in public speaking or solving math problems on a deadline) were 2 to 3 times more likely to suffer a heart attack or progressive chest pain in the future (Jiang et al., 1996).

# STRESS MANAGEMENT

Although many Americans report that stress has had some effect on their health, it is less likely to be reported by older adults (about a third) than younger adults (about half) (USDHHS, 1991). Similarly, in response to the broader question of how much stress they feel in their daily life, older adults were less likely to report considerable stress (about half) than younger adults (almost two thirds) (American Board of Family Practice, 1987).

It is possible that older adults manage their stress better than do younger adults, either through managing their perceptions of stress better, more frequent prayer, or the practice of other informal stress-management techniques. One study reported that stress changes with age and that older adults get better at managing it (Almeida et al., 2002). Young adults focus more on tension in relationships; middle-aged adults are over-loaded by demands on them; and older adults primarily face health problems. Almeida and colleagues reported at the American Psychological Association conference, in Chicago in August 2002, that the older adults in their sample reported more stress-free days than middle-aged and younger adults.

It is also possible that older adults are less willing to report stress. They may find it more of a stigma than do younger adults and are reluctant to admit to it. Or they may be less able to recognize it, either due to lack of knowledge about what stress is or because the stress is masked by depression, which older adults are more likely to exhibit symptoms of.

Regardless of age, many adults report a great deal of stress from time to time, and the great majority of them consciously take informal steps to control or reduce it. Only a few, however, try formal stress management techniques. The most popular stress management measures are the informal strategies of physical exercise, psychological denial, and avoidance (H. Taylor & Kagay, 1985).

Regarding exercise, a group of older adults with knee arthritis significantly lowered their depressive symptoms as a consequence of aerobic exercise. The subjects also reduced their disability and pain, and increased their walking speed (Penninx et al., 2002). Another study used a variety of more formal stress management techniques (anger coping, muscle relaxation, deep-breathing, etc.) and individualized them according to the needs and preferences of subjects with high blood pressure. The researchers reported that blood pressure level was reduced through stress management, in comparison to a control group where blood pressure was unchanged (Linden et al., 2001). Another study implemented a group stress management program and reported clinically significant benefits for patients with type II diabetes (Surwit et al., 2002).

An interesting study examined the effects of writing on stressful experiences, and subsequent symptom reduction in patients with asthma or rheumatoid arthritis (Smyth et al., 1999). This randomized trial reported significantly greater symptomatic improvement (lung function and disease activity) in the intervention groups compared with the control groups that wrote about emotionally neutral topics. It is possible that the participants' immune function improved after they unburdened themselves or that they learned ways to cope better with the current stresses in their life after they completed the exercise.

Journal writing is a popular method for stress management and personal growth. For information on techniques and workshops, contact the Center for Journal Therapy at www.journaltherapy.com or call toll-free 888-421-2298; or Dialogue House Associates at www.intensivejournal.org or toll-free 800-221-5844.

## A POSITIVE ATTITUDE

The Harvard Study of Adult Development is a 60-year longitudinal study of 824 persons from adolescence to late life, conducted for the purpose of learning about successful aging (Vaillant, 2002). In addition to looking at privileged men and women from Harvard University and from California, the study examined healthy aging among inner-city men (Vaillant & Western, 2001). The psychiatrist George Vaillant, director of the study, concluded that good mental health with aging involves a capacity for gratitude, forgiveness, and love; a desire to connect with people and replenish social networks; an interest in play and creativity; and a commitment to lifelong learning.

A longitudinal study of 23 years' duration reported that older individuals with more positive self-perceptions of aging lived 7.5 years longer than those with less positive self-perceptions of aging (Levy et al., 2002). This advantage remained after controlling for a number of potentially confounding variables. In other words, a positive perception of aging demonstrated a better survival outcome regardless of whether participants were young-old or old-old, men or women, higher income or lower income, lonely or not, or better or worse off in functional health. This finding was not only robust, but appeared to be a more powerful predictor of longevity than blood pressure level, cholesterol level, smoking, and exercise.

In 1991–1992, the psychologist Leonard Poon of the University of Georgia interviewed about 100 centenarians through the Georgia Centenarian Study and concluded that mental health is more important to survival than the longevity of your parents or what you have eaten over a lifetime. Poon reports that survivors over the age of 100 appear to be optimistic, to be passionately engaged in some activity, and to have the ability to adapt to repeated losses over time.

Alice Day's (1992) interviews of American women in their 70s and 80s uncovered similar qualities among women who were aging successfully: they tended to have a positive attitude, to stay involved, and to foster social support. These factors can even override barriers to physical health and threats to financial well-being.

The epidemiologist Glen Ostir and his colleagues reported that positive affect predicted subsequent functional independence and survival after a major health event among older Mexican Americans (Ostir et al., 2000), and among older Blacks and Whites (Ostir et al., 2002). Scheier and colleagues (1999) reported that optimism predicted a lower rate of rehospitalization after coronary artery bypass graft surgery.

Conversely, negative attitudes like anger, pessimism, and gloomy self-perceptions of aging can lead to a host of unpleasant consequences. A high level of anger is associated with subsequent heart disease (Chang et al., 2002; Williams et al., 2001) and stroke (Williams et al., 2002b; Ostir et al., 2001). A 30-year follow-up study of 723 patients revealed that those with pessimistic personalities had a 19% increased risk of mortality (Maruta et al., 2000). And a 23-year longitudinal study of older adults reported that negative self-perceptions of aging will diminish life expectancy (Levy et al., 2002).

The protective effect of a positive attitude on physical health may work in a variety of ways. Positive emotions can work directly on physiologic homeostasis, or on enhancing a person's social support system, or on stimulating motivation for self-care and adherence to treatment regimens, or on engaging in more social and physical activities that help to maintain the fitness level necessary for higher level functioning (Penninx, 2000).

## THE PLACEBO EFFECT

The placebo effect is often referred to as the power of positive thinking. Placebo is Latin for "I shall please" and refers to a dummy substance or treatment that is designed to look like the real thing. People may respond favorably to a sham substance or treatment if they do not know it is phony and if they think it is a credible attempt at helping them. A placebo, therefore, provides a standard of comparison for evaluating a new drug or intervention, which must then significantly outperform the placebo.

Placebos often produce positive change among a substantial minority of those who take them. Among 183 subjects taking a placebo pill for high blood pressure, for instance, 25% achieved normal blood pressure (Materson et al., 1993). A positive response to a placebo was obtained from 45% of those who were depressed less than a year, and from 23% of those who were more chronically depressed (Khan et al., 1991). The power of the placebo is frequently extolled in health newsletters (e.g., "The power of the placebo effect," 2000; "The surprising power of placebos," 2000).

And then along came two contrarian Danish researchers to dispute the conventional wisdom (see the section on mammograms in chapter 3 on Clinical Preventive Services for another attempt by the same Danish researcher, Gotzsche, who relishes a dispute with conventional wisdom). The two researchers examined 114 studies and concluded that with the exception of subjective outcomes, particularly pain outcomes, there was no such thing as a placebo effect (Hrobjartsson & Gotzsche, 2001). They argued that instead of positive attitudes producing positive physical results, spontaneous remission—which occurs naturally in many diseases—accounts for the placebo effect.

This single study is not the definitive word on the power of the placebo. If it is substantiated, though, there is an upside to debunking the placebo effect, as well as the purported medical advantages in general that are associated with a positive attitude: Those who do not achieve successful medical outcomes do not need to feel guilty about their inability to stimulate the placebo effect.

## THE BOTOX ALTERNATIVE

The Botox (botulinum toxin type A) craze came along in 2002 when the Food and Drug Administration approved use of the drug to smooth out aging faces. Small doses of the toxin are injected into the forehead every few months to temporarily paralyze the injected muscle. The drug is expensive, requires repeated application, may have adverse side effects, and can make one look more zombie-like than youthful, but that has not discouraged the generation that has already accepted hair transplants, hair coloring, breast augmentation, liposuction, nose jobs, and Viagra.

Botox and the cosmetic revolution to keep us looking young were on my mind when I read an essay by Gwenda Blair (2001) called "The Many Faces I See." She wrote about the *matryoshka* doll that comes from Russia: a wooden doll that is hollowed out, with a smaller version of the doll inside, which is also hollowed out with a smaller version inside, and so forth. Ms. Blair wrote about feeling like a matryoshka, with all her earlier *me's* inside and fitted into one another. The rest of the world may only see the wrinkled older woman on the outside, but she knew all the earlier selves still inside her.

Instead of making her external face look younger, Ms. Blair accepted herself as a little girl, a young mother, a middle-aged woman, and an older woman—all rolled into one. Instead of ignoring the old lady with wrinkles and gray hair, she and society can admire the woman who not only knows what it is like to be an old person, but also knows what it is like to be a child, a teenager, a parent, a worker, a mortgage holder, a grandparent, and a retiree.

I have heard strong arguments that mental health can improve with age if those who so choose change their looks to be more youthful in their appearance. I make the opposite argument: that mental health can improve more with age if we accept the appearance of old age and all that goes with it, and feel positive about it. This argument would be strengthened, I admit, if there was more societal support of a new genre of elder images (Schachter-Shalomi, 1995), where positive visions of older adults are portrayed frequently in movies, television, theatre, books, popular lyrics, and the fine arts.

Instead of William Shakespeare's description of old age as "second childishness and mere oblivion/sans teeth, sans eyes, sans taste, sans everything," artists could discover and reinforce the image of old age as one that embodies more than physical diminishment, but wisdom, joyfulness, spirituality, resiliency, and integrity.

Integrity versus despair is the challenge of the last stage of Erik Erikson's theory of development (Erikson et al., 1987). The task of the elder at this stage of existence is to reflect on one's life, to review experiences and accomplishments, and to integrate these memories into the feeling that one has led a meaningful life. Those who accept the aging process and find integrity rather than despair in late life may not only find it personally satisfying, but they may also become positive role models for succeeding generations.

Or, there is always the botox alternative.

# MENTAL HEALTH AND AGING RESOURCES

AARP offers a variety of mental health programs and resources to the general public. Two of their programs are the Reminiscence Program, in which trained volunteers help isolated elders in institutions and community settings regain touch with significant past experiences in order to improve their self-worth; and the Widowed Persons Service, a peer support program of trained volunteers, themselves widowed, who assist the newly widowed to recover from their losses and rebuild their lives. To access these programs, contact AARP, Social Outreach and Support, 601 E Street, NW, Washington, DC 20049.

To find out more about AARP's grief and loss programs, go to the Web site griefandloss@aarp.org. Or call AARP's Grief Support Line at 866-797-2277, which is open to everyone, not just AARP members. AARP's primary booklet for the newly widowed is called *On Being Alone*. Both the English and Spanish versions can be ordered online or by calling 800-424-3410. A list of other AARP mental health resources, including organizations, publications, and audio programs, is available free of charge, from AARP Fulfillment, Mental Health/Wellness/Older Adults Resource List, 601 E Street NW Washington, DC 20049.

To borrow a Reminiscence Video Training Kit (stock number D13403) at no charge, or to obtain a free 11-page booklet on creative uses of life review in a variety of settings (stock number D14930), contact AARP Fulfillment, 601 E Street, NW, Washington, DC 20049.

The National Alliance for the Mentally Ill provides information on mental illness and its treatment, including the publication *Mood Disorders, Depression and Manic Depression*. Referrals are also made to local support groups. Contact the National Alliance for the Mentally Ill, Colonial Place Three, 2107 Wilson Boulevard, Suite 300, Arlington, VA 22201; 800-950-6264.

For additional information on mental illness, access the following two Web sites: the National Institute of Mental Health at www.nimh.nih.gov and the National Mental Health Association, www.nmha.org. The National Institute of Mental Health provides literature and other resources designed for older adults.

Fostering creativity in older adults can also improve their mental health. "There is some degree of creativity in every person, and the [health practitioner's] function is to assist the aged person to recognize and believe in his or her full potential. Products of creativity are less important than fostering a creative attitude. Curiosity, inquisitiveness, wonderment, puzzlement, and craving for understanding are creative attitudes. [It is possible to help older persons] to break free" (Ebersole & Hess, 1990).

To obtain information about the following creative arts therapies or to identify certified therapists near your location, contact the following non-profit organizations: the American Music Therapy Association at 301-589-3300 or www.musictherapy.org; the American Dance Therapy Association at 410-997-4040, or www.adza.org; the American Art Therapy Association at 847-949-6064, or www.arttherapy.org; and the National Association for Poetry Therapy at 202-966-2536, or www.poetrytherapy.org.

A monograph by McMurray (1990) provides a good source of information for sparking creativity in older persons. Ebersole and Hess (1990) refer to several other guides that encourage creative expression in older adults, including art, music, poetry, humor, and self-actualization. Koch's (1977) account describing how he taught poetry to nursing home residents is a particularly enjoyable and useful resource guide. For an assortment of mental health treatment protocols used by nurses in a variety of practice settings, see Kurlowicz (1997).

The National Center for Creative Aging, founded by Susan Perlstein in 2001, is a clearinghouse throughout the United States for information, research, and training on arts and aging. The mission of the center is to promote creative expression and healthy aging. For additional information, go to www.creativeaging.org.

## QUESTIONS FOR DISCUSSION

1. Given the emotional and physical losses that accumulate in late life, why is depression not considered a normal part of the aging process?
2. Find additional reading material on conducting a life review and then conduct a life review with an older adult. What did you learn about the aging process that was most important to you?
3. When research studies reach a more advanced stage of completion, do you expect cognitive stimulation to be an important factor in postponing dementia? Why do you believe that?
4. Aside from research projects, is it ethical to give someone a placebo? Why do you believe that?
5. Do you think continued research will demonstrate that you can manipulate a positive attitude and extend longevity? Or do you

think long-lived people are more likely to have a positive disposition and that this is a trait that cannot be manipulated for the purpose of extending longevity?

6. Do you believe older adults who deny stress in their lives would be better off if they acknowledged their stress? Explain your answer.

7. Do you agree with the assertion that stress is primarily a matter of perception? Why?

8. Is trying to look younger in old age an ageist reaction to a natural process, or can it be an effective way to cope in a youth-oriented society? Explain your answer.

9. Eleanor Roosevelt once said "Beautiful young people are accidents of nature, but beautiful old people are works of art." What do you think she meant by that?

# 12

## Community Health

## COMMUNITY ORGANIZATIONS

Unless they live in remote rural settings, older persons are likely to have a wide array of community-based health-promoting programs, resources, and services available to them. Moreover, neither frailty nor disability automatically prevents older adults from gaining access to them. Programs and services for older adults are housed at religious institutions, senior centers, AARP chapters, hospitals, and other community sites, and they are becoming increasingly responsive to the health needs and limitations of older adults.

A logical place for older persons to begin to locate relevant community health resources is the local Area Agency on Aging (AAA). These agencies are responsible for providing aging information, as well as coordinating the more than 20,000 organizations around the country that provide services for the aging. Unfortunately, the 672 AAAs do not have uniform names and can be difficult to locate in a telephone directory. The National Association of Area Agencies on Aging (927 15th Street, NW, 6th floor, Washington, DC 20005; 202-296-8130) provides current local AAA information through its *Directory of State and Area Agencies on Aging*.

### SENIOR CENTERS

Older adults seek health information more actively than younger adults. A major source of information for about 20% of older adults is the neighborhood senior center. A national survey revealed that every one of the more than 10,000 senior centers around the country provided some type of health education or screening program (Leanse, 1986). In addition, most senior centers provided a combination of general health education seminars, exercise and nutrition classes, self-help groups, self-care programs, or referrals to appropriate health services.

Senior centers exist in almost every community, provide a broad spectrum of health education offerings, and many have good connections with the medical community. More than 80% are linked to physicians, hospitals, or public health departments (Leanse, 1986).

According to one survey, though, health education and health promotion opportunities are not primarily associated by community health practitioners with senior centers (Campanelli, 1990). Community practitioners who were asked where they would locate information on health education or health promotion for older adults identified a wide array of sites, giving no specific emphasis to senior centers. Identified sites included state and local health departments, institutes of higher education, hospitals, public service agencies, and voluntary organizations.

Nevertheless, many of the senior centers around the country are the best place to go to access a wide range of health-promoting activities, and I provide summaries of a few of the innovative senior centers that I visited in Texas. The Maurice Barnett Geriatric Wellness Center offered a wide array of health programs, including health assessments, medical screenings and immunizations, health education, caregiving programs, and support groups. In addition, this senior center was unique in two ways. It identified itself as a comprehensive wellness center to the community, and it provided a leadership role for older adults on its board of directors: Maurice Barnett Geriatric Wellness Center, 401 W. 16th Street, P.O. Box 861492, Plano, TX 75086.

Retirees not only crafted the native stone wall outside of the Comal County Senior Citizens Center, but also disassembled, hand-sanded, and reassembled into squares thousands of inch-long pieces of wood for the parquet tile floor. Retirees continued to make contributions to this senior center, including the operation of a thrift shop that provided considerable revenue for center activities: Comal County Senior Citizens Center, 655 Landa Street, New Braunfels, TX 78130.

The Galveston County Multipurpose Senior Center offered a variety of health programs, including exercise and country-western dance classes. The most innovative aspect of this senior center was an effort to develop leadership among the attending older adults through a senior leadership training program (Grasso & Haber, 1995): Galveston County Multipurpose Senior Center, 2201 Avenue L, Galveston, TX 77550.

## RELIGIOUS INSTITUTIONS

The church, synagogue, or mosque has the potential to be one of the most important sources of health-promoting programs in the country. Congregational members share values, beliefs, traditions, cultural bonds, and the trust and respect that these engender. Among minority groups, religious institutions may be the only community organizations deemed trustworthy of providing health information and social support (R. Davis et al., 1994; S. Thomas et al., 1994; M. Williams, 1996). In addition, religious institutions are able to connect with hard-to-reach older adults, who may be isolated from other sources of health care.

Religious institutions are often called upon to provide a wide array of educational, counseling, and social support services for those persons who are least served by health care institutions: minorities and the poor. It would entail only a small additional step—collaboration with health professionals—for many of these institutions to be able to implement medical screenings and health education programs. Yet the immense potential contribution of religious institutions toward the health promotion of individuals remains substantially untapped (Neighbors et al., 1995; Wind, 1990).

More than 80% of Americans past age 65 claim their religious faith is the most important influence in their lives (Moberg, 1983). Of the 5 million persons aged 65 and over who do unpaid volunteer work, fully 43% perform most of their work at religious organizations. These older volunteers tend to put in more hours per week and more weeks per year than do younger volunteer workers (U.S. Department of Labor, 1989). Many of these older volunteers could be trained to provide health-promoting services to their peers.

Health programs implemented at religious institutions have contributed to the health of congregation members in a variety of ways. These programs, for example, have improved mammography adherence (Duan et al., 2000), reduced hypertension (Smith et al., 1997), increased fruit and vegetable intake (Resnicow et al., 2001), decreased weight (Kumanyika et al., 1992), and produced an array of other physical and mental health benefits (Ransdell, 1995).

Many religious institutions have broadened their mission to include mental health-promoting services. A survey of 2,500 self-help groups, for instance, revealed that 44% of these groups had met in churches or synagogues, more than had met in any other community site (Madara & Peterson, 1986).

Finally, there is the growing role of parish nurses. Typically, parish nurses are members of a congregation who are either volunteers or salaried part-time, and who engage in health screening, health counseling, grief support groups, and community referrals. Though most parish nurses report prior work experience in health settings, one survey reported that only 50% had at least a baccalaureate degree in nursing (McDermott & Burke, 1993). Many parish nurses focus on the relation between faith and health, and their congregational clients are disproportionately over the age of 55.

## THE SHEPHERD'S CENTERS OF AMERICA

The Shepherd's Centers of America is a national association of nonprofit organizations, typically housed in local neighborhood congregations that offer older persons an array of educational courses, services, and resources with a wellness approach. Formed in Kansas City, Missouri, in 1972 by Dr. Elbert Cole, this organization originally consisted of 6 men who delivered hot meals to 7 homebound women. In 2002 the organization had almost 100 centers, with leadership primarily in the hands of older persons. The center reached more than 200,000 persons and provided health education, life enrichment and life review classes, caregiver seminars, bereavement support, exercise and nutrition classes, medical screenings, medication seminars, peer support groups, transportation services, respite care programs, advocacy, and other activities.

The empowerment philosophy of the Shepherd Center is embodied in the saying, "No one should do for older persons what they can do for themselves." For information on how to join or start a program, contact the Shepherd's Centers of America, One W. Armour Boulevard, #201, Kansas City, MO 64111; contact Dr. Elbert Cole at 816-960-2022 or 800-547-7073; or go the Web site www.shepherdcenters.org.

## OTHER NATIONAL RESOURCES WITH A FOCUS ON RELIGION AND AGING

Starting in 1983 as the Interfaith Volunteer Caregivers Program (Haber, 1988b), and continuing in 1993 as the Faith in Action (FIA) program, this Robert Wood Johnson Foundation initiative supports community projects that are designed to expand and support the caregivers of the nation's elders. FIA shares a step-by-step approach to link members of multiple congregations in a specific geographic area into a single association in order to meet specific caregiving needs of older congregation members and others in need. The goal of the project is to enhance the quality of life of older persons in the community who want to avoid premature institutionalization.

With the aid of start-up grants from the Robert Wood Johnson Foundation, along with continued support and advice, about 1,000 interfaith volunteer caregiver programs have been implemented nationwide. To obtain more information, contact Faith in Action, Wake Forest University School of Medicine, Medical Center Boulevard, Winston-Salem, NC, 27157-1204; 877-324-8411 (toll-free); or go to www.fiavolunteers.org.

The Forum on Religion, Spirituality and Aging is a constituent group of the American Society on Aging. The Forum distributes a newsletter, *Aging and Spirituality,* and assists members of this professional organization who want to address their concerns about spirituality and aging. To obtain more information, contact the American Society on Aging, 833 Market Street, #511, San Francisco, CA 94103-1824; 415-974-9600; or www.asaging.org.

## WORKSITE WELLNESS

In 1987, in Omaha, Nebraska, the Wellness Councils of America (WELCOA) was founded for the purpose of developing community-based wellness councils to encourage health promotion activities at the worksite. The growth of these councils in cities across America peaked in 1993 with 40 such councils, but was reduced in number to 11 in 2002. The focus of WELCOA the past few years has been on membership rather than councils, with 2,000 member organizations signed up. These organizations receive a newsletter and may also purchase consultation or how-to books for starting or strengthening worksite health-promoting activities. Organizations are also eligible for being recognized with a Well Workplace Award. WELCOA's membership fee in 2003 was $365 a year.

Over the past 15 years there has been little emphasis on the health of the *older* worker at WELCOA, despite this author's efforts to encourage such a focus (Haber & Wicht, 1987). Beginning in 2003, however, WELCOA included a column in their newsletter that has focused on the wellness of aging workers. For additional information on WELCOA, contact David Hunnicutt, President, Wellness Councils of America, 9802 Nicholas Street, #315, Omaha, NE 68114; 402-827-3590; www.welcoa.org.

In general, corporate leaders believe wellness programs have both health benefits for their employees and financial benefits for their organization. They have become more knowledgeable about the studies that have correlated participation in worksite wellness programs with lower absenteeism and tardiness, fewer medical insurance and disability compensation claims, increased productivity due to higher morale, and lower turnover rates (Kizer, 1987). Among 31 worksite wellness programs evaluated in terms of cost-effectiveness, only one failed to indicate a positive return on investment (Stokols et al., 1995). Another 20 worksite health programs were evaluated, and only one was not associated with reduced costs or increased benefits (Pelletier, 1996).

One of the pioneers in worksite wellness was Johnson & Johnson, the nation's largest producer of health care products. It began its Live for Life program in 1978 to improve the health of more than 10,000 employees. Compared with employees at Johnson & Johnson companies who did not have access to the program, the participating employees became more active, lost more weight, smoked less, showed greater improvement in applying stress management techniques, and lost less time due to sickness (Nathan, 1984).

A similar program, Control Data Corporation's Staywell Program, was started about the same time. As with Live for Life, Staywell began with a health screening profile, then followed up with professionally run programs and support groups called action teams. Both programs led to corporate-wide environmental changes, such as the provision of nutritious foods in the cafeteria and in vending machines, no-smoking areas, and on-site exercise facilities (Naditch, 1984).

When the cost of corporate medical plans rose 25% in 1991 (Meyer, 1991), some companies took a punitive approach. Turner Broadcasting Systems, for instance, attempted to lower insurance costs by firing or refusing to hire smokers and overweight people. A less extreme response was instituted by companies that raised health care costs for employees who engaged in lifestyle risk behaviors and provided programs to help them reduce risk factors. Hershey Foods employees, for instance, were required to pay $1,400 more in insurance costs per year if they became obese (I presume this penalty accrued even if the excess weight was a result of eating Hershey chocolate bars), smoked, remained sedentary, or had high blood pressure or high cholesterol levels.

A more positive perspective was taken by Southern California Edison (SCE), which gave premium reductions or reimbursements to employees who underwent screenings or joined risk reduction programs. SCE was motivated by the finding that employees with three risk factors averaged insurance claims that were twice as high as those with no risk factors (Meyer, 1991).

One of the major shortcomings of worksite wellness programs has been the tendency for those who need these programs the least—the younger and healthier workers—to utilize them the most. This is due, in part, to the youth of staff members according to Levin (1987). "At General Electric, Campbell Soup and Johnson and Johnson, the average age of staff members is less than 30. This is typical for fitness center staff; it is rare to find instructors over the age of 40." Levin questioned whether youth-oriented fitness staff members understood the special needs and interests of older employees and retirees.

Retirees may be excluded from wellness programs deliberately, for such reasons as space limitations, added staff costs, and possible legal liability. In 1985, only 15% of companies with wellness programs permitted retirees to participate ("Year End Update," 1985). On the positive side, however, an estimated three fourths of major employers offered preretirement programs, and many of these programs included a wellness component. Even more encouraging, many of these companies reached out to employees in their 40s, rather than waiting for the more traditional preretirement eligibility age of 55 or 60.

## HOSPITALS

About half the patients in American hospitals are geriatric patients, so it is not surprising that many hospitals in the United States host health programs for older persons and their families. In addition to fostering good public relations, these programs are considered beneficial marketing strategies. These hospital-based senior membership programs typically offer a variety of health education and health promotion services, including a newsletter, educational seminars, senior exercise classes, medical screening programs, and assistance with health insurance.

One such program, affiliated with the hospitals at the University of Texas Medical Branch (UTMB) in Galveston, Texas, is called SageSource. This program sponsors luncheons and dinners for adults aged 55 and over, with faculty and clinicians from the UTMB hospitals providing community health education. There is also a weekly radio show on senior activities and health issues, land- and water-based exercise classes, a quarterly newsletter called *SageSource News,* and the sponsorship of a variety of medical screenings and health fairs. There is no membership fee, but a modest fee is charged for each individual activity. For more information, contact the UTMB Senior Services Office, P.O. Box 35081, Galveston, TX 77555-5081; 409-747-2142; www.utmb.edu/aging.

## EDUCATIONAL INSTITUTIONS

Elderhostel is an international program that provides low-cost room and board and specially designed classes for adults aged 55 and over on college campuses. In 2002, about 250,000 older adults participated in 10,000

Elderhostel programs at more than 1,600 universities, museums, state and national parks, and other community sites throughout the United States and 100 other countries.

There are no homework assignments, no examinations, and no grades. Elderhostel's emphasis is on thought-provoking and challenging programs. Typically, noncredit college courses are 1 to 3 weeks long. Expenses tend to average about $100 a day and are all-inclusive. The elder students may live in dormitories and eat in college dining halls, or they may reside in a variety of other community settings. Classes frequently are taught by college faculty and cover many different types of subjects such as music, art, religion, history, health, and astronomy. Free catalogs of national and international programs are available. For information, contact Elderhostel, 11 Avenue de Lafayette, Boston, MA 02111-1746; or call toll-free at 877-426-8056; or go to www.elderhostel.org.

Many of the Elderhostel programs are quite innovative. An interesting example that takes place at Texas A & M University at Galveston is a sea camp that focuses on the coastal environment and endangered species. During the 5-day residential learning program, the students attend classes, take sailing trips, and go netting aboard the *Roamin' Empire,* a 48-foot research vessel. Elderhostelers who want to share their experience with their grandchildren (ages 9 through 12) can join an intergenerational program. The intergenerational participants share firsthand, on-the-water experiences during 5 days in the summer, and reside in dormitories on campus at night. For information, contact Elderhostel Program, Texas A & M University, Galveston, TX 77550.

Community colleges around the country also offer low-cost educational and health promotion programs for senior adults. One excellent program is the College of the Mainland Senior Adult Program, which provides a variety of educational programs for adults aged 55-plus, including arts, crafts, aerobics classes, weight-training classes, computer education, area trips, and long-distance travel. For information, contact Carol Looney, Director, College of the Mainland Senior Adult Program, 1200 Amburn Road, Texas City, TX 77591; 409-938-1211.

## SHOPPING MALL-BASED PROGRAMS

OASIS (Older Adult Service and Information System) provides shopping mall-based educational programs at May Company department stores in 26 cities, serving about 340,000 adults aged 55 and over. Oasis began in 1982 through its founder and president, Marylen Mann, in collaboration with Margie Wolcott May of the May department stores. The founding site and national headquarters is at the May department store in St. Louis, Missouri.

There is only one paid administrator at each OASIS site, with considerable administrative responsibility assumed by older adult volunteers. The array of courses focus on mental and physical health, intellectual stimulation on a wide scope of subjects, and fun. Contact OASIS, 7710 Carondelet Avenue, Suite 125, St. Louis, MO, 63105; Marylen Mann, President, 314-862-2933; or at www.oasisnet.org.

Given that there is a Jim Smith Society (for men named Jim Smith) and a National Association for the Advancement of Perry Mason, it is possible that America has a national organization for just about everyone—including shopping mall walkers. The National Organization of Mall Walkers once claimed 3 million members who were racking up miles in malls across America. Some of the shopping mall owners were enticing walkers to their malls with gifts, provided they accumulated sufficient mall mileage.

Not all has been bliss in mall walking America, however. The National Organization of Mall Walkers, alas, appears to have bit the dust. And there was a *New York Times* article ("Sneaker-clad army," 2001) that reported on a mall owner in suburban Chicago who was attempting to get rid of its older mall walkers. He complained that they rarely did any shopping and, to boot (so to speak), he believed that the walkers got in the way of the real shoppers. This story had a happy ending, though, as the mall walkers successfully advocated for their right to walk in this mall. And they accomplished this victory without the benefit of a national mall walking organization.

## COMPUTER EDUCATION

Ball State University's Fisher Institute for Wellness and Gerontology runs a community center for older adults in downtown Muncie, Indiana. This center is a learning laboratory for its graduate students, who organize and implement a variety of wellness and learning programs at the Community Center for Vital Aging (CCVA) (contact www.bsu.edu/wellness). The first program implemented at the Center was SeniorNet Computer Training, a class for older adults to learn how to use the computer. Each of the computer classes at the CCVA has met its maximum enrollment over the first 2 years of the center's existence, and the older students who completed their classes reported that they felt more connected with family members by learning to use e-mail, and more connected in general through access to the Internet.

SeniorNet is an award-winning national program, and the largest trainer of adults aged 50 and older on computers. The organization began in 1988 with 22 members and now has 39,000 members at 220 learning centers in communities around the country. SeniorNet provides training for teaching staff; offers hardware, software, and course curricula; and shares strategies with community organizations for effective marketing to seniors. SeniorNet also provides online computer courses, discussion rooms for computer users, discounts on computer hardware and software, and newsletters. For more information, contact SeniorNet, 121 Second Street, 7th floor, San Francisco, CA 94105; 800-747-6848; or www.seniornet.org.

# MODEL HEALTH PROMOTION PROGRAMS

Although there is no certain method for determining the quality of a health promotion program, there has been no shortage of attempts to identify model health promotion programs, develop a catalog that includes a summary of these exemplars, and distribute the catalog around the country in order to encourage their replication. Many of these model health promotion programs have been developed over the years with the aid of federal grants and other funding sources, have gone through multiple program evaluations, and can be helpful to health professionals who are interested in launching or improving their own program.

National directories of model health programs for older adults began in the 1980s when a directory of 40 programs was compiled by the Administration on Aging and distributed by the National Council on the Aging. Another directory was published in 1992 and included 24 model health promotion programs that were selected by a panel of experts through a cooperative project between AARP and the U.S. Public Health Service's Office of Disease Prevention and Health Promotion.

One of the more recent efforts in this regard began in 1999 by the Health Promotion Institute (HPI) of the National Council on the Aging. HPI started by summarizing 16 model programs or best practices and compiling them into a loose-leaf directory. The summaries included information on the planning process, implementation of the program, and program evaluations. Each year, new best practices have been added to this directory. If interested in obtaining a copy, contact The National Council on the Aging, Health Promotion Institute, 409 3rd Street, SW, #200, Washington, DC 20024; 202-479-1200; or www.ncoa.org.

The author of this book has had two programs listed in HPI's best practices manual: the Healthy Aging Exercise and Health Education program that has taken place in churches, senior centers, and other community sites, and is described in chapter 5 on Exercise; and the Health Assessment and Intervention program that uses health contract/calendars and has taken place in conjunction with geriatric primary care clinics, and is described in chapter 4 on Health Behavior.

The 5 model programs that were added to the best practices directory by HPI in 2002, reveal the diversity of settings and content that these programs represent. Brief summaries of the 5 programs follow:

1. Wellness Works, a health counseling and Internet assessment program that is a collaboration between the Milwaukee County Department of Aging and the University of Wisconsin, contact Linda Cieslik, Lcieslik@milwaukeecounty.com, 414-289-6633;
2. Prime Time, a wellness resource center located at Catholic Medical Center in New Hampshire, contact Connie Jones, cjones@cmc-nh.org, 603-663-6333;
3. Mather Café, three cafes in Chicago that promote the health of older adults, contact Kate Schreiber, kschreiber@matherlifeways.com, 773-622-9770;
4. LaPlanche Clinic, a medical/nursing practice that promotes wellness at Midstate Medical Center in Connecticut, contact Lynn Faria, lynfaria@hotmail.com, 203-639-8030; and
5. Wellness Makes S.E.N.S.E., a Greenfield Council on Aging program in Massachusetts that includes a wellness tool kit and service learning programs, contact Hope Macary, hopmacary@aol.com, 413-772-1517.

Another directory entitled: *Promoting Older Adult Health* (DHHS publication SMA 02-3628) was published in 2002 by the Substance Abuse and Mental Health Services Administration, in conjunction with the National Council on the Aging. This directory focuses on model mental health programs, including programs that focus on problems with mental disorders, alcohol abuse, and medication abuse. These 15 model programs are divided among four sections: education and prevention; outreach; screening, referral, intervention, and treatment; and service improvement through coalitions and teams. For more information, go to www.samhas.gov.

## HEALTHWISE

The best-known older adult *medical self-care* program is a model program called Healthwise, located in Boise, Idaho. The Healthwise program relies mostly on the *Healthwise Handbook,* which provides information and prevention tips on 190 common health problems, with information periodically updated. There are physician-approved guidelines in this handbook on when to call a health professional for each of the health problems that are covered. Some Healthwise programs supplement the distribution of the handbook with group health education programs or nurse call-in programs. There is a Spanish language edition of the *Healthwise Handbook,* called *La Salud en Casa.* There is also a special self-care guide for older adults called *Healthwise for Life.*

With the assistance of a $2.1 million grant from the Robert Wood Johnson Foundation, Healthwise distributed its medical self-care guide to 125,000 Idaho households, along with toll-free nurse consultation phone service and self-care workshops. Thirty-nine percent of handbook recipients reported that the handbook helped them avoid a visit to the doctor (Mettler, 1997). Blue Cross of Idaho reported 18% fewer visits to the emergency room by owners of the guide.

Elements of the Healthwise program have been replicated in the United Kingdom, South Africa, New Zealand, Australia, and Canada. In British Columbia, *Healthwise Handbooks* were distributed to every household, and all 4.3 million residents had potential access to the Healthwise content through a Web site and a nurse call center.

Additional information can be obtained from Healthwise, Inc., P.O. Box 1989, Boise, ID 83701; 208-331-6963; or go to www.healthwise.org.

## CHRONIC DISEASE SELF-MANAGEMENT PROGRAM

Kate Lorig and colleagues at the Stanford University School of Medicine have been evaluating community-based, peer-led, chronic disease self-management programs for many years, beginning with the Arthritis Self-Management Program (Lorig et al., 1986). This program has since evolved into a curriculum that is applicable to a wide array of chronic diseases and conditions.

Typically, each program involves about a dozen participants, led by peer leaders who have received 20 hours of training. The peer leaders, like the students, are typically older and have chronic diseases that they contend with. The program consists of seven weekly sessions about 2½ hours long, with a content focus on exercise, symptom management, nutrition, fatigue and sleep management, use of medications, managing emotions, community resources, communicating with health professionals, problemsolving, and decisionmaking.

The theoretical basis of the program has been to promote a sense of personal efficacy among participants (Bandura, 1997) by using such techniques as guided mastery of skills, peer modeling, reinterpretation of symptoms, social persuasion through group support, and individual self-management guidance. In addition to improving self-efficacy, Lorig and colleagues (2001) reported reduced emergency room and outpatient visits, and decreased health distress.

## SENIOR WELLNESS PROJECT

Senior Services of Seattle/King County began the Senior Wellness Project (SWP) in 1997 at the North Shore Senior Center in Bothell, Washington. SWP is a research-based health promotion program that includes a component of chronic care self-management that was modeled after Kate Lorig's program (Lorig et al., 1999). The program also includes health and functional assessments; individual and group counseling; exercise programs; a personal health action plan with the support of a nurse, social worker, and volunteer health mentor; and support groups. A randomized controlled study of chronically ill seniors reported a reduction in number of hospital stays and average length of stay, a reduction in psychotropic medications, and better functioning in activities of daily living (Leveille et al., 1998).

SWP represents a demonstration of a partnership among a university, an Area Agency on Aging, local and national foundations, health departments, senior centers, primary care providers, older volunteers, and older participants. Versions of this model program are being replicated at senior wellness sites around the country (56 sites in the United States and two sites in Sweden) to test its effectiveness in a variety of communities, in an assortment of sites, serving a diversity of clientele. Initial findings have demonstrated higher levels of physical activity and lower levels of depression among its participants (Dobkin, 2002).

In order to sustain this program in good times and bad and to sustain activities when there is little reimbursable support in the way of Medicare, Medicaid, and other health insurance companies, the SWP has cultivated a diversified funding base. In descending order of financial amount, SWP receives support from the following sources: senior center; Area Agency on Aging; foundation; health department; fees from technical assistance and software licensing; income from clients, health providers, and insurers; university funding; and funds from United Way and general fund-raising.

To learn more about SWP, contact Susan Snyder, Program Director at Senior Services, 1601 Second Avenue, #800, Seattle, WA, 98101; 206-727-6297); susans@seniorservices.org.

## ORNISH PROGRAM FOR REVERSING HEART DISEASE

Dr. Dean Ornish, a physician at the University of California at San Francisco and founder of the Preventive Medicine Research Institute, has developed a program for reversing heart disease that has been replicated at several sites around the country. Dr. Ornish (1992) has recommended a vegetarian diet with fat intake of 10% or less of total calories, moderate aerobic exercise at least 3 times a week, yoga and meditation an hour a day, group support sessions, and smoking cessation.

Dr. Ornish and his colleagues (Gould et al., 1995) have reported that as a result of their program, blockages in arteries have decreased in size, and blood flow has improved in as many as 82% of their heart patients. A 5-year follow-up of this program reported an 8% reduction in athero-sclerotic plaques, while the control group had a 28% increase. Also during this time, cardiac events were more than doubled in the control group (Ornish et al., 1998). These types of results have attracted the attention of Medicare, which funded a demonstration project to evaluate the Ornish program. Mutual of Omaha and other health insurance vendors have funded the program as well.

The applicability of this program to nonheart patients, however, is still of uncertain utility. It may take highly motivated individuals (e.g., patients with severe heart disease) and significant medical and health support (requiring significant resources) for the program to be useful to others. For additional information, contact Dean Ornish, MD, Preventive Medicine Research Institute, 900 Bridgeway, Suite 1, Sausalito, CA 94965; DeanOrnish@aol.com.

## COMMUNITY-ORIENTED PRIMARY CARE

Over a 4-year period (1992–1996) I participated in two Community-Oriented Primary Care (COPC) interdisciplinary teams, one housed in a Public Health Service Section 330 community health clinic for patients who are indigent and the other in a university-affiliated outpatient clinic (Thompson et al., 1996, 1998). COPC refers to the activities of primary care health care professionals who go out into the community on their own initiative to gain more understanding of clients as well as the community from which they come. This contrasts with a traditional primary care practice where individual patients seek medical primary care at a clinic site.

Thus, in addition to the traditional focus on the individual patient, COPC also makes the family and the community the focus of diagnosis, treatment, and ongoing surveillance (Nutting, 1987). The practitioner of COPC moves from the narrow, biomedical, physician-led, clinic-based, one-to-one form of medical care, to a new vision of providing health care that includes the social environment that shapes an individual's health and behavior choices.

The two most popular definitions of a community are a) individuals who share a geographical area, and b) a group of persons who share values and/or lifestyles. The concept of community from a COPC perspective, however, typically focuses on clients of a health professional or a health facility who have a specific type or set of health problems (e.g., diabetes, noncompliance, cancer, alcohol abuse, teenage pregnancy). A COPC project also tends to take a broad view of community and to systematically examine the status or perceptions of the wide variety of persons who represent the community of interest (e.g., spouse, minister, *curandero*, pharmacist, peers, etc.).

In addition to identifying relevant persons in the community who can shed light on a specific health problem, the COPC practitioner reviews extant data or collects new data. The county health department or other city and county agencies may provide relevant demographic, social, economic, mortality, and morbidity data. Other sources of data include chart reviews of clients or surveys of clients or residents in the community.

Often, health or disease data at the local community level are compared with data from similar populations in other parts of the country or with Healthy People 2010 baseline data or projections. Health problems in a local community that are not only documented through data but are also of unusual magnitude tend to stimulate COPC projects.

The goals of a COPC project are to a) identify measurable objectives for reducing a health problem or the risk factors that contribute to it; b) include a focus on health education, disease prevention, or health promotion; c) inform providers and consumers that they have the opportunity and the responsibility to be advocates of change and to make the health care system more responsive to their needs; and d) recognize that health professionals can be more effective in teams, including relying on such health professionals as primary care physicians, clinical nurses, community health nurses, physician's assistants, epidemiologists, public health specialists, social workers, medical sociologists, and health educators.

Some of the COPC projects that we completed were a) the development of a health screening instrument to help homeless shelter staff assess the medical status of their clients, and to provide the staff with referral telephone numbers for dealing with a wide range of health problems; b) implementation of a health fair at another homeless shelter site with the assistance of homeless shelter residents in the planning process; and c) completion of 80 interviews with former patients of a recently closed Public Health Service Section 330 community health clinic for those who are indigent, in order to determine how they had been receiving medical care since the closing of the clinic, and to identify the barriers to health care that were generated by the closing. The findings were compiled, and the resulting report distributed to community leaders and government officials as the first step in an attempt to reopen this much-needed medical clinic.

Without a mechanism for reimbursement of its activities, the COPC model may have only a modest impact on the average clinical practice in the community. At least two abbreviated elements of the COPC model, however, can supplement traditional clinical practices in a cost-effective way: a) define a health problem that affects a significant number of clients, and b) develop a small project in the community that systematically addresses this problem (Nutting, 1987).

## A MODEL HEALTH PROGRAM IN A CHINESE COMMUNITY

I observed what may have been the best example of a model health promotion program—a self-led tai chi class—while on an early morning jog in China in 1978. Tai chi is a nonstrenuous sequence of physical movements derived from the ancient Chinese martial arts. Tai chi attempts to increase energy, improve balance, and enhance mental and spiritual health. The participants I observed in the community, over half of whom were older adults, had maximum accessibility to this program—they had only to exit their front doors. There were no fees to be paid and no professionals to depend on. See Figure 12.1, which shows people practicing tai chi.

I later observed similar groups of older persons in China practicing tai chi in community parks (Haber, 1979). Since that time, several studies have reported that tai chi is beneficial for older adults with balance problems (Wolf et al., 1996; Wolfson et al., 1996), and it is now being taught at many senior centers and other community sites throughout the United States.

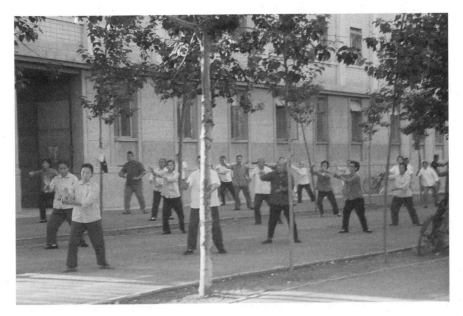

FIGURE 12.1 Tai chi in China.

## PROFESSIONAL ASSOCIATIONS

Health promotion and health education programs are sponsored by many disease-specific professional associations. The Arthritis Foundation, for example, offers a wide array of health education programs, among them several self-help and peer support programs, including the Arthritis Self-Help Course, PACE Exercise, arthritis clubs, and aquatic programs. All programs are taught by trained volunteer instructors, many of whom cope with arthritis.

It is estimated that everyone over the age of 60 has some degree of osteoarthritis, and about 40% of older Americans recognize some of its symptoms. Osteoarthritis, the most common form of arthritis, is the gradual wearing away of tissue around the joints of the hands, feet, knees, hips, neck, or back. Arthritic pain may vary from mild to severe, and it may come and go. Arthritis cannot be prevented nor cured but the function of arthritic joints can be improved and the pain often can be alleviated.

More than 100 local chapters of the Arthritis Foundation offer a 6-week course that provides information on medications, exercise, nutrition, relaxation techniques, coping skills, and the practical concerns of daily living. Practical information can range from the identification of places to purchase Velcro-modified clothing, to the location of aquatic exercise programs.

Many of the Arthritis Foundation programs were developed and evaluated at the Stanford Arthritis Center over many years and are offered around the country. Participants are typically asked to pay a small fee for courses and instructional materials. Besides health education programs, local arthritis chapters distribute free booklets on arthritis as well as information about most arthritis medications.

For additional information, contact the Arthritis Foundation, P.O. Box 7669, Atlanta, GA 30357-0669; 800-283-7800; www.athritis.org.

Many other professional associations also offer health education programs and materials. If you cannot locate a state or local chapter of a specific professional association, contact one of the following national headquarters for information on local educational opportunities and support groups, as well as for resource materials:

- Alzheimer's Association (24-hour toll-free telephone link to access information about local chapters and community resources, free catalog of educational publications, and research program): 919 North Michigan Avenue, Suite 1100, Chicago, IL 60611–1676; 800-272-3900; www.alz.org.
- American Cancer Society (education and support programs, workshops, transportation programs, publications, and financial aid): 1599 Clifton Road NE, Atlanta, GA 30329; 800-227-2345; www.cancer.org.
- American Diabetes Association (local chapters for support and referrals, outreach programs for minority communities): 1701 North Beauregard Street, Alexandria, VA 22311; 800-342-2383; www.diabetes.org.
- American Heart Association (cookbooks, guides on treatment and prevention, and research funding program): 7272 Greenville Avenue, Dallas, TX 75231; 800-242-8721; www.americanheart.org.
- American Lung Association (education, advocacy, and research on asthma, emphysema, tuberculosis, and lung cancer): 61 Broadway, 6th Floor, New York, NY 10006; 800-LUNG-USA; www.stroke.org.
- American Parkinson's Disease Association (local chapters, educational materials, referrals, and research): 1250 Hylan Boulevard, Suite 4B, Staten Island, NY 10305; 800-223-2732; www.apdaparkinson.org.
- Better Hearing Institute (information on medical, surgical, and rehabilitation options): 5021-B Backlick Road, Annandale, VA 22003; 800-327-9355; www.betterhearing.org.

- National Association for Continence (advocacy, education, and support): P.O. Box 8310, Spartanburg, SC 29305–8310; 800-252-3337; www.nafc.org.
- National Association for the Mentally Ill (support groups, education, advocacy, and research): Colonial Place Three, 2107 Wilson Boulevard, Suite 300, Arlington, VA 22201; 800-950-6264; www.nami.org.
- National Council on Alcoholism and Drug Dependence (advocacy, information, and referrals): Inc., 20 Exchange Place, #2902, New York, NY 10005; 800-622-2255; www.ncadd.org.
- National Digestive Disease Information Clearinghouse (support groups, referrals, and fact sheets on gastroesophageal reflux disease, hemorrhoids, constipation, ulcers, and irritable bowel syndrome): NIH, 2 Information Way, Bethesda, MD 20892–3570; 800-891-5389; www.niddk.nih.gov.
- National Mental Health Association (referrals and publications): 2001 N. Beauregard Street, 12th Floor, Alexandria, VA 22311; 800-969-6642; www.nmha.org.
- National Osteoporosis Foundation (research, education, and advocacy): 1232 22nd Street, NW, Washington, DC 20037; 202-223-2226; www.nof.org.
- National Stroke Association (support groups, local resources, and information about prevention, treatment, recovery, and rehabilitation): 9707 E. Easter Lane, Englewood, CO 80112; 800-STROKES; www.stroke.org.

## COMMUNITY VOLUNTEERING

"The United States finds itself with two parallel phenomena that invite convergence. On the one hand the country has vast unmet community service needs; on the other hand, the United States draws only partially on the large and growing productive potential of older people." (Caro & Morris, 2001).

Although many analysts see the rapidly growing older adult population in the United States in terms of being a financial burden on future generations, others see a vast, untapped social resource for improving the health and well-being of older adults and society itself. An AARP survey in 2002 reported that over half of Americans ages 50 to 75 are planning to incorporate community service into later life (M. Freedman, 2002). The Bureau of Labor Statistics of the U.S. Department of Labor, however, reported that in 2002 the volunteer rate for people aged 65 and older was less than half of that (22.7%).

If the potential tidal wave of community volunteering could be unleashed, there would likely be greater fulfillment in, and purpose to, the latter part of the life cycle. A meta-analysis of 37 independent studies reported that the sense of well-being among older volunteers was consistently enhanced as a consequence of their volunteer efforts (J. Wheeler et al., 1998). The authors also noted that while this mental health phenomenon was taking place, significant experience and energy was being directed at the service needs of society's more vulnerable groups.

About a century ago, many services in America—education, law enforcement, fire fighting, hospital care, social service—relied upon volunteers. Over time, however, community services began to be dominated by paid personnel, with the more affluent obtaining services privately and the less affluent relying on inferior publicly funded services. As a consequence, volunteering in the public sector became less attractive and peripheral to the main work of paid staff. Volunteer responsibilities were not only becoming peripheral to the mission of public organizations, but when volunteers were utilized, they were oftentimes lacking in volunteer training, supervision, and recognition (Caro & Morris, 2001).

Marc Freedman, president of Civic Ventures, describes the volunteer opportunities available to older adults as "incapable of capturing the imagination of a new generation of older Americans." In his book *Prime Time: How Baby Boomers Will Revolutionize Retirement and Transform America,* Freedman (1999) argues that we need to "learn how to tap the time, talent, and civic potential of the group that is our country's only increasing natural resource."

The following community volunteer programs represent model programs that do provide training, supervision, and recognition. Program evaluations, though limited, support the contention that these types of programs not only enhance the lives of the persons they serve, but also the mental health of the older volunteers themselves (Morrow-Howell et al., 2003).

## FEDERAL VOLUNTEERISM

The National Senior Services Corps (also known as SeniorCorps) was established in 1973 and is the principal vehicle for federal volunteerism for Americans aged 55 and older. About 500,000 older Americans participate in the corps, most of whom are low-income and accept a small stipend for their effort. Volunteers serve primarily through one of the following three programs:

1. The Retired Senior Volunteer Program (RSVP) matches the personal interests and skills of older Americans with opportunities to solve community problems.
2. The Foster Grandparent Program trains low-income adults aged 60 and over to serve 20 hours a week to help children with special needs (for example, a seriously ill child with cancer).
3. The Senior Companion Program trains low-income adults aged 60 and over to support their peers who are frail and disabled (for example, a stroke victim who is confined to a wheelchair and suffering from depression), in order to help them remain independent.

For additional information on these programs and other federal volunteer opportunities, contact: www.seniorcorps.org.

There are two intergenerational programs that receive substantial federal support: Experience Corps and the National Mentoring Partnership Program. The goal of the Experience Corps is to place adult volunteers aged 55 and older in elementary schools and youth-focused organizations, particularly in the innercity. Experience Corps has more than 1,000 volunteers in 14 cities, with the goal of going nationwide. Older adults who serve at least 15 hours a week receive a stipend ranging from $100 to $200 a month. For additional information, contact www.experiencecorps.org.

Unlike the Experience Corps, the National Mentoring Partnership program is not focused exclusively on the training and placing of older volunteers. However, many older adults participate in this program. The National Mentoring Partnership provides the information and tools that volunteers need to mentor young people in their communities. This organization has seeded and nurtured programs in 23 states. For additional information, contact www.mentoring.org.

The Service Corps of Retired Executives (SCORE), in conjunction with the Small Business Administration, helps retired executives and business owners who have the time to counsel younger entrepreneurs who are launching America's small businesses. There are 389 SCORE chapters with 10,500 older volunteers, who provide free counseling and low-cost workshops in local communities. SCORE consultants are in the 55-plus age range and average 40 years of business experience. If you are interested in obtaining additional information, go to the Web site www.score.org.

## AARP

More than 70 years ago, the founder of AARP, Ethel Percy Andrus, said that the way to lead a life with purpose and meaning was "to serve, and not to be served." This tradition can be found among the half of AARP's

35 million members who volunteer annually. In addition, AARP has more than 3,200 local chapters dispersed among the 50 states, through which more formal community service programs are implemented. These programs reach about 3.5 million people annually. To locate one of these local chapters contact AARP at the toll-free number 800-424-3410.

Four of the most popular AARP community volunteer programs are:

1. The 55 Alive Driver Safety Program is implemented by volunteers who are trained to provide instruction. This program makes older drivers safer and can significantly lower their automobile insurance rates. Over 600,000 drivers graduated in 2001. Contact the toll-free number 888-227-7669.
2. The Grief and Loss program provides resources and information to those who are bereaved. Volunteers are trained to provide one-to-one and group support for the newly bereaved. Contact the e-mail address griefandloss@aarp.org.
3. The Tax-Aide program provides free tax counseling and preparation service for middle- and low-income taxpayers aged 60 and older. Volunteer tax counselors are trained and certified by the Internal Revenue Service. Tax-Aide assisted almost 2 million people during the 2001 tax season and was staffed by more than 30,000 AARP volunteers. Contact the toll-free number 888-227-7669.
4. The Senior Community Service Employment Program is implemented in conjunction with the Department of Labor. This program trains and transitions low-income older people into paid employment. There were about 100 sites in the United States and Puerto Rico, and the program had a 54% placement rate in 2001.

In a major initiative prompted by the terrorist attacks of September 11, 2001, AARP partnered with 8 other national organizations to enhance volunteer opportunities across the country. These eight organizations are the American Hospice Foundation (www.americanhospice.org); America's Second Harvest (domestic hunger relief, www.secondharvest.org); Big Brothers Big Sisters of America (youth mentoring, www.bbbsa.org); Meals on Wheels Association of America (www.mowaa.org); National Mentoring Partnership (youth mentoring, www.mentoring.org); Points of Light Foundation (community volunteering, www.pointsoflife.org); and Rebuilding Together (revitalizing low-income housing, www.rebuildingtogether.com).

For an overview of AARP's volunteer programs, to link with a local AARP chapter, to review the benefits of volunteering, or to obtain a guide for developing your own volunteer initiatives, go to www.aarp.org/connect.html.

## CYBER VOLUNTEERING

In addition to the Web sites previously provided, there is a wealth of information on volunteering in cyberspace. One comprehensive online volunteer recruitment tool provides summaries of volunteer programs, and it can directly match volunteer interests with opportunities in specific areas. Contact www.impactonline.org.

Another Web site to promote and facilitate collaboration, volunteerism, and community building throughout the world is www.idealist.org. This site also contains the largest directory of nonprofit organizations in the world.

# COMMUNITY HEALTH ADVOCACY

The best-known role model for community health advocacy in aging was Maggie Kuhn, founder of the Gray Panthers, an intergenerational advocacy group. I took this photograph of Maggie in 1978 (see Figure 12.2), literally, on a slow boat to China, when Chinese relations with the Soviet Union were very strained. Ever the feisty one, Maggie thought posing in a Russian hat might amuse our Chinese guides. The expressions on the faces of our guides, however, were inscrutable.

## ENVIRONMENTAL ADVOCACY

Environmental advocacy is a strong interest among many older adults, perhaps as part of their quest to leave planet Earth in as good a shape as when they were born into it. In 1991, 35 national organizations recognized that many local and national efforts existed in the environmental protection arena, and they organized an alliance to coordinate these efforts. The Environmental Alliance for Senior Involvement (EASI) attempts to facilitate the efforts of older adults to accomplish such goals as monitoring and improving water and air quality, reducing pollution from local growth and transportation, implementing noise abatement, and diminishing the hazardous use of toxic chemicals.

In 1999, 20,000 elders from the Retired Senior Volunteer Programs (RSVP) became involved with the EASI coalition. These RSVP participants contributed 4 million volunteer hours to 310 local projects around the nation. In Montana, they tackled water pollution and cleaning up a toxic site. In Texas, older volunteers provided environmental education programs to thousands of students. For more information about EASI, contact the organization headquarters in Virginia at 540-788-3274; or the Web site www.easi.org.

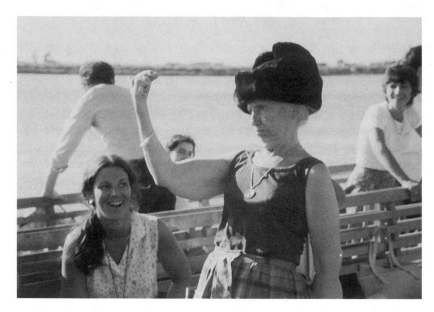

**FIGURE 12.2    Maggie Kuhn, founder of the Gray Panthers advocacy group.**

There are local environmental organizations, unrelated to EASI, that originated because of the unique efforts of one individual. One such program was launched by Susan Tixier of Escalante, Utah, who began the Great Old Broads for Wilderness in 1989. She was concerned about motorized vehicles in designated wilderness areas, and rampant grazing and mining that were scarring the Utah landscape. She organized an annual hike (the Broadwalk), published a newspaper (the Broadside), declared that women members younger than 45 would have to be called "Great Old Broads-in-Training," and organized a variety of environmental advocacy efforts. In 2003, the organization had moved to Durango, Colorado, with Veronica Egan as its interim executive director. For more information, contact: www.greatoldbroads.org.

## THE LONG-TERM CARE OMBUDSMAN PROGRAM

Long-term care ombudsmen are advocates for residents of nursing homes, board and care homes, assisted living facilities, and similar adult care facilities. Roughly two thirds of ombudsmen are older adults (based on conversations with state ombudsmen directors and my own experience), and about 90% of the persons served by ombudsmen are older adults.

Begun in 1972 as a demonstration program and continued under the federal Older Americans Act, every state is required to have an ombudsman program that addresses resident complaints, and advocates for improvements in the long term care system. In 2002, there were 14,000 certified volunteer ombudsmen who investigated 230,000 complaints made by 135,000 individuals. The most frequent complaint was lack of care due to inadequate staffing.

For additional information contact the National Long Term Care Ombudsman Resource Center at www.ltcombudsman.org; 1424 16th Street, NW, #202, Washington, DC 20036; 202-232-2275 or the National Citizens' Coalition for Nursing Home Reform at www.nccnhr.org.

## BENEFITSCHECKUP

BenefitsCheckUp was launched nationally in June 2001 by the National Council on the Aging. It is the first national Web site for older adults that helps consumers look for federal and state program benefits that they are entitled to but are not currently receiving. The site includes information on more than 1,000 public benefit programs and has 40,000 local entry points. For example, seniors may be eligible for Supplemental Security Income, food stamps, utility bills assistance, home weatherization, vocational rehabilitation, in-home services, caregiving support services, legal services, nutrition programs, and training and education opportunities. In 2003, BenefitsCheckUpRx was launched, a national Web site to allow older adults to find out which of 250-plus programs can help them save money on their prescriptions.

Users receive a printed report that tells them which programs they may likely qualify for and where to enroll. What may have taken the older consumer or their helper days or weeks to ascertain, BenefitsCheckUp may do in minutes. To access this service, go to the Web site www.benefitscheckup.org or call 202-479-6616.

# QUESTIONS FOR DISCUSSION

1. Provide information about two health programs oriented toward older adults (in sufficient detail to satisfy the curiosity of an interested older adult). Choose programs that are located at two of the following sites: hospital, senior center, AARP chapter, religious institution, retirement community, university, community college, area agency on aging, or shopping mall.

2. Chose one of the model health promotion programs summarized in this chapter, and find out something of interest to you about that program that is not mentioned in this chapter.
3. Describe any volunteering experience you have had. Were you trained, supervised, and recognized? Was it a satisfying experience? How could your experience have been improved?
4. Devise a plan for realizing the expressed desires of the 50% of baby boomers who wish to include community service in their retirement years. Which baby boomers would you target, where would you reach out to them, when would you approach them (before retirement, early into their retirement, or anytime), and how would you reach out to them?
5. If you were to start up an advocacy group in retirement, what would you focus on and how would you go about it?
6. Contact the Web site of one of the professional associations listed in this chapter, and report on the most innovative program that involves older adults that you can find.

# 13

# Diversity

Over a lifetime, people of similar ages can be expected to become increasingly diverse. As they age, some people will become ever more learned and wise, while others will make little progress in these areas. Some will discover fitness to be a rewarding hobby and persist in it as they grow older, while others will become increasingly sedentary and frail. Some will appreciate each day more and more as the number of remaining days become fewer and fewer, while others will view aging as a depressing decline into decrepitude.

Despite the increasing diversity with age, much of the content of this book reports on what we can expect will happen to most of us as we age. If the author qualified every statement with "depending on a person's age, race, socioeconomic status, gender, geographical location, etc." this would be a ponderous book indeed. (Pardon the author's assumption that it is not). This chapter, therefore, is intended to draw this diversity with aging to the attention of the reader, and to allow the reader to contemplate how difficult it is to make general statements about how we age.

## AGE

The very definition of being old is not obvious. The onset of old age can range in age from at least age 40 to age 75. At age 40, workers are old enough to be deemed in need of protection from age discrimination as defined by the 1967 Age Discrimination in Employment Act. At age 50, people become eligible for membership in AARP. At age 60, individuals are eligible to participate in activities at most senior centers. At age 62, residents can live in public housing for elders and receive early Social Security retirement benefits. At age 65, retirees qualify for normal Social

Security benefits. At age 75, a patient is eligible for treatment at some geriatric primary care clinics, including the one that the author used to be affiliated with in Texas.

Nonetheless, the more or less official starting point for old age in America is 65. Apparently this tradition had its roots in Germany when Chancellor Otto von Bismarck established age 65 as the standard retirement age in 1884. (Actually, he initially set 70 as the retirement age—hoping, perhaps, that few if any would qualify for benefits. The qualifying age was eventually reduced to 65 in 1916). When Social Security was enacted in the United States in 1935, the precedent of establishing age 65 as the eligibility age for requirement was continued. Thus, age 65 was instituted as a quasilegal and de facto national definition of old age.

Gerontologists began to realize, however, that few meaningful statements can be made about the population in general over age 65. They began to argue about the tendency to write about adults aged 65 and over as if they were all the same when, in fact, "age is becoming increasingly irrelevant as a predictor of lifestyle or need" (Neugarten, 1979, page 50).

Gerontologists then began to divide the older adult population into two groups, the young-old and the old-old with age 75 as the dividing point at first; then age 80; and now it is not unusual to use age 85. Perhaps as the number of centenarians increase to a million or more when the baby boomers become of age, another dividing line will be added at age 100, in order to differentiate among the young-old, middle-old, and old-old.

Dividing the older population into two or more categories is helpful for making more specific statements about being older. The old-old are different physically and cognitively than the young-old, even if these differences are affected by changes in physical status or public policy from one decade to the next.

Take, for example, the decline in nursing home use among the old-old over the past 15 years. Using age 85 as the dividing line for being old-old, 25% of the 85-and-over population resided in nursing homes in 1985; by 1999 this percentage had been reduced to 18%. Though the percentage may have been reduced, the 85-and-over age group was still 18 times more likely to be institutionalized than those aged 65 to 74 in 1999; the same ratio as in 1985.

Thus, while the old-old were less likely to be institutionalized over a 15-year period, the old-old in comparison to the young-old continued to be vulnerable to institutionalization at the same ratio. Economic, political, and lifestyle realities may change over time, but differentiating between the young-old and the old-old is likely to remain consistently useful for researchers and clinicians.

Among those aged 85 and older, about 96% of the population have at least one chronic condition, disability, or functional limitation, versus 76% among those aged 65 to 69 (AARP, 2002). Among those aged 85 and older, about 30% to 45% have Alzheimer's disease, versus 2% among those aged 65 to 69 (D. Evans et al., 1989; Jorm et al., 1987). Among those noninstitutionalized, the average health care expenditures for those aged 85 and over is $7,500, versus $4,000 for those aged 65 to 74 (AARP, 2002). The old-old are considerably more physically, mentally, and financially vulnerable than the young-old.

Before the reader gets too carried away with the differences between the old-old and the young-old, we end with the reminder that even when we divide older adults into more specific age groups, we still fail to account for the considerable variability that remains. As noted in chapter 1 in the section on extraordinary accomplishments and aging, some nonagenarians are recording new works of music and producing hit singles, while others are completing marathons and climbing mountains. Some sexagenarians, on the other hand, are looking forward to becoming decreasingly active as they enter retirement.

# GENDER

As the population ages, it also becomes decidedly more female. The life expectancy of a boy born in the United States in 2001 is 74 years, and that of a girl is 79.5 years. Women represent 56% of the population aged 65 to 74, and 72% of those over age 85. Though women are more likely to become older, the prevalence of disability is consistently higher in women as well. More than half of women aged 70 and older report difficulty with mobility, such as walking across a room or climbing stairs, compared to 36% of men. Women aged 70 and older are more than twice as likely (57% to 28%) as men to have difficulties with strength activities.

In addition, older women have higher rates of illness, physician visits, drug prescription use, acute illnesses, and chronic conditions. Among the chronic conditions that both women and men can acquire, osteoporosis is the most unfair to women, with 80% of those who have this condition being women. Men, however, are more likely to encounter life-threatening acute conditions and to require hospitalization (Hooyman & Kiyak, 1999). Thus, Medicare insurance with its emphasis on hospital coverage, and its weaknesses in providing nursing home, community care, and home care, favors the profile of older men's medical status more than older women's.

Older women are more likely to be unpaid caregivers. Older wives are more likely to care for their spouses than older husbands are. Among adult children who care for their elderly parents, about 75% are daughters. And about two thirds of the 2.4 million grandparents who are raising grandchildren are women (HRSA, 2002). The greater responsibility for caregiving is due primarily to cultural expectations. Society expects women to leave the workforce when family obligations beckon. Not only have women been viewed as less essential than men in the workforce, they have been expected to accept substantially less money in the workforce than men do. For most of the life cycle, the current cohort of older women have been considered the primary caregivers for family members while men have been considered the primary breadwinners.

Unpaid caregiving responsibilities and lower wages for women are then complicated by widowhood. Because women generally marry men older than themselves, live longer than men, and infrequently remarry in their 50s and older, it follows that 52% of women aged 65 and over are widowed in contrast to 14% of men. Consequently, it is not surprising that women are more likely to experience economic insecurity in old age than are men.

The median income of female older adults was 56% of that of male older adults, and the poverty rate of older women was almost twice as high as for older men (13% versus 7%) (year 2000 data accessed through www.agingstats.gov). In 1994, the average monthly Social Security benefit was $601 for women, compared to $785 for men (Butler et al., 1998). As noted by the late Tish Sommers, founder of the Older Women's League, "Motherhood and apple pie may be sacred, but neither guarantees economic security in old age." This economic disparity, however, will diminish in the future as the labor participation of women in general continues to become more equivalent to that of men and as wage disparities continue to lessen.

Despite the physical and financial disparities, older women are more health conscious and more resilient. They are twice as likely as men between the ages of 45 and 64 to have a regular physician, almost three times more likely to have seen a physician in the past year, and more likely to seek immediate medical care if they are sick or in pain (D. Shelton, 2000). They are also more likely to eat a healthful diet and more likely to take a supplementary vitamin pill. In addition, older women have more frequent social contacts and more intimate relationships than do older men.

Perhaps some combination of these factors contributes to a lower likelihood of committing suicide. Between the ages of 65 and 69, male suicides outnumber female suicides by 4 to 1; by age 85, this ratio increases to 12 to 1.

It seems ironic that for many years clinical research trials sponsored by the National Institutes of Health focused almost exclusively on male subjects, while men in general demonstrated such little interest in their own health. This practice of excluding women from clinical trials was ended in 1991 by Dr. Bernadine Healy, the first woman to head the National Institutes of Health. Dr. Healy also created the Office on Women's Health in the Department of Health and Human Services. There has been little interest in creating a counterpart office for men. And while women's health centers are commonplace in the community, men's health centers are a rarity.

A final note on the gender and age issue: not only do differences between men and women increase with age, but also aging women are becoming more diverse. An article in the *Journal of the American Medical Association* reports that there is now no medical reason for excluding women in the sixth decade of life from attempting pregnancy on the basis of their age alone (Paulson et al., 2002).

# RACE AND ETHNICITY

## DEFINITION

There are several terms that overlap in meaning and are often used without definitions: minority groups, racial groups, ethnic groups, and disadvantaged. *Minority groups* tend to refer to subgroups within a population that are subject to discrimination, usually on the basis of race, ethnicity, or national origin. *Racial groups* are categories based on parentage and physical appearance and are increasingly problematic because of widespread genetic diversity. *Ethnic groups* are individuals who share a sense of race, religion, national origin, or other cultural category. And *disadvantaged* refers to subgroups with fewer resources than the mainstream, oftentimes associated with minority groups, racial groups, or ethnic groups.

Perhaps in deference to the difficulty of defining racial or ethnic categories, the census form in 2000 allowed Americans to select more than one racial or ethnic category. Nearly 7 million Americans took this opportunity to identify themselves as a blend of two or more races. This category, available for the first time in 2000, already contains 2.4% of the country's population.

Although Americans are allowed to select more than one racial category, confusion still reigned in the 2000 census. People of Middle Eastern descent were considered White by federal counters, while people from India, once classified as White, were placed into the Asian category. C education professor at the University of Phoenix wondered why a Pakistani in America is not considered Black, but a biracial adult with blond hair and blue eyes can check Black on the census form (Briggs, 2002).

Though most biologists and anthropologists now deny the legitimacy of creating distinct racial categories, the reality for older adults in America is quite different. Most minority elders have grown up without equal rights and protection under the law. Job discrimination over the years has left minorities "with less resources to cope with their old age and a legacy of poverty, poor nutrition, and living in substandard housing that generally translates into poorer health in old age" (Yee, 1990). This history of discrimination also affects the minority older adult's willingness to access the health care system, though the advent of Medicare corrected that problem to a large degree.

During their work years, many minority elders had labor-intensive jobs, inadequate access to health care, poor diets, and substantial stress (Krause & Wray, 1991). Not surprisingly, therefore, elderly minorities experienced greater health problems than elderly Anglos. One consequence is that many minority elders consider "old age" as beginning in the early 50s or even younger (National Indian Council on Aging, 1984; Lopez & Aguilera, 1991).

## RACIAL DISPARITIES IN HEALTH CARE

The Institute of Medicine, an independent research institution that advises Congress, reported in March 2002 on the first comprehensive examination of racial disparities in health care among people who have health insurance. Previous studies had reported on the lack of access to health care by minorities, as well as on how the lifestyles of minorities contribute to poor health. This study tackled the delicate issue of racial prejudice in health care.

The report reviewed more than 100 studies conducted over the past decade and concluded that racial disparities contribute to higher death rates among minorities. It cited that minorities are less likely to be given appropriate medications for heart disease; less likely to be offered bypass surgery, angioplasty, kidney dialysis, or transplants; less likely to receive the most sophisticated treatment for HIV; and more likely to have lower limbs amputated as a result of diabetes (Stolberg, 2002).

The authors believe that a racial bias, perhaps subconscious, contributes to a reduced opportunity for minority patients to receive the latest and most sophisticated treatments. The explanation of why this takes place is complex and may include the fact that there are disproportionately fewer minority physicians, that minorities are less likely to have a long-lasting relationship with a primary care physician, and that physicians may assume that minority patients are less likely to comply with follow-up care.

## RACIAL AND ETHNIC DISTRIBUTION

The United States older adult population is becoming more racially and ethnically diverse, as evidenced by Table 13.1. In six decades, American minorities will increase from 16% to 36% of the total population.

Although African Americans constitute the largest group of minority elders in the United States, persons of Hispanic origin are the fastest growing minority group and will surpass African Americans some time around 2028.

## AFRICAN AMERICAN ELDERS

African Americans have higher overall cancer rates and significantly lower survival rates than any other population group in the United States (Baquet & Gibbs, 1992). At every age, Blacks are at higher risk of developing diabetes than Whites (Johnson, 1991). Stroke deaths among Black males are nearly twice as high as those among White males, and coronary heart disease rates are twice as high in Black women as in White women. Black women over age 65 are at greater risk of hypertension than any other group in the United States (Report of the Special Committee on Aging, 1996; Hildreth & Saunders, 1992).

Older Blacks are much more likely to rate their health as fair or poor (48%) than older whites (28%), and are almost 50% more burdened by illness or injury that restricts daily activities (44 days per year versus 30

**TABLE 13.1 Percentage of Persons Age 65+ in U.S. by Race and Hispanic Origin**

| Population Category | 1990 | 2050 (Projected) |
|---|---|---|
| White | 84% | 64% |
| African-American | 8% | 12% |
| Hispanic-American | 6% | 16% |
| Asian/Pacific Islander | 2% | 7% |
| American Indian/Eskimo | 0.4% | 0.6% |

From U.S. Census Bureau, Population Projections of the United States, January, 2000 days) (AARP, 1989). For reasons not clearly understood, however, some analysts find evidence for a "crossover" phenomenon once Blacks reach age 75, that is, that remaining life expectancy is higher than that of Whites.

Although it is important to acknowledge and support ethnic food preferences, Black elders are susceptible to eating foods high in fat and sodium, including products such as bacon, sausage, pork, pig's feet, foods fried in animal fat, smoked foods, and pickled foods (AARP, 1989). Because Blacks are more likely than others to be salt-sensitive and have high blood pressure, it is important that sodium intake be limited. African Americans need to change more of their seasoning to products such as herbs, spices, lemon juice, garlic, pepper, and ginger.

African Americans are also disadvantaged by neighborhood grocery stores that are more likely to be well stocked with processed foods and short on fruits and vegetables. A high number of neighborhood fast-food restaurants do not offer low-income older Blacks very many healthy alternatives to high-fat and high-salt diets.

On the bright side, caregiving appears to be less of a mental health burden on Black grandmothers who are raising grandchildren in their households than White grandmothers. A study of 867 grandmothers reported that Black grandmothers are more likely to embrace raising grandchildren and consider this to be an important role in holding kin networks together (Pruchno & McKenney, 2002). Grandparent caregivers are increasing rapidly in the United States, reaching 2.4 million persons in 2000.

## HISPANIC AMERICAN ELDERS

Hispanic Americans comprise the second largest minority group in the United States, but they are soon to become the largest. They include Mexican Americans (54%), Cuban Americans (14%), Puerto Ricans (9%), and people from Central America, South America, and Spain (24%). Although the Hispanic populations share the Spanish language, there is much diversity in their dialects, their ability to speak English, and length of time spent in the United States.

Hispanics in general have high rates of heart disease, diabetes, and cancer, and certain subgroups disproportionately fall prey to poor eating habits, smoking, lack of exercise, and alcohol excess. Hispanics would benefit from eating a higher proportion of traditional foods that are rich in fiber and complex carbohydrates, such as chickpeas, fava, pinto beans, plantains, cassavas, sweet potatoes, taniers, mangoes, guavas, papayas, d corn tortillas (AARP, 1989).

In 1998, 29% of the Hispanic population aged 65 and older had finished high school, compared to 67% of the total older population; 5% of Hispanic older Americans had a bachelor's degree or higher, compared to 15% of all older persons.

AARP's National Eldercare Institute on Health Promotion (now defunct) conducted a study that examined the barriers to community health-promotion programs among primarily Spanish-speaking Hispanic elders. A list of significant barriers follows:

1. Many Hispanic elders are unfamiliar with senior citizens centers, while others who visit the centers find the programs to be culturally insensitive to Hispanic elders.
2. Hispanic physicians, followed by Spanish-speaking or bilingual health professionals, are preferred but are in short supply. The belief in folk medicine and the healing power of God can often result in the postponement of timely doctors' visits.
3. Lack of knowledge of, and experience in, the American health care system, compounded by financial limitations and lack of transportation, constitute a major barrier to timely health care services.
4. The most credible source of health information for Hispanic elders is Spanish-language television and radio—40% of Hispanic elderly speak Spanish only—followed by the extended family, churches, community groups, and Hispanic social clubs and organizations.

Health education programs need to involve the extended family, both in program development and implementation. Program presenters need to be sensitized to the spiritual beliefs and folk medicine of Hispanic elders and, when possible, to focus on ideas from both folk and Western medicine. The role of the *curandero,* a traditional healer who provides physical, psychological, social, and spiritual support for the Hispanic family (not just the individual), also needs to be understood and incorporated into health education programs. Curanderos believe that morbidity and mortality are associated with strong emotional states, like *biles* (rage) and *susto* (fright).

## ASIAN AND PACIFIC ISLANDER ELDERS

Asian and Pacific Island Americans encompass at least 16 ethnic and cultural groups, often with little in common in terms of language, culture, religion, and immigration history. The largest group of Asian old Americans is Chinese, followed by Japanese, Filipino, and other (Kor Asian Indian, Vietnamese, Cambodian, Laotian, Hmong, Thai, Pak and Indonesian). The largest group of Pacific Island Americans are Hawaiian and Samoan, followed by Polynesian, Micronesian, and Melanesian. There are many other smaller islands that could be included as well.

It is difficult to generalize within this diverse group. The poverty rates for older Japanese, Filipino, and Asian Indian Americans are low, while the poverty rates for older Southeast Asians are very high, reaching as high as 47% among the Hmong elders. Within this diverse group is the highest proportion of people with less than a ninth-grade education, and the highest proportion of those with a bachelor's degree or more.

Among Southeast Asian Americans, only 2% of the population is elderly because the refugee experience limited the number of elders who could immigrate, and as relative newcomers to America most have not reached age 65 since their arrival. At the other end of the spectrum are the Japanese elders, who currently constitute 7% of their population. The percentage of Japanese elders in America is expected to grow due to the current limitation on the immigration of younger persons from Japan.

After the Japanese attack on Pearl Harbor in 1942, 110,000 Japanese Americans living in the Western states were incarcerated. It is believed that many of these now elderly Japanese Americans tried to suppress their Japanese ancestry, often teaching their children to do the same. This is one example of the dramatic differences in the life experiences of older adults among the various Asian American and Pacific Islander ethnic groups.

Asian and Pacific Islander cultures traditionally emphasize the importance of family bonds and the unquestioned authority of elder family members. The extent to which younger family members abide by these traditional values and beliefs, however, is varied at best. In fact, among Southeast Asian American elders the traditional family roles are reversed. More than 85% of the elders live with younger family members who provide almost all of their economic and social support. This transfer of authority to the younger generation is one example of the difficulties that these elders have had in adapting to American culture.

In general, though, it appears that Asian American baby boomers still provide more caregiving support for their parents than other ethnicities, as evidence by Table 13.2. And yet the erosion of family caregiving support over the past decade has been revealed in other ways. Vietnamese elders, for example, are now being placed in nursing homes in America, something that was not condoned 15 years ago.

## NATIVE AMERICAN ELDERS

ive Americans are defined by the Bureau of the Census as American
ns, Eskimos, and Aleuts. As members of approximately 500 nations,

TABLE 13.2  Percentage of Persons Age 45–55 Caring for Parents by Ethnicity

| Ethnicity | % Providing Care |
| --- | --- |
| White | 19% |
| African American | 28% |
| Hispanic American | 34% |
| Asian American | 42% |

From In the Middle: A Report on Multicultural Boomers Coping with Family and Aging Issues, July 2001. AARP, Washington, DC.

tribes, bands, or villages, Native Americans are exceptionally diverse both culturally and linguistically.

Native Americans have the smallest percentage of adults living to age 65—only 5.4%, among all cultural groups. A 1981 study by the National Indian Council on Aging found that at age 45, reservation-dwelling Native Americans had the health characteristics of the average American at age 65. Urban-dwelling Native Americans had these elderly characteristics at age 55.

Because many do not live long enough to develop them, Native Americans have less heart disease and cancer than the general population, but more pneumonia, influenza, diabetes, accidents, chronic liver diseases, septicemia, gall bladder disease and hypertension (Butler et al., 1998). Since 1955 the Indian Health Service has focused its resources on treating infectious and acute diseases that occur in infancy through young adulthood, with few resources available for managing the chronic diseases of aging.

There is widespread poverty among Native Americans, and as late as 1984 25% of them lived in households without plumbing. Elderly Native Americans have had a work history of high levels of unemployment and low-wage jobs, with 65% having worked as semiskilled workers, unskilled workers, or farm workers. Only about 22% graduated from high school, and 12% have no formal education at all.

## NATIONAL ORGANIZATIONS WITH AN EMPHASIS ON MINORITY AGING

- AARP, Minority Affairs Program, 601 E Street, NW, Washington DC 20049; 800-424-3410; www.aarp.org.

- American Society on Aging, Diversity Programs, 833 Market Street, #511, San Francisco, CA 94103; 415-974-9630; www.asaging.org.
- Asian & Pacific Islander Health Forum, 942 Market Street, #200, San Francisco, CA 94102; 415-954-9988; www.apiahf.org.
- Asociacion Nacional Pro Personas Mayores, 234 E. Colorado Boulevard, #300, Pasadena, CA 91104; 626-564-1988.
- Association of Asian Pacific Community Health Organizations, 439 23rd Street, Oakland, CA 94612; 510-272-9536; www.aapcho.org.
- National Caucus and Center on Black Aged, Inc., 1220 L. Street, NW, #800, Washington, DC 20005; 202-637-8400.
- National Center on Minority Health and Health Disparities, NIH, 6707 Democracy Boulevard, MSC 5465, Bethesda, MD 20892–5465; 301-402-1366.
- National Hispanic Council on Aging, 2713 Ontario Road NW, Washington, DC 20009; 202-265-1288; www.nhcoa.org.
- National Indian Council on Aging, 10501 Montgomery Boulevard, NE, #210, Albuquerque, NM 87111; 505-292-2001; www.nicoa.org.
- Office of Minority Health Resource Center, P.O. Box 37337, Washington, DC 20013–7337; 800-444-6472; www.omhrc.gov.

# CULTURE

Culture has been defined as our entire nonbiological inheritance. Among those who believe that cultural differences among older adults are at least as important as socioeconomic differences are the academicians who refer to themselves as ethnogeriatricians. The field of ethnogeriatrics in health care focuses on the ability to provide health care in ways that are acceptable to older adults because they are congruent with their cultural backgrounds and expectations.

One topic of particular interest to ethnogeriatricians is the degree to which the acculturation of the older person—the incorporation of mainstream cultural values, beliefs, language, and skills—affects health care and health behavior. In other words, to what extent does identification with one's ethnicity or racial category, versus identification with mainstream culture, affect one's belief in allopathic medicine and the efficacy of scientific treatments; one's ability to work with a health care provider of a different cultural background; one's need for dependence on family for decision making in health care; one's belief in the control over health outcomes; and one's willingness to negotiate with a complex medical bureaucracy?

Communication between persons with different cultural identifications can be problematic. Some people prefer a slower pace of conversation in a health care setting, while others prefer a fast-paced conversation and expect to be interrupted. Some patients prefer close physical proximity when communicating with their health care provider, while others prefer the provider to be an arm's length away. Some cultures prefer eye contact, while others may consider this disrespectful. Some cultures value stoicism or mask their emotions with laughter or a smile, while others encourage open expression of pain, sorrow, and joy. The etiquette of touch, hand gestures, and finger pointing is highly variable across cultures. There is also a diversity of attitudes toward the subjects of death and dying, ranging from a preference for direct communication to the stance that these topics are inappropriate for discussion.

Communication is also hampered by the lack of appropriate foreign language access in medical clinics and health care settings around the country, as cited in the 2002 Institute of Medicine's Report on Unequal Treatment. This situation is particularly burdensome for Hispanic elderly because 40% do not speak English.

When offering health care, health education, disease prevention, or health promotion *programs* to minority or ethnic older adults, the following precautions are recommended by Dorfman (1991):

1. Ethnic communities need to establish their own health priorities and be involved in program development and implementation.
2. Factors affecting accessibility within a community must be identified and addressed.
3. Language should be familiar, nontechnical, concise, factual, and specific.
4. Nonprint formats, such as videotapes, audiotapes, slide shows, songs, games, and plays, should be encouraged.
5. Printed materials should use large type, be attractive, and make generous use of photographs and drawings of older peers.
6. Communication should acknowledge and incorporate cultural beliefs, and visual images should include familiar people, settings, and symbols.
7. Efforts toward cultural sensitivity must be sustained and reinforced over time

Just as there is diversity among cultural groups, there is diversity within cultural groups. A Spanish-speaking grandmother with little formal education may have little in common with an English-speaking, co educated, gay older male, though both came from Cuba and are present-ly living in Miami. Cultural insensitivity can just as easily come from stereotyping the older person's cultural affiliation as from ignoring their cultural affiliation completely. One's ethnic or minority identification may be tempered by education level, the primary language, religion, gen-der, year of immigration, and so forth.

When *communicating* with diverse older persons in a medical or com-munity health setting, cultural sensitivity may be enhanced by asking a series of questions:

1. In times of illness or need, to whom do you turn for health infor-mation or care?
2. What help or assistance do you expect from your family members?
3. Are there ideas that you grew up with that help you to explain your specific illness or health problem?
4. What types of traditional medicine, or alternative medicine, do you use?
5. Do your health beliefs or practices differ from what you find in medical care or community health settings?
6. What are your attitudes toward medicine in this country, and how soon in the course of an illness do you seek to access it?
7. What roles do traditional foods play in your health? Are these foods accessible and affordable?
8. What advice would you give to health care providers about your health care?

Nurses in particular appear to be paying attention to how to incorpo-rate cultural considerations into the health care they provide (Giger et al., 1997) and into the patient education materials they create (F. Wilson, 1996). For additional information on how culture and language affect the delivery of health care, go to the Web site www.diversityrx.org.

The Commonwealth Fund issued a report on Cultural Competence in Health Care (Betancourt & Carrillo, 2002), highlighting exemplary prac-tices. The Family Practice Residency Program at White Memorial Medical Center in Los Angeles provides 30 hours of cross-cultural training for all family practice residents that includes topics like the role of traditional healers. The state of Washington provides reimbursement for certified interpreters and translators for Medicaid beneficiaries, with eight lan-guages readily available. The Kaiser Permanente Medical Center in San Francisco encourages workplace diversity, on-site interpreters, and an emphasis on culturally competent care delivery. The Sunset Park Family Health Center Network at the Lutheran Medical Center in Brooklyn,

New York, trains Chinese-educated nurses to upgrade their clinical skills in order to pass state licensing exams, provides language and interpretation services, and celebrates various religious and cultural holidays.

## SOCIOECONOMIC STATUS

At retirement, the Black median household income is only 48% of the White median household income, and the Hispanic median household income only 40%. Social security benefits account for more than half of Black and about two thirds of Hispanic median household retirement income, in comparison to a little more than a third of white median household retirement income. Viewed another way, 8% of White older adults live in poverty, versus approximately 25% of Hispanic and Black older adults. This leads to a major question in sociology and health, as yet unanswered. In terms of health care and health behavior, which has more explanatory power, racial or ethnic differences or socioeconomic status?

One study, for instance, reported that regardless of ethnicity poor patients with less education do poorly after heart surgery. They are less likely to survive it or, if they do survive, will have a lower quality of life than persons more advantaged in terms of income and education level (V. Elliott, 2000). Persons of lower income and educational level seek treatment later in the course of the disease, are less likely to follow the treatment plan, and are more likely to cut back or discontinue medication because of its cost.

Type II diabetes patients who are disadvantaged by education and income are more likely to have problems reading prescription bottles, educational brochures, and nutrition labels. Consequently, they have more difficulty with blood-sugar control and more diabetes-related complications than persons with higher income and literacy levels (Schillinger et al., 2002).

Another study reported that lower socioeconomic status was more important than race in determining the quality of medical care for women with breast cancer (Bradley et al., 2002). A similar finding was cited in a different study, with more than half of the racial disparity in breast cancer screening of older adults explained by income and education (E. Schneider et al., 2002).

This same study, however, reported that racial differences were more important than socioeconomic differences when it came to eye examinations for patients with diabetes, administering beta-blocker medications after heart attacks, and following up after hospitalizations for menta' illness (E. Schneider et al., 2002). A study of Medicare patients reported that when patient income, education, and attitudes were controlled, only 46% of Black Medicare patients received flu shots, versus 68% of White Medicare patients (E. Schneider et al., 2001).

Yet a survey of 1,599 poor urban residents ("Urban Obstacles," 1996) revealed that economic factors alone impinge on good health habits. Twice as many low-income adults reported feeling worried about the safety of walking in their neighborhood as did higher-income adults, and they reported less access to safe parks or recreational facilities. Twice as many low-income respondents reported that fresh fruits and vegetables were not readily available where they shopped, and when they were available they cost too much. Another study of low-income versus high-income families reported that low-income families eat more processed foods and less fruits and vegetables, and pay more for what they eat ("Vanishing Inner-City Grocery Stores," 1996).

Although there are research studies on health care patterns and health behavior change that attempt to compare the influence of income and education levels versus racial and ethnic differences, they are definitely the exception rather than the rule.

## RURAL

In 1996, 52 million people, or 20% of the U.S. population, lived in rural areas. Among older adults the percentage is higher, with 25% residing in rural areas. Living in a rural area increases the probability of living in poverty; income levels for older rural families are about one third lower than those for older urban families.

The combination of lower income and rural living is associated with substandard and dilapidated housing; a larger number of health problems; greater likelihood of living in a community without a doctor, nurse, or medical facility; inadequate caregiving support complicated by the migration of children to cities in search of work; challenging transportation issues due to longer distances to drive to needed services, lack of public transportation, and poor roads; and greater likelihood of having an attitude of distrust toward the health care system, or to have been instilled with an attitude of independence and self-reliance and a reluctance to demand needed health services (HRSA, 2002).

Nurses, social workers, physicians, and other health professionals are in short supply in rural settings. This is due in part to health policies, such as lower reimbursements for health providers in rural settings, but also due to a lack of community and health care resources in many rural locations. Health professionals are concerned about locating in rural areas that may lack quality public schools, cultural opportunities, and sophisticated hospital equipment. Consequently, there are 10 internists per 100,000 population in rural areas, compared to 52 per 100,000 in urban areas (V. Elliott, 2001b).

Elderly persons who live in rural areas receive fewer services per home health care visit, and they have poorer health outcomes than their city-dwelling older adult counterparts (Schlenker et al., 2002). These findings may represent accommodation of rural home health providers to rural realities, such as the lower availability of certain health care personnel like physical therapists or longer travel distances.

On a variety of measures, rural populations are in poorer health and at higher risk for poor health due to harmful health behaviors. Adults living in rural areas are more likely to smoke and have limited activity levels due to chronic conditions (HRSA, 2002); be overweight ("Wisconsin Study," 1996); have a higher rate of self-reported depression and have a more negative self-appraisal of health (Thorson, 2000) than their counterparts in urban areas.

Rural elderly exhibit a larger number of medical problems than urban elderly, problems that also tend to be more severe (Coward & Lee, 1985). Rural elders are more likely than their urban counterparts to rate their health as poor or fair, to be heavy drinkers, and to *not* be "uniquely advantaged by embeddedness in strong, supportive kin networks" (Lee & Cassidy, 1986, p. 165), even though the rural stereotype of strong kin support suggests the contrary.

Inadequate accessibility of health care services makes it especially important that rural residents engage in prevention and health-promoting behavior. The adoption of health-promoting practices by older adults in rural areas may be enhanced through the encouragement of health care professionals. A survey of family and general practice physicians in rural Mississippi revealed that such encouragement is more likely if a staff person is assigned by the physician to preventive medicine education and if flow charts are used to direct physician attention to needed prevention activities (Bross et al., 1993).

## RURAL RESOURCES

The National Resource Center for Rural Elderly at the University of Missouri-Kansas City produces informational materials and a newsletter Contact Dr. Share Bane, Graduate Social Work Program, 4825 Troos Kansas City, MO 64110; 816-235-1026.

The Rural Assistance Center (RAC) makes referrals to federal and state agencies, provides publications, and serves as a clearinghouse for rural information. The RAC will be the repository of rural information on more than 225 different federal health programs and additional private programs. Searchable databases, Congressional bill tracking, and quarterly newsletters will be added by 2004. Contact the Rural Assistance Center, PO Box 9037, Grand Forks, ND 58202; 800-270-1898; or go to info@raconline.org. Inquiries can also be directed to the Health Resources and Services Administration's Office of Rural Health Policy at http://ruralhealth.hrsa.gov.

One Web site that provides information on rural health is sponsored by the National Rural Health Association: www.nrharural.org.

# GLOBAL

The major source of diversity in global aging is based on whether a country is economically developed or not. For example, there is almost a 20-year difference in life expectancy in Sweden versus India. In the more developed countries of the world, the population aged 65 and above rose from 8% to 14% of total population between 1950 and 2000 and is projected to rise to 26% by 2050 (AARP, 2001).

Population aging is occurring even more rapidly in some of the developing world. Due to a significant decline in fertility and an improvement in adult mortality in China, persons aged 65 and over now constitute about 7% of the population but are projected to rise to 13% by 2025 and to 25% by 2050. The population increase in other developing countries is much more modest. Nearly 5% of Indians are now aged 65 or older and are projected to rise to 8% in 2025 and 15% in 2050. Nearly 60% of the world's older population lives in less developed countries today, but this percentage is expected to rise to almost 80% in 2050 (AARP, 2001).

The increase in the percentage of older adults in developing countries may present additional challenges for the future. The economist Young-Ping Chen noted that "the developed countries got rich before they got old; the less developed countries are getting old before they have a chance to get rich" (AARP, 2001). Thus, the rise in the number of countries with old-age disability or survivors programs—from 33% in 1940 to 74% in 1999—may not keep pace with the growing number of older adults in developing countries. Conversely, these developing countries may have ɔ rely even more heavily on a less prosperous informal network of fam- and community to support their burgeoning older adult population.

In China, for instance, 70% of older adults are supported by their families, and only 16% rely on the government's troubled pension system. Yet China's traditional extended family is dispersing more rapidly than ever before, and adult children are now leaving their elderly parents to fend for themselves.

In 2001, Japanese life expectancy was the highest in the world. Women could expect to live to 85 years, and men to 78 years. About a quarter of the population was over the age of 60. Many other developed countries are not too far behind. As the number of working-age people for every older adult shrinks, we will learn about the magnitude of the economic strains this increasing dependency ratio will produce in developed countries. There is a potential, for instance, for conflict over funding for social security and health care for older adults versus a country's need to support public schools and unemployment benefits for younger adults.

In the United States, women could expect to live to 79.5 years, and men to 74 years in 2001. Though the country has been getting older, the United States is still absorbing many young immigrants. As a consequence, the dependency ratio of workers to older adults in the United States is declining more slowly.

## QUESTIONS FOR DISCUSSION

1. What makes the most analytical sense to you: One category for persons age 65 and above, or a separate category for the old-old? If there are to be separate categories after age 65 for analytical purposes, at what chronological age(s) would you separate older age group(s)? Explain your answer.
2. Women live longer, are better connected socially, and commit suicide less often in late life. On the other hand, they appear to have more health burdens and more financial burdens. Who is better off in America: older women or older men?
3. What are the advantages and disadvantages of the blurring of racial and ethnic categories that is now taking place in America?
4. Black elders appear to have the greatest amount of homogeneity among the four minority categories recognized by the U.S. Census Bureau. What advantages or disadvantages does this pose for researchers, clinicians, and community leaders?
5. In terms of the health care and health behavior of older adults, which do you believe has more explanatory power: racial or ethnic differences, or socioeconomic status? Justify your opinion.

6. If you were launching a health promotion program for older adults, what are some of the details you will need to consider that are unique to a rural setting?

7. Are there lessons that developed and developing countries can offer each other when it comes to the role of older adults in society? To the care of older adults in society?

8. Vietnamese elders are now being placed in nursing homes in America, something that was not condoned 15 years ago. From the perspective of Vietnamese adult child caregivers do you think this trend is a positive or negative contribution to their lifestyle? Why do you believe that?

# 14

# Public Health

Americans live about 30 years longer than they did a century ago, and most of this accomplishment is due to triumphs in public health, such as improvements in sanitation, water quality, air quality, hygiene, health education, and immunization. Public health differs from medicine in that it focuses on preventing disease and promoting health in whole populations rather than treating disease and injury in a single patient.

Most Americans today, however, have much less awareness of public health care in this country than they do of medical care. The best-known aspects of public health relate to the goals of maintaining clean water and a clean environment, food safety, and control of communicable disease. But these public health roles come to the attention of the public only when there is a threat to water or food safety or there is an outbreak of a drug-resistant infection.

Even less well-known to the public is the role that public health plays in gathering health information, conducting screenings and immunizations, providing health education, and conducting health interventions. These types of activities reflect public health's concern with a broad range of health factors that influence the quality of life of individuals, families, groups, and communities.

The public's lack of awareness of these endeavors is probably due to the fact that relatively little funding (miniscule in comparison to what we spend on medical care) is targeted to support these types of public health activities. Ironically, in 2003 when there was a modest infusion of federal funds into public health departments for bioterrorism preparedness cash-strapped state and local governments were forced to reduce the public health budgets for health education and health interventions.

Another factor that contributes to the anonymity of public health efforts in the areas of community health education and intervention is that its diminutive budget is focused on low-income young mothers, adolescents, and children. Public health has largely ignored aging adults, despite the steady increase in the average age of the American population. A recent report concluded that "The new challenge for public health is to develop a focus on healthy aging. . . . Inadequate resources and attention are focused on health promotion and prevention of disease or secondary disability for older adults, the very population that experiences the highest rates of chronic disease and disability" (Palombo et al., 2002).

The study authors also noted the lack of collaboration between public health departments that attempt to improve overall health in the community and the small network of practitioners in aging agencies who strive to improve the quality of life for aging persons. This raises the question: What if this collaboration between public health and aging was strengthened as well as backed by substantial resources?

Additional questions are then raised: How would public health foster healthy aging in American society? What policies and practices would it attempt to implement? How would additional funding be generated, and how would existing medical expenditures be reduced?

I will examine these questions next, beginning with the section that proposes the establishment of a Wellness General of the United States.

At the end of the previous edition of this book, in the final chapter, the concluding subsection is entitled "President Haber." In the last two paragraphs I proposed my health promotion platform for the country. It consisted of four sentences on three moderately controversial priorities: universal health care, reimbursement for health promotion that has proven to be effective, and federal resources to help promote more physical activity among Americans.

For this edition of my book, I expand my platform to dozens of proposals and escalate the controversial nature of some of them. I attribute this change to the aging process. I may or may not be growing wiser with age, but it does appear that I am growing bolder.

# WELLNESS GENERAL
# OF THE UNITED STATES

My first task as president will be to convert the position of the Surgeon General of the United States to Wellness General of the United States. The designation, *surgeon general*, refers to the chief medical officer of a military, state, or federal public health service. At the federal public health service level, the position of Surgeon General of the United States is filled by a physician selected by the President for the purpose of leading the nation toward better health. The physician primarily uses this office as a bully pulpit, exhorting policy makers, community leaders, and citizens toward healthier lifestyles.

The Wellness General of the United States will have new resources and responsibilities (Haber, 2002). The resources for wellness will be generated by a junk food tax. The responsibilities of the Wellness General will be: a) to strengthen wellness research, and b) to increase wellness utilization at the community, family, and individual level.

Before examining these two responsibilities, the term *wellness* and the generation of resources through a controversial junk food tax will be reviewed.

## WELLNESS

*Surgeon general* is a military term that can be disconcerting to advocates of wellness. The "general" part of the term may be accepted within the narrow definition of a leadership position. The word "surgeon," however, is not as easily salvageable. It is derived from the domain of medicine and narrowly linked to an operation or a manual procedure relating to physical disease or injury. *Wellness,* on the other hand, is a broader term that includes not only disease and injury, but health promotion and disease prevention; not only the physical realm, but the emotional, social, intellectual, and spiritual domains.

Although the term *wellness* has had many supporters in the health professions over the past 25 years (Jonas, 2000), it tends to be less recognized than the terms *health promotion* and *disease prevention.* Health promotion, also referred to in the medical domain as primary prevention, refers to mainstream interventions like exercise, nutrition, and stress management that have relevance to a variety of diseases or disabilities, and to immunizations that are targeted to prevent specific diseases.

Wellness, however, conveys one additional important message—that good health is more than physical well-being and that it is more than a response to actual or potential disease or disability. Ardell's (2000) definition is the most cogent: optimal health and life satisfaction that includes physical elements (exercise and nutrition), psychological aspects (stress management and emotional intelligence), social and intellectual elements (connectedness to significant others and passionate ideas) and spiritual components (seeking meaning and purpose in life).

Although exercise, nutrition, and stress management are the most familiar and practiced components of wellness (and its cousin, health promotion), it tends to be the more alternative activities—herbal medicine, chiropractic, acupuncture, massage therapy, spiritual healing, aroma therapy, relaxation techniques, self-help groups—that are associated with wellness. Perhaps this is due to the tremendous growth in these activities over the past decade and the significant amount of media attention devoted to them.

Because a wellness general will cover more territory than a surgeon general and have more responsibilities (to be examined later), it will be necessary to increase the stature and resources of the position. Stature can be increased by elevating the position to cabinet-level status, complementary to the Secretary of Health and Human Services. Resources can be increased by legislating a wellness budget.

## JUNK FOOD TAX

One way to create a budget for the Wellness General is to craft federal legislation that mandates a small tax on junk food—candy bars, cookie packages, cakes, pastries, ice cream, soda, corn chips, tortilla chips, potato chips, and the remaining high-fat, high-sugar or high-salt junk foods that constitute over 20% of Americans' calories. Jacobson and Brownell (2000) estimate that a national tax of one cent per 12-oz soft drink would generate about $1.5 billion annually, and one cent per pound of candy, chips, and other snack foods would raise more than $100 million annually.

This is not a strategy without controversy. The main argument against junk food taxes is that the government should not pry into people's personal business. A *Washington Post* editorial (11/15/99), for instance, belittled then Agriculture Secretary Dan Glickman, who had reported "it is the government's role to guide Americans into adopting a healthier lifestyle." The editor of the *Post* argued that we should tackle obesity and inactivity with common sense and self-discipline, rather than expecting government to do it for us. The editor also asserted that a tax on unhealthy foods "sounds like something the government-always-knows-best social engineers in Washington, D.C., could feast upon." Other newspaper editors have agreed that a tax on junk food is a bad idea (J. Jacoby, 1998).

Civil liberty concerns are raised as well. Wellness advocate Donald Ardell asks "Don't we have a right to choose what we eat? Should we also tax those who do not exercise enough? What about those with no sense of humor? Now there's a group to sock with a big tax hit! (personal communication)."

Those opposed to junk food taxes ask: If government gets more involved with promoting individual health will it interfere with individual freedom and personal responsibility (D. Callahan, 2000)? Those in favor of junk food taxes respond: If government gets involved successfully, the resulting wellness outcomes will enhance individual freedom and responsibility as well as the interests of society. These opinions and values are difficult to reconcile.

Philosophical concerns aside, there are 'sin' taxes that work. As noted in chapter 9 on Other Health Education Topics, cigarette taxes reduce smoking and are followed by a reduction in lung cancer rates ("Voters allow hefty cigarette tax," 2000; "State tobacco programs are effective," 2000; Pechacek, 2000). It may be unreasonable to also assume, however, that junk food taxes will reduce the consumption of junk foods. There is little doubt that these foods are unhealthy and costly to our health care system—with a conservative estimate of $70+ billion annually for diet-related diseases (Frazao, 1999). But food consumption habits are probably shaped more by advertising dollars than by food taxes. And unlike tobacco products, there are no regulations to curb food product advertising.

Quite the opposite situation exists, in fact. McDonald's marketing budget in 1999 was $1.1 billion. Coca cola's was $866 million (Jacobson, 2000). Many billions of advertising dollars encouraged the consumption of high-fat, high-sugar, and high-salt products in 1999. In contrast to this spending spree, the National Cancer Institute spent $1 million in 1999 to promote its 5-a-Day (fruits and vegetables) campaign (Jacobson & Brownell, 2000).

Even if a junk food tax could counter the effect of advertising and lower the consumption of junk food, wholesalers and retailers could regain sales levels by absorbing the tax burden through price reductions. And if the taxing authority countered these price reductions with additional tax increases, low-income persons would bear the highest tax burden (Marshall, 2000).

The implementation of small, not very burdensome taxes on junk food, however, could be instituted for the purpose of raising revenue rather than curbing consumption. Nineteen states and cities in the United States and seven provinces and the federal government of Canada levy taxes on nutritionally deficient foods such as soft drinks, candy, chewing gum, potato chips, and so forth. (Jacobson & Brownell, 2000). Nationally, these special taxes on junk foods generate about $1 billion a year.

Much of these tax revenues, though, are spent on non-health activities. Another problem is that raising taxes on junk food at the state, county, or city level—no matter how modest—can provoke junk food industries to fight back. In response to industry threats or incentives (e.g., not build, or to build, manufacturing or distribution centers), 12 cities, counties, or states have reduced or repealed their junk food taxes (Jacobson & Brownell, 2000).

It makes more sense, therefore, to implement junk food taxes at the federal level, rather than at a lower level of government. It also makes more sense to implement junk food taxes for the purpose of implementing community wellness programs that have undergone research scrutiny (Reger et al., 2000), than for the purpose of reducing the consumption of junk food or raising revenue for nonhealth purposes.

## STRENGTHEN WELLNESS RESEARCH

One of the two primary responsibilities of the Wellness General will be to strengthen wellness research (left side of Figure 14.1). Wellness, health promotion, and disease prevention have not been high research priorities in the American research community (Woolf & Johnson, 2000). Moreover, the research that has taken place has been scattered among the various institutes of the National Institutes of Health and other funding sources. The wellness movement will benefit, therefore, if funding for research is not only increased through a budget generated by a junk food tax, but consolidated into and coordinated through one of the institutes of health.

A good candidate to house wellness research is the National Institutes of Health's National Center for Complementary and Alternative Medicine (see chapter 8 on Complementary and Alternative Medicine), which should be renamed the National Center on Wellness.

## THE NATIONAL CENTER ON WELLNESS

The Wellness General of the United States will play the leadership role in the conversion of the National Center for Complementary and Alternative Medicine into the National Center on Wellness (NCW). The NCW will continue to fund research on complementary and alternative medicine therapies like acupuncture, dietary supplements, and homeopathy. It will place additional emphasis, however, on research to improve the utilization of more proven mainstream therapies like exercise, nutrition, immunizations, and smoking cessation. These interventions are still not practiced widely enough (McGinnis & Foege, 1993).

## UNITED STATES PREVENTION SERVICES TASK FORCE

The National Wellness Center will not only fund mainstream and alternative research topics, it also will be coordinated with the United States

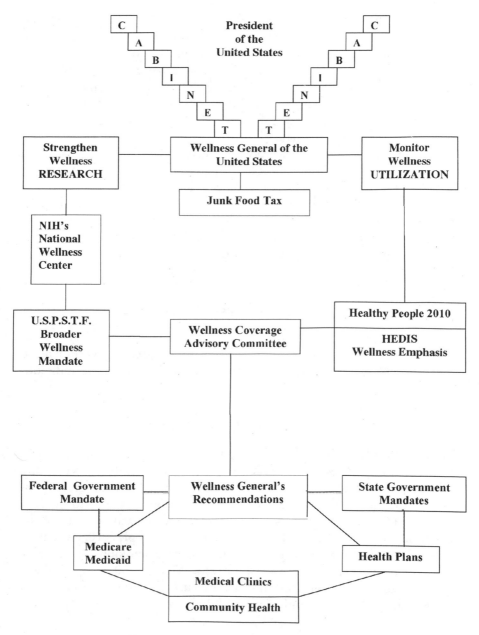

FIGURE 14.1   Wellness General of the United States.

Preventive Services Task Force (USPSTF). The USPSTF published *The Guide to Clinical Preventive Services* (USDHHS, 1996), the definitive resource manual on evidence-based recommendations for prevention services (see chapter 3 on Clinical Preventive Services). The Wellness General will expand the content of this guide from a focus on prevention services to a broader range of wellness interventions, will summarize their research findings in general every 4 years and, most important, will help link research recommendations to practice.

The link between research recommendations and practice has been lacking ("Medicare patients," 2000; Firman & Holmes, 1999; USDHHS, 1998), despite the fact that *The Guide to Clinical Preventive Services* has been a well-respected evidence-based document for decisionmaking. To correct this oversight, the Wellness General will link the recommendations of the *Guide* to the practical reimbursement decisions recommended by the Wellness Coverage Advisory Committee (this committee will be examined later as a wellness utilization strategy).

## INCREASE WELLNESS UTILIZATION

The second goal of the Wellness General of the United States will be to increase wellness utilization at all levels of society, from government, to insurance, to work, to community, to clinics, to family, and to individuals (right side of Figure 14.1).

## HEALTHY PEOPLE 2010

Healthy People 2010 (USDHHS, 2000) is a public-private effort to promote health over the decade 2000 to 2010 (see chapter 1, Introduction). Although health goals are established, data compiled, and progress monitored, the financial support to achieve Healthy People 2010 goals is missing. This same limitation was an obstacle to the achievement of the ambitious goals set by the earlier initiative, Healthy People 2000. Percentage rates of physical inactivity, obesity, and cigarette smoking stayed fairly constant or even increased over the decade 1990 to 2000. The Wellness General will need to set priorities that are *backed by financial support* in order to help Healthy People 2010 achieve its wellness goals.

## HEDIS

In the private sector the National Committee for Quality Assurance (NCQA) is a nonprofit watchdog of managed care organizations that also provides them with accreditation. Each year NCQA issues a report card on the quality of managed health care plans that is derived from its Health Plan Employer Data and Information Set (HEDIS).

HEDIS is based on 50 performance measures, only a few of which are wellness activities. The Wellness General will encourage NCQA to expand the number of wellness services to be evaluated under HEDIS and to measure whether managed care organizations are effectively reaching out to beneficiaries and increasing the utilization rate of these wellness services (Asch et al., 2000).

## WELLNESS COVERAGE ADVISORY COMMITTEE

The Wellness Coverage Advisory Committee (WCAC) will make reimbursement recommendations to the Wellness General based on: a) the strength of the research findings supported by the National Wellness Center, b) the summary of these research findings and the recommendations made by the United States Preventive Services Task Force, and c) the percentage of persons engaged in specific wellness activities as documented by the Healthy People 2010 initiative and the HEDIS performance measures.

The WCAC will be derived from the Medicare Coverage Advisory Committee (MCAC). MCAC was created in 1998 to evaluate new therapies and to recommend to the Centers for Medicare and Medicaid Services (formerly the Health Care Financing Administration) whether to reimburse new treatments as part of the Medicare program (Cys, 2000). The Wellness General will convert the MCAC into the WCAC, and will expand their mandate to evaluate a broader base of wellness interventions. Reimbursement decisions for specific interventions will be mandatory at the federal level, but recommendations will also be forwarded to state governments and to the private sector, particularly to managed care organizations.

The WCAC will employ an additional innovation—the recruitment of consumers into advocacy roles on its committee. These consumer advocates will make sure that the research on a new wellness therapy has relevance to low-income individuals and other underserved elements of the population, including the assessment of a wellness therapy's potential for utilization by the underserved in the government and private sectors.

## WELLNESS GENERAL REPORTS

The Wellness General will continue in the tradition of the Surgeon General and attempt to publish a major report each year or two in order t heighten America's awareness of important public health issues. The *Surgeon General's Report on Tobacco* in 1964, for instance, summarized the research on the health hazards of tobacco use and many analysts believe it was a major factor in the 50% reduction in tobacco use that took place over the next three decades. The 1979 *Surgeon General's Report on Health Promotion and Disease Prevention* became one of the most, if not *the* most, widely cited documents on the role that risk factors play in morbidity, mortality, and medical costs. This report also helped launched the Healthy People 1990 initiative and subsequently the Healthy People 2000 and 2010 initiatives.

In 1996 the *Surgeon General's Report on Physical Activity and Health* did an excellent job of summarizing the research on the importance of moderate-intensity physical activity or exercise, the value of accumulating activity or exercise over the course of a day, the importance of resistance training along with aerobic exercise, and the utility of establishing an exercise habit of 30 minutes a day, most days of the week. (I hope this recommendation will outlast the federal guideline promoted by the Institute of Medicine in 2002, which recommended an unrealistic—for most persons—60 minutes of exercise every day of the week).

The *Surgeon General's Report on Mental Health* in 1999 reported on the surprising prevalence of depressive symptoms among older adults and the inability of health professionals to identify and treat this problem. It also highlighted the reimbursement discrepancy between mental health and physical health problems. (For additional information on these Surgeon General's reports, access the Web site www.surgeongeneral.gov).

The Wellness General will not only continue this important educational mission, but it will also disseminate these reports to academic faculty who are training health care professionals, to health insurance administrators who are establishing health insurance policies, and to health practitioners who are implementing programs in medical clinics and community health organizations.

## WELLNESS IN MANAGED CARE

Fee-for-service health insurance plans may continue to resist coverage for wellness services. Physicians, in turn, may continue to routinely lie on insurance forms, claiming that patients who saw them for prevention and health promotion purposes were being treated for medical problems so that the insurer would cover the cost of the visit (Brody, 2000b). Managed care health insurance, on the other hand, with its tremendous growth at the end of the last millennium and an alleged emphasis on disease prevention and health promotion, ought to be more receptive.

The Wellness General of the United States, however, needs to restore the promise of a wellness emphasis in managed care. During much of the 1990s, the promise was partially realized while enrollment greatly expanded. Between 1991 and 1997, Medicare beneficiary enrollment in managed care plans rose from 6% to 16%. Between 1992 and 1996 managed care enrollment among U.S. workers increased by 35% ("Managed care strives," 1998). By 1997, 85% of all United States workers were enrolled in some form of managed care.

Since 1997, though, the promise of wellness in managed care has been diminished under the shadow of medical costs that are rising rapidly once again. Wellness, health promotion, and preventive care programs have not expanded beyond token offerings. Prescription coverage has also been greatly curtailed. And managed care plans have been losing money or terminating business. Of 506 HMOs examined in 1997, 57% lost money (Jacob, 1998). Managed care organizations that had been making a profit for years reported their first losses ever in 1997. By 2000, managed care insurance companies claimed that payment rates were increasingly inadequate and bureaucratic obstacles remained high (Landers, 2000).

Regarding Medicare managed care, federal payments were not adequate to cover the cost of caring for older adults. Consequently, between 1998 and 2003, 2.4 million Medicare managed care beneficiaries had to find other sources of health care coverage. The Wellness General will need to restore wellness services to managed care in order to help offset its image as the management of costs and profits, rather than the management of quality care.

## STATE MANDATES

Based on studies documenting the cost-effectiveness of wellness interventions (Colditz, 1999), the Wellness General will encourage state governments to follow the federal government's lead and mandate wellness insurance benefits. One such study, a national survey of community-dwelling Medicare beneficiaries, reported that improved client health behaviors lowered Medicare costs (Stearns et al., 2000). Similar results have been obtained in the managed care sector. Positive changes in physical activity, weight management, and smoking cessation among beneficiaries significantly lowered health plan expenditures within 18 months (Pronk et al., 2000).

Insurance companies may remain unconvinced, however, that wellness interventions can take effect quickly enough to benefit their bottom line, given the instability of beneficiaries (Brody, 2000b). Insurance plans do not want to invest in the health of clients who become healthier members of a save money for, their next health care plan. The Wellness General can circumvent this barrier by recommending state mandates that require *all* health plans to include comprehensive *or* specific types of wellness coverage.

The first and only state-mandated comprehensive wellness program, the New Jersey Health Wellness Promotion Act (NJHWP), was implemented on November 6, 2000. The NJHWP required most managed care and fee-for-service insurers in New Jersey to provide health and wellness treatments. Health plans in New Jersey initially opposed the legislation, attempting to mandate extra fees for plans that adopt wellness activities. Their opposition stalled the program for 7 years until they were successful in establishing a financial cap of $220. The state was expected to adjust this cap based on inflation, new scientific evidence, and the decision of an advisory board.

Other state health insurance mandates have primarily taken the form of mandatory coverage for specific cancer-screening tests (Schauffler, 2000). In 1999, 43 states and the District of Columbia mandated coverage for cancer screenings (Rathore et al., 2000). In contrast to the enthusiasm for cancer screenings, few states mandate coverage of counseling or behavioral interventions to address unhealthy behaviors like tobacco use, alcohol use, sedentary behaviors, and poor nutritional habits (D. Nelson et al., 2002).

State mandates that are narrowly focused on medical screenings for cancer are influenced more by medical lobbyists rather than by evidence-based guidelines and recommendations (Schauffler, 2000). Even within the arena of medical screenings for cancer, questionable state mandates have been implemented. It is unclear why more states (n = 27) mandate coverage of prostate cancer screening than of colorectal cancer screening (n = 17), despite the fact that there is stronger evidence for the benefits of screening for colorectal cancer.

To counteract medical lobbyists who encourage federal and state legislators to cover medical screenings with minimal additional health benefits, the Wellness General's recommendations to both public and private health plans will be based on the recommendations of the Wellness Coverage Advisory Committee.

## LINKING MEDICAL CLINICS AND COMMUNITY HEALTH

Health insurance primarily covers treatments in hospitals and medical clinics. Unfortunately, the link between these medical institutions and community health programs barely exists. The Wellness General of the United States will strengthen this relationship.

American adults visit or consult with their physician on a regular basis, and the older they get the more frequent the contact. In 1998 the average Medicare beneficiary visited or consulted with physicians 13 times during the year (Federal Interagency Forum on Aging-Related Statistics, 2000). On the basis of access alone, therefore, it is a good idea to involve medical clinics in the wellness of Americans.

In addition, medical personnel can be persuasive when it comes to recommending lifestyle changes. An attempt to quit smoking, for instance, is "twice as likely to occur among smokers who receive nonsmoking advice from their physicians compared with those who are not advised to quit" (Glynn, 1990). If every primary care provider offered a smoking cessation intervention to smokers, it is estimated that an additional one million persons would quit each year.

Unfortunately, clinic staff rarely find the time for even brief wellness counseling, much less to provide adequate patient education and sufficient follow-up. In this era of health care cost containment, patient health education at the medical clinic site is a scarce commodity. It is more feasible and affordable, therefore, if clinicians refer clients to less expensive health education specialists or even trained peer leaders who conduct community-based health programs.

These community-based programs are likely to be more accessible, affordable, and effective when embedded in trusted institutions like the church, the school, and the senior center; and more likely to be affordable and sustained when led by trained peers who provide ongoing social support. One model program named the Chronic Disease Self-Management Program was evaluated through a 6-month randomized controlled trial. Almost 1,000 adults at churches, community centers, and other sites completed a 15-hour, 6-week wellness program. The program cost $70 per participant and saved $750 per participant, primarily through fewer days in the hospital (Lorig et al., 1999).

Another model program, the Senior Wellness Project, involved 201 adults and was also tested through a randomized controlled trial. The program cost $300 per participant and saved $1,200 per participant (Leveille et al., 1998). Given the government's emphasis on revenue-neutral legislation, "evidence of effectiveness should be supplemented when possible by information on cost-effectiveness (USDHSS, 1996, p. xcii).

The Wellness General will establish guidelines for medical clinics and community health programs on not only which services are reimbursable, but also on client eligibility for wellness services, criteria for provider expertise, and intervention content—including length and periodicity of interventions (Haber, 2001a). Coverage policies will be updated to reflect the latest scientific evidence and to emphasize the need to reach low-income and other underserved components of the patient population.

The link between community health programs and medical settings is essential. Even seemingly benign wellness interventions, such as a walking program, can impact on medications and alter physiological parameters that affect medical treatment.

## AN OPPOSING POINT OF VIEW (SORT OF)

Fire the Wellness General! Get government off our backs! If the government is going to be involved in health promotion at all, let it focus on the social, environmental, and particularly the economic contexts in which health behaviors are shaped. Improve living conditions, and health behaviors will follow suit. Give individuals freedom and self-responsibility instead of creating a backlash against health-promoting initiatives through government meddling.

Hire a Wellness General and where will Big Brother intrude next? Should government encourage a downhill skier to take a 30-minute walk instead? Should government add to the stigmatization of overweight Americans by singling them out for ineffective interventions? Should government encourage insurance plans to be punitive toward smokers? If so, should it add overweight people, sedentary people and, oh yes, those pesky downhill skiers to the list of scofflaws?

If this argument and these questions appeal to you, read Daniel Callahan's (2000) *Promoting Healthy Behavior: How Much Freedom? Whose Responsibility?*

Shortly after reading Callahan's book, I read *Food Politics* (Nestle, 2002) and *Fast Food Nation* (Schlosser, 2001). And another set of questions rose in my mind: Is it fair that the food and drink industries spend billions of dollars a year advertising high-fat, high-sugar, and high-salt products, and yet the federal government spends a few million on nutrition education? Or as stated by Kelly Brownell, Director of Yale University's Center for Eating and Weight Disorders "The entire federal budget for nutrition education is equal to one-fifth of the advertising costs for Altoids mints."

Is it fair that diet-related diseases result in $70 billion in annual medical expenditures (Frazao, 1999), and that sedentary behaviors may cost even more, while more than 41 million Americans cannot afford health care insurance? Is it fair that research on increased physical activity and exercise reports an almost miraculous effect on disease protection and improved functionality, and yet we do so little to dislodge Americans from sitting in front of their television sets and computer screens?

And was it *un*fair that the federal government played such an important role (or meddled, depending on your point of view) in reducing the number of Americans who smoked cigarettes by 50%, in less than three decades?

Clearly, this is no longer an opposing view. Read on if you are willing to be politically incorrect (in the era of "get big government off of our backs") and endorse a big-government role in the promotion of healthy aging in our society.

## AND NOW FOR THE REST OF THE WELLNESS GENERAL'S PLATFORM

### UNIVERSAL HEALTH CARE COVERAGE

In 2001, 41.2 million Americans, or 15% of the population, lacked health care coverage. Apparently we treat health care as a privilege in this country and are willing to tolerate a huge number of uninsured people. Ironically, the only Americans who are guaranteed health care coverage (even Medicare beneficiaries must be able to afford premiums and deductibles) are prison inmates. One California inmate, in fact, received a million dollar heart transplant. The right to access health care, however, does not extend toward nonconvicts.

I believe health care coverage should be a right for all Americans, not just prisoners, and that the federal government should provide universal health care. In my opinion, the major barrier to accomplishing this goal is more financial than it is philosophical or political. It is hard to contemplate an expansion of health care coverage to all Americans when spending on health care nationwide almost doubled during the 1990s without universal coverage. This growth in health care costs during the decade topped out at $1.3 trillion in the year 2000, and the increase in health care costs in the last year of the decade was the largest 1-year jump in 12 years (Landa, 2002).

Despite the rapid growth in health care costs during the 1990s, it was a pretty good decade compared to the previous one, in terms of health care cost containment. There was double-digit growth in the 1980s, while the highest growth rate in the 1990s was "only" 7% from 1999 to 2000.

But there is still much to be concerned about. Outpatient prescription drug spending increased at double-digit growth throughout much of the

1990s, peaking at a 17.3% increase from 1999 to 2000. Also, health care spending is now outpacing the growth of the economy, which was not the case throughout much of the 1990s. And Medicare, which now consumes 12% of the federal budget, is projected to rise to 25% by 2025 (and this does not include costs that would be associated with a new prescription drug benefit), thanks to the escalating eligibility of baby boomers.

In order to provide universal health care, medical care spending must be brought under control. The problem of escalating medical costs is not only getting worse, but the baby boomers are poised for retirement in less than a decade and the problem will soon be of catastrophic proportions. Our political leaders, however, create policies that allow us to limp along until the end of their term, ignoring the growing problem of higher health care costs and fewer citizens covered by health insurance.

As we wait for political leaders who will implement universal health care, I suggest the following actions in the near-future: a) Because people live longer and healthier, we need to accelerate raising the retirement age (scheduled to rise to age 66 in 2008, and age 67 in 2017) to age 70 by 2017; b) In order to increase revenues, wealthier retirees should pay higher premiums and cost-sharing; c) To cover low-income and uninsured patients, we need to increase community health center funding so that it provides a minimum package of medical care for all citizens. This action can be supplemented at the state or federal level with policies that waive liability insurance and registration fees for retired physicians who are willing and able to help out at these 3,300 community health centers, or at the estimated 250 free clinics nationwide; d) To reduce the fastest growing expenditure area—pharmaceutical costs—we need to reduce the cost of pharmaceuticals rather than focus most of our attention on prescription drug coverage under Medicare.

In this last regard, an eight-state survey of community-dwelling older adults reported that 23% spent at least $100 per month on their medications in 2001, and 22% reported skipping medications or not filling prescriptions due to costs (Safran et al., 2002). I propose the following steps: 1. Eliminate loopholes for patented medications that delay the cost-effective generics from coming to the market. 2. Follow the actions of West Virginia and Michigan and encourage states to hire their own counterdetailers to visit physicians and persuade them to prescribe generics whenever possible. 3. Prohibit the advertisement—to the tune of $2.5 billion in 2001—of (expensive, new) prescription drugs, based on the evidence that advertising promotes the purchase of unnecessarily expensive medications (as well as unnecessary medications) over generics (Bell et al., 1999; Landers, 2001). 4. Instead of offering rebates to pharmacy benefit managers to promote large-scale consumer usage of their medications, have drug manufacturers redirect the rebates to consumers rather than to the middlemen.

Paradoxically, instead of a movement to reduce medical costs and close the gap between the insured and the 41.2 million uninsured in America, progress is being made toward increasing medical costs and creating another tier of medical care for the well off. Boutique medicine, also referred to as a concierge-style practice, is being developed in places around the country in order to offer higher-level care (such as additional health promotion and disease prevention services, quicker access or even same day service, and more time allowed with the physician) to patients who can afford higher fees.

## MANAGED CARE

Managed care organizations are prepaid medical organizations with fixed budgets that rely on incentives or controls for providers and patients in order to contain costs. In exchange for the limitations that are placed on their choice of health providers and health institutions, and for their willingness to have their need for more expensive specialized medical care monitored, managed care patients expect to be the beneficiaries of higher quality care at lower cost. Another aspect of managed care associated with higher quality care and lower cost, theoretically at least, is a greater emphasis on health promotion, disease prevention, and early detection of disease.

Managed care was given much of the credit for the decline in health care costs in the 1990s. Annual inflation of health care costs had reached a high of 16% in 1981 and stayed in double-digits for the rest of the 1980s. However, as the era of managed care took hold in the 1990s there was a steady decrease in the medical inflation rate, reaching a low of 4.4% in 1996 ("Managed Care Cited," 1998), the lowest rate since health spending trends were first compiled in 1960. Managed care enrollment rose steadily from 1992 to 1999, more than doubling during that time frame.

By the end of 1999, however, managed care costs were steadily increasing, and the number of managed care organizations and enrollees were on the way back down. Over the next 2 years, there was a 16% drop in the number of managed care organizations and a 3% drop in managed care enrollees. By 2003, the fortunes of managed care organizations were starting to cycle back, and they were becoming profitable again. This was accomplished by substantially increasing the cost burden to employees through increased premiums and copayments. There were similar disturbing trends in Medicare managed care.

Medicare managed care began with the 1982 Tax Equity and Fiscal Responsibility Act, which allowed Medicare enrollees to join federally accredited managed care alternatives. Enrollment growth in Medicare managed care was quite slow in the 1980s, and only began to increase rapidly between 1993 and 1996, averaging about a 30% increase per year. Medicare managed care appeared to be working, offering limited prescription medication coverage and a smidgen of prevention to attract new converts, while holding costs. There was considerable speculation, though, that these results were being maintained only as long as Medicare managed care focused on the youngest and healthiest of the older population.

The speculation proved to be accurate. The association between Medicare managed care and cost containment was short-lived. By 2002, as beneficiaries aged and prescription costs skyrocketed, Medicare managed care was costing more than traditional Medicare, and the beneficiaries were feeling the financial pinch as well. Out-of-pocket costs for Medicare managed care enrollees increased by 50% between 1999 and 2001. The number of older adults in Medicare managed care was reduced by 1.7 million during this time.

Most managed care plans, Medicare or otherwise, are investor-owned, and executives are required to maximize profits within the limits of the law. This fiduciary responsibility created an incentive for managed care plans to seek healthier enrollees, and to limit services to those with serious disease and functional limitations (Angell, 1997).

As I noted in an earlier book (Haber, 1989), "Adverse selection occurs when a disproportionate percentage of Medicare enrollees require medical services. The negative impact of adverse selection may be even greater in the future when Medicare managed care enrollees no longer tend to be healthier than the general Medicare population" (p. 11). And so it went.

As beneficiaries aged and costs escalated, the vision of managed care as a population-based preventive care strategy dimmed as well. Managed care businesses became increasingly concerned about short-term profits, while preventive medicine became an increasingly irrelevant long-term strategy.

Almost 2.5 million beneficiaries were dropped by Medicare managed care organizations between 1998 and 2003. And many of the remaining beneficiaries were finding out that managed care was becoming no different than traditional Medicare—no coverage for prescription drugs, minimal prevention benefits, and rising premiums.

Managed care versus fee-for-service care is, in my opinion, a red herring issue: it distracts attention from the real issue. Instead of focusing on the advantages and disadvantages of managed care versus fee for service health care systems, we should concentrate on one unified health care system that is available to all. The trick of course is to develop a system with an ongoing focus on improvement in quality care and monitoring and controlling costs.

A free market health care system does not accomplish these goals. Additional costs for advertising competing health care plans or for maximizing profits does not spur improvement in quality. It does stimulate even greater costs—for the administration of diverse health care plans. In this regard, Sweden, with its single payer system, can provide cost-savings for physicians who link to its one system for implementing electronic medical records. Thus, 90% of their physicians do so. In the United States, however, which lacks a single payer system, only 17% of physicians use a cost-effective electronic medical record (Chin, 2002b). Instead, we have hundreds of payment systems requiring untold costs in training and deployment of personnel to sort through all the unique regulations.

Not only does competition raise costs in the health care industry, it is impossible for the health consumer to figure out which plan among the competing health care plans is the best one to suit their needs. Even if consumers were given educational assistance in this regard, they would have to be clairvoyant to know which health care plan will best meet their upcoming medical needs.

Finally, how do you get competitive health plans to provide coverage for the sickest and oldest people? Though it may be possible to design such a free-market solution guaranteeing coverage to the most vulnerable citizens, no one has done it yet.

The question is not whether health care needs to be managed, but how to manage it well. Universal health care coverage will be an important milestone in this journey.

## LONG-TERM CARE

Long-term care is part of the final chapter in most people's life histories. It refers to the personal care and assistance needed on a chronic basis due to disability or illness that limits the ability of the individual to function independently. Perhaps the ideal goal for long-term care was articulated best by William Thomas, the founder of the Eden Alternative, who stated that we should seek community-based long-term care developed on a cornerstone of love (Thomas, 1996).

The actuality of long-term care, however, is predicated on institutional care, which is based on rigid control over resident routines and on safety regulations. As noted by Kane (2001), the "bulk of [long-term care] public dollars go where older people do not want to go." Despite the overwhelming preference of older Americans to remain in their own homes, we spend 80% of public dollars on the care provided by nursing homes. Regarding the perception of the quality of the care provided in these nursing homes, almost 30% of a sample of seriously ill older persons reported that they would rather die than move permanently to a nursing home (Mattimore et al., 1997).

Two thirds of the nation's 17,000 nursing homes are for-profit homes, which tend to be less concerned about quality of care and more concerned about keeping costs down and profits up (Harrington et al., 2001). One example of this is the Evergreen Gridley Health Care Center in Northern California. In 2002, an investigation reported that they spent an average of $1.91 per day to feed residents, about $1 a day less than California spent on food for inmates in state medical prisons. It is also about $2 a day less than the U.S. Department of Agriculture cites as the minimum necessary for a nutritious diet for older adults (Schmitt, 2002).

What *are* the options? Remaining in one's own home is probably the ideal way to provide long-term care for most people, but it is predicated on in-home assistance that is hard to find and even harder to afford. In the absence of this gold standard for long-term care, there are three congregate options that may be more realistic than home care and more humane than nursing home care. They too are not without their challenges.

1. Assisted Living. Assisted living is long-term housing with *private* bedrooms and the provision of meals, social activities, and assistance with activities that residents can no longer perform themselves. Assisted living is growing rapidly and consists of many ways to combine housing options and needed services. The attraction of assisted living is that it allows consumers to maintain what they prize most: to organize their day with as much autonomy and dignity as possible. The owners of assisted living facilities have more autonomy too. And while this can lead to more innovative care options, it can also lead to deficiencies in the quality of care and consumer protection.

The challenge for assisted living is that it needs to be an affordable option to those who want to choose it over a more institutionalized nursing home setting. There also needs to be a way to discourage assisted living facilities from transferring residents when the first signs appear that their health care needs are becoming increasingly burdensome.

2. Nursing *Homes* (not institutions). There are long-term care settings that emphasize quality of life over regulations and safety. The Eden Alternative, with its emphasis on pets, plants, and caring relationships (Thomas, 1996), is at the forefront of this movement. A radical remake of

the nursing home industry along the lines of the Eden Alternative, however, will be slow and difficult. Over the past decade about 300 nursing homes, less than 2%, have adopted some aspects of the Eden Alternative.

Pets, plants, and children will not only make nursing homes more attractive to residents, but they should also make them more attractive to staff. And the recruitment and retention of good staff is at the heart of quality care in nursing homes. Unfortunately, there is a crisis in this regard in nursing homes today. About 90% of nursing homes have too few workers per patients (Pear, 2002).

3. PACE (Programs of All-Inclusive Care for the Elderly). This integrated model of care targets individuals who are eligible for nursing home care, but are able to live in the community with the help of PACE supportive services. By combining Medicare dollars, state Medicaid funds, and individual personal resources, a more comprehensive range of services is provided, including prevention. Services and resources can be targeted toward the home (like grab bars and ramps), or provided at adult day health centers.

The adult day health center is the heart of the PACE program. It includes a health care clinic, occupational and physical therapy services beyond what traditional Medicare or Medicaid would provide, and various other resources. The average PACE participant attends the center 2.5 days a week, with some spending 5 days a week if they live with a family member who works, and others attending only a few times a month (Greenwood, 2002a).

The upside to the PACE program is that more individualized care may be provided at lower costs. The downside to this innovative program is that state governments must be active partners, and the financial risks of starting and maintaining a program are still not well understood (Greenwood, 2002b). For more information about PACE, contact the National PACE Association at www.npaonline.org; or call 703-535-1517.

Perhaps the beginning of a solution, or solutions, to a system of long-term care that maximizes the health and independence of older adults will take place when the Wellness General of the United States (or perhaps a lieutenant general that she hires) spearheads an initiative to revolutionize long-term care. The goal of this office will be to make the final chapter in most people's life histories as autonomous, dignified, and loving as possible. Along the way toward accomplishing this goal, some of the principles upon which California's Aging With Dignity Initiative is based, may provide a sense of direction:

- long-term care tax credits for families caring for seniors at home
- additional resources for staff training for in-home, assisted living, and nursing home options
- increased wages for paid caregivers
- substantial financial awards distributed to exemplary long-term care settings
- punitive responses to owners of long-term care settings that perform poorly
- establishment of state information and support clearinghouses

For additional information about long-term care, contact the National Center for Assisted Living, 202-842-4444, www.ncal.org; the National Citizens' Coalition for Nursing Home Reform, 202-332-2275, www.nccnhr.org; or Eldercare Locator for information about caregiving in a particular ZIP code area, 800-677-1116.

## OTHER PUBLIC HEALTH POLICY ISSUES

Erring on the side once again of a too-strong federal or state government role in promoting the health of an aging society, I recommend the following additional public policies:

1. Tobacco: Tobacco should be regulated, including tobacco advertising, through the U.S. Food and Drug Administration. Smoking in enclosed workplaces and in public places that allow children to visit should be banned. Federal and state taxes on tobacco products should continue to increase.

2. Alcohol: Establish uniform drinking and driving laws for all states, including a legal blood alcohol content for drivers that is no more than .08%. Increase the federal excise tax on alcoholic beverages, and use the additional revenue to promote responsible drinking practices. Prohibit television networks from flirting once again with the prospect of alcohol advertising.

3. Physical Activity or Exercise: For the benefit of future cohorts of older adults, require daily physical education classes in high schools. Give recognition to shopping malls that promote walking and stairway use, communities that promote bicycle and walking paths, and worksites that promote exercise for sedentary employees, perhaps through certification as a heart-friendly location. Require commercial building codes to include safe, attractive, and accessible stairways (i.e., build stairwells in the centrally located sites where most elevators are now situated).

Reward transportation planners who shift their focus from cars to bike paths and sidewalks.

4. Nutrition: For the benefit of future cohorts of older adults, limit fast foods and ban soft-drink vending machines in public schools. Prohibit the marketing of junk foods directed at children. Add a one-cent tax on high-fat, high-sugar, and high-salt junk foods, and use the resources for health-promoting initiatives. Require restaurant menu boards and menus to state the caloric content of all foods and drinks. Set limits on the amount of salt allowed in processed foods and restaurant meals. Change nutrition labels so that sugar and trans fatty acid (when introduced in 2006) are included in the percentage of the daily value that it represents. Limit the sugar content of certain products such as breakfast cereals.

5. Research: Increase funding for research that evaluates the effectiveness of counseling and other behavior-changing strategies that are focused on smoking cessation, reducing problem drinking, increasing physical activity, improving nutrition, and helping older adults become public health advocates (particularly in the areas of environmental protection and strengthening elementary school education). And, when deemed effective, incorporate these strategies into Medicare and encourage their adoption by state legislatures or private health care plans.

6. Officially Declare Oregon as the Model State for Health Promotion: Prior to 2003 (when Oregon and most other states experienced a budget catastrophe) Oregon was the model state for testing innovative health promotion practices that may some day be adopted by other states, or on a national basis. Examples of this state's health-promoting innovations include recycling, the development of health care rationing criteria, the Oregon Death With Dignity Act, home and community-based alternatives to nursing homes, availability of hospice services, and a state ballot measure for a one-payer health care system. Oregon has been likely to lead the way on health promotion—so why not make it their official role?

Regarding the last innovation—the one-payer health care system—it should be noted that in November 2002, the citizens of Oregon rejected this initiative by 79% to 21%. It should also be noted that opponents of the ballot measure spent 99.99523% of all money raised to educate the public on this issue.

Which brings us back to the question that began this book: "Did you know that the federal government establishes goals for healthy aging?" My response is three-fold: Make universal health care one of the goals. Select and support a Wellness General. Redefine health care in America so that the focus is on medical care *and* health promotion.

# QUESTIONS FOR DISCUSSION

1. Discuss the pros and cons of the idea to tax junk foods.
2. In addition to your views on taxing junk foods, what do you like and not like about the proposal to appoint a Wellness General?
3. Access the surgeon general's reports on physical activity and mental health. Describe one important age-related finding in each report.
4. Clearly the author promotes a (too?) strong government role in promoting the health of an aging society. State the advantages and disadvantages of such an approach, and then state your own opinion.
5. Where will we be 10 years from now: universal health care, widespread boutique medicine, or something else? Why do you believe that?
6. The author is clearly against a market-driven, fee-for-service, profit-oriented health care system. And yet markets, profit, competition, and other elements of capitalism have proven their worth over the years in contributing to quality products at affordable costs. Are these elements of capitalism incompatible with universal health care? Explain your answer.
7. Why is long-term care more of a health promotion issue than a medical care issue? Or, if you believe otherwise, support your position.
8. Review the section "Other Public Health Policy Issues" in this chapter and then propose another change that you believe will be for the better.
9. Can you relate the following quotation by Henry Wadsworth Longfellow to improving the quality of the American health care system? "Age is opportunity no less than youth itself, though in another dress, and as the evening twilight fades away, the sky is filled with stars, invisible by day."

# References

A world of information beckons. (1998, February). *AARP Bulletin, 39*(2), 1.

AARP. (2002). *Beyond 50: A report to the nation on trends in health security.* Washington, DC: AARP.

AARP. (2001). *Global aging: Achieving its potential.* AARP Public Policy Institute report. Washington, DC: AARP.

AARP. (1991). *Healthy people 2000: Healthy older adults.* Excerpted from Healthy People 2000 National Health Promotion and Disease Prevention Objectives, U.S. Department of Health and Human Services, Public Health Service, Washington, DC.

AARP. (1989). *Health risks and preventive care among older hispanics. Health risks and preventive care among older blacks.* Health Advocacy Services Program Department, Minority Affairs Initiative. Washington, DC: AARP.

*AARP Bulletin.* (1991). *32*(5), p. 2.

*AARP Bulletin.* (1990). *31*(3), p. 2.

Abete, P. et al. (2001). High level of physical activity preserves the cardioprotective effect of preinfarction angina in elderly patients. *Journal of the American College of Cardiology. 38,* 1357–1367.

Abramson, J. et al. (2001). Moderate alcohol consumption and risk of heart failure among older persons. *Journal of the American Medical Association, 285,* 1971–1977.

Accidents don't just happen. (1995, March 20). *American Medical News,* 10–14.

ACTION. (1985). *Senior Companion Program impact evaluation.* Alexandria, VA: SRA Technologies.

ACTION. (1984). *Descriptive evaluation of RSVP and FGP Volunteers working with Headstart.* Washington, DC: Office of Policy and Planning Evaluation Division.

Adachi, M. et al. (2002). Effect of professional oral health care on the elderly living in nursing homes. *Oral Medicine. 94,* 191–195.

Adams, W. et al. (1993). Alcohol-related hospitalizations of elderly people. *Journal of the American Medical Association, 270,* 1222–1225.

Adelman, R. et al. (1989). Concordance between physicians and their older and younger patients in the primary care medical encounter. *Gerontologist, 29,* 808–813.

Age, hearing loss and hearing aids. (2000, November). *Harvard Health Letter,* 4–5.

Ahlquist, D. et al. (2000). Colorectal cancer screening by detection of altered human DNA in stool: Feasibility of a multitarget assay panel. *Gastroenterology, 119,* 1219–1227.

Ai, A. et al. (2002). Private prayer and optimism in middle-aged and older patients awaiting cardiac surgery. *Gerontologist, 42,* 70–81.

Ajzen, I. (1988). *Attitudes, personality, and behavior.* Chicago: Dorsey Press.

Albert, M. et al. (1995). Predictors of cognitive change in older persons: MacArthur studies of successful aging. *Psychology and Aging, 10,* 578–586.

Alberts, D. et al. (2000). Lack of effect of a high-fiber cereal supplement on the recurrence of colorectal adenomas. *New England Journal of Medicine, 342,* 1156–1162.

Alexander, C. et al. (1996). Trial of stress reduction for hypertension in older African Americans. *Hypertension, 28,* 228–237.

Alexopoulos, G., & Salzman, C. (1998). Treatment of depression with heterocyclic antidepressants, monoamine oxidase inhibitors, and psychomotor stimulants. In C. Salzman (Ed.), *Clinical geriatric psychopharmacology* (pp. 184–244). Baltimore: Williams & Wilkins.

Alexy, B. (1985). Goal-setting and health reduction. *Nursing Research, 34,* 283–288.

Allukian, M. (2000). The neglected epidemic and the Surgeon General's Report: A call to action for better oral health. *American Journal of Public Health, 90,* 843–845.

Almeida, D. et al. (2002). The daily inventory of stressful events: An interview-based approach for measuring daily stressors. *Assessment, 9,* 41–55.

Altman, L. (2001, November 14). Cholesterol fighters lower heart attack risk, study finds. *The New York Times,* p. A14.

AMA urges awareness of dehydration in elderly. (1995, November 20). *American Medical News,* p. 15.

AMA reports hidden epidemic of elderly alcoholism. (1995, September 25). *American Medical News.*

Ambady, N. et al. (2002). Surgeons' tone of voice: A clue to malpractice history. *Surgery, 132,* 5–9.

American Board of Family Practice. (1987). *Rights and responsibilities: Part II, The changing health care consumer and patient/doctor partnership.* A National Survey of Health Care Opinions. Lexington, KY.

American Cancer Society. (1994). *A survey concerning cigarette smoking.* Princeton, NJ: Gallup Organization.

American Cancer Society. (1990). *Cancer facts and figures.* Atlanta, GA: American Cancer Society.

American College of Sports Medicine. (1995). *ACSM's guidelines for exercise testing and prescription* (5th ed.). Baltimore: Williams and Wilkins.

American Dietetic Association. (1990). ADA-IFIC Gallup Poll. *American Dietetic Association Courier, 29,* 2.

*American Medical News.* (1993, February 8). p. 31.

*American Medical News.* (1992, March 16). p. 37.

*American Medical News.* (1992b, May 11). p. 8.

American Psychiatric Association. (1994). *Diagnostic and statistical manual of mental disorders* (4th ed.). Washington, DC: Author.

Amery, A. et al. (1986). Efficacy of antihypertensive drug treatment according to age, sex, blood prssure and previous cardiovascular disease in patients over the age of 60. *Lancet, 2,* 589–592.

Anderson, J. et al. (2001). Long-term weight-loss maintenance: A meta-analysis of US studies. *American Journal of Clinical Nutrition, 74,* 579–584.

Anderson, R. et al. (1999). Effects of lifestyle activity vs. structured aerobic exercise in obese women. *Journal of the American Medical Association, 281,* 335–340.

Angell, M. (1997). Fixing Medicare. *New England Journal of Medicine, 337,* 192–194

Ansell, B. (2002). Should physicians be recommending statins for most older Americans? *Clinical Geriatrics, 10,* 33–40.

Appel, L. et al. (2003). Effects of comprehensive lifestyle modification on blood pressure control: Main results of the PREMIER clinical trial. *Journal of the American Medical Association, 289,* 2131–2132.

Applegate, W. (1992). High blood pressure treatment in the elderly. In G. Omenn (Ed.), *Clinics in geriatric medicine* (pp. 103–117). Philadelphia: W. B. Saunders.

Arday, D. et al. (2002). Smoking patterns among seniors and the Medicare Stop Smoking Program. *Journal of American Geriatrics Society, 50,* 1689–1697.

Ardell, D. (2000, November 10). The hierarchy of wellness. *Ardell Wellness Report,* pp. 1–3.

Arean, P. et al. (1993). Comparative effectiveness of social problem-solving therapy and reminiscence therapy as treatments for depression in older adults. *Journal of Consulting and Clinical Psychology, 61,* 1003–1010.

Are Natural Fen-Phens Safe? (1998, March). *Health,* p. 30.

Are You Eating Right? (1992, October). *Consumer Reports,* pp. 644–655.

Asch, S. et al. (2000). Measuring underuse of necessary care among elderly Medicare beneficiaries using inpatient and outpatient claims. *Journal of the American Medical Association, 284,* 2325–2333.

Astin, J. (1998). Why patients use alternative medicine: Results of a national study. *Journal of the American Medical Association, 279,* 1548–1553.

Astin, J. et al. (2000). Complementary and alternative medicine use among elderly persons: One-year analysis of a Blue Shield Medicare supplement. *Journal of Gerontology: Medical Sciences, 55A,* M4–M9.

Aston, G. (2002, July 1). Medicare's mindfield. *American Medical News,* pp. 5–6.

Atchley, R. (1998). Long-range antecedents of functional capability in later life. *Journal of Aging and Health. 10,* 3–19.

Atkins, R. (1997). *Dr. Atkins' new diet revolution.* New York: Avon.

Atkinson, S. (1998, April). Calcium: Why get more? *Nutrition Action Healthletter,* pp. 3–5.

Attracted to magnets? (2000, June). *Consumer Reports on Health,* p. 2.

Baby boomers turning to yoga for spiritual workouts. (2000, October 12). *Houston Chronicle,* pp. 1D, 3D.

Baer, D. et al. (2002). Moderate alcohol consumption lowers risk factors for cardiovascular disease in postmenopausal women fed a controlled diet. *American Journal of Clinical Nutrition, 75,* 593–599.

Bailey, C. (1996). *Smart eating.* Boston: Houghton-Mifflin.

Bailey, C. (1994). *Smart exercise: Burning fat, getting fat.* London: Aurum Press.

Baker, K. et al. (2001). The efficacy of home based progressive strength training in older adults with knee osteoarthritis: A randomized clinical trial. *Journal of Rheumatology, 28,* 1655–1665.

Baker, L., & Wilson, F. (1996, March/April). Consumer health materials recommended for public libraries. *Public Libraries,* 124–130.

Ballard, C. et al. (2002). Aromatherapy as a safe and effective treatment for the management of agitation in severe dementia: The results of a double-blind, placebo-controlled trial with Melissa. *Journal of Clinical Psychiatry, 63,* 553–558.

Bandura, A. (1997). *Self-efficacy: The exercise of control.* New York: W. H. Freeman.

Bandura, A. (1977). *Social learning theory.* Englewood Cliffs, NJ: Prentice-Hall.

Banks, M., & Banks, W. (2002). The effects of animal-assisted therapy on loneliness in an elderly population in long-term care facilities. *Journal of Gerontology: Biological and Medical Sciences, 57,* M428–M432.

Baquet, C., & Gibbs, T. (1992). Cancer and Black Americans. In R. Braithwaite & S. Taylor (Eds.), *Health issues in the Black community* (pp. 106–112). San Francisco: Jossey-Bass.

Barlow, J. et al. (1996). How are written patient-education materials used in out-patient clinics? Insight from rheumatology. *Health Education Journal, 55,* 275–284.

Barnes, D. et al. (2003). A longitudinal study of cardiorespiratory fitness and cognitive function in healthy older adults. *Journal of American Geriatrics Society, 51,* 459–465.

Barrett, B. et al. (2002). Treatment of the common cold with unrefined Echinacea. *Annals of Internal of Medicine, 137,* 939–946.

Barrett-Connor, E. et al. (2002). Raloxifene and cardiovascular events in osteoporotic postmenopausal women. *Journal of the American Medical Association, 287,* 847–857.

Bassuk, S. et al. (1999). Social disengagement and incident cognitive decline in community-dwelling elderly persons. *Annals of Internal Medicine, 131,* 165–173.

Bauldoff, G. et al. (2002). Exercise maintenance following pulmonary rehabilitation: Effect of distractive stimuli. *Chest, 122,* 948–954.

Baxter, N. (2001). Preventive health care, 2001 update: Should women be routinely taught breast self-examination to screen for breast cancer? *Canadian Medical Association Journal, 164,* 1837–1846, 1851–1852.

Beck, R. et al. (2002). Physician-patient communication in the primary care office: A systematic review. *Journal of the American Board of Family Practice. 15,* 25–38.

Becker, M. (1974). The health belief model and personal health behavior. *Health Education Monographs, 2,* 236.

Beekman, A. et al. (2002). The natural history of late-life depression: A 6-year prospective study in the community. *Archives of General Psychiatry, 59,* 605–611.

Beers, M., & Berkow, R. (2000). *The Merck manual of geriatrics* (3rd ed.). Whitehouse Station, NJ: Merck Research Laboratories.

Beisecker, A. (1990, November). The older patient's companion. Paper presentation at the 43rd Annual Scientific Meeting of the Gerontological Society of America, Boston, MA.

Bell, R. et al. (1999). Direct-to-consumer prescription drug advertising and the public. *Journal of General Internal Medicine, 14,* 651–657.

Benner, J. et al. (2002). Long-term persistence in use of statin therapy in elderly patients. *Journal of the American Medical Association, 288,* 455–461.

Benson, H. (1984). *Beyond the relaxation response.* New York: Times Books.

Bent, S. et al. (2003). The relative safety of ephedra compared with other herbal products. *Annals of Internal Medicine, 18,* 138, 468–471.

Berkman, L. (1983). *Health and ways of living: Findings from the Alameda County study.* New York: Oxford University Press.

Berry, M. et al. (1989). Work-site health promotion: The effects of a goal-setting program on nutrition-related behaviors. *Journal of American Dietary Association, 89,* 914–920.

Beta Carotene Pills. (1997, June). *Mayo Clinic Health Letter: Supplement,* p. 4.

Betancourt, J., & Carrillo, J. (2002). *Cultural ompetence in health care: Emerging frameworks and practical approaches.* New York: The Commonwealth Fund.

Beutler, L. et al. (1987). Group cognitive therapy and alprazolam in the treatment of depression in older adults. *Journal of Consulting and Clinical Psychology, 55,* 550–556.

Biesada, A. (2000, June). Rx for trouble. *Texas Monthly,* pp. 72–76.

Birch, B. (1995). *Power yoga: The total wellness workout for mind and body.* New York: Fireside.

Birren, J., & Cochran, K. (2001). *Telling the stories of life through guided autobiography groups.* Baltimore: The Johns Hopkins University Press.

Birren, J., & Deutchman, D. (1991). *Guiding autobiography groups for older adults.* Baltimore: Johns Hopkins University Press.

Birren, J. et al. (1996). *Aging and biography: Explorations in adult development.* New York: Springer.

Blackman, M. et al. (2002). Growth hormone and sex steroid administration in healthy aged women and men: A randomized controlled trial. *Journal of the American Medical Association, 288,* 2282–2292.

Blair, G. (2001, Fall/Winter). The many faces I see. *Newsweek* [Special Issue], p. 64.

Blair, S. et al. (1996). Influences of cardiorespiratory fitness and other precursors on cardiovascular disease and all-cause mortality in men and women. *Journal of the American Medical Association, 276,* 205–210.

Blair, S. et al. (1989). Physical fitness and all-cause mortality: A prospective study of healthy men and women. *Journal of the American Medical Association, 262,* 2395–2401.

Blendon, R. et al. (2001). Americans' views on the use and regulation of dietary supplements. *Archives of Internal Medicine, 161,* 805–810.

Blittner, M. et al. (1978). Cognitive self-control factors in the reduction of smoking behavior. *Behavior Therapy, 9,* 553–561.

Blondal, T. et al. (1999). Nicotine nasal spray with nicotine patch for smoking cessation: Randomised trial with six year follow up. *British Medical Journal, 318,* 285–288.

Blumenthal, J. et al. (1999). Effects of exercise training on older patients with major depression. *Archives of Internal Medicine, 159,* 2349–2356.

Blumenthal, J. et al. (1991). Long-term effects of exercise on psychological functioning in older men and women. *Journal of Gerontology, 46,* 352–361.

Blumenthal, R. (1996, September). The many benefits of fiber. Johns Hopkins Medical Letter. *Health After 50,* p. 4.

Bogden, J. et al. (1995). Studies on micronutrient supplements and immunity in older people. *Nutrition Reviews, 3,* S59–S64.

Boldt, M., & Dellmann-Jenkins, M. (1992). The impact of companion animals in later life and considerations for practice. *Journal of Applied Gerontology, 11,* 228–239.

Boling, R. (2000, March-April). A shot of youth. *Modern Maturity,* pp. 70–71.

Bonita, R. et al. (1999, Summer). Passive smoking as well as active smoking increases the risk of acute stroke. *Tobacco Control, 8,* 156–160.

Borg, G. (1982). Psychophysical bases of perceived exertion. *Medicine and Science in Sports and Exercise, 14,* 377–381.

Borkman, T. (1982). Where are older persons in mutual self-help groups? In A. Kolker & P. Ahmed (Eds.), *Aging.* New York: Elsevier.

Braddock, C. et al. (1999). Informed decision making in outpatient practice. *Journal of the American Medical Association, 282,* 2313–2320.

Bradley, C. et al. (2002). Race, socioeconomic status, and breast cancer treatment and survival. *Journal of National Cancer Institute, 94,* 490–496.

Bratton, R. et al. (2002). Effect of "ionized" wrist bracelets on musculoskeletal pain: A randomized, double-blind, placebo-controlled trial. *Mayo Clinic Proceedings, 77,* 1164–1168.

Brennan, P. et al. (1995). The effects of a special computer network on caregivers of persons with Alzheimer's disease. *Nursing Research, 44,* 166–171.

Brett, A. (2002). How common is undiagnosed dysfunction? *Journal Watch,* pp. 51–52.

Briggs, B. (2002, April 7). What is race? Color lines are blurring as more Americans proclaim mixed heritage. *The Denver Post,* pp. 1L, 4L.

Brimer, E. et al. (1991). Why do some women get regular mammographies? *American Journal of Preventive Medicine, 7,* 69–74.

Broadening your view of health. (2000, November). *Dr. Andrew Weil's Self Healing,* p. 2.

Brody, J. (2002, July 16). How to eat out without tipping the scales. *The New York Times,* Science section.

Brody, J. (2000a, September 17). American diets dangerously awash in sugar. *The New York Times,* p. 2J.

Brody, J. (2000b, March 20). HMOs have maintenance problem on their hands. *New York Times,* Personal Health section, p. 1.

Brody, J. (1998, February 15). Cretan diet rich in fruits, vegetables, grains proves heart-healthy. *Houston Chronicle,* p. 5F.

Brody, J. (1996, February 28). Good habits outweigh genes as key to a healthy old age. *The New York Times* Health section, p. 12.

Brookfield, S. (1990). *Understanding and facilitating adult learning.* San Francisco: Jossey-Bass.

Bross, M. et al. (1993, November). *Health promotion and disease prevention: A survey of rural family physicians.* Presentation at Society of Teachers of Family Medicine, Orlando, FL.

Brown, C., & Kessler, L. (1988). Projections of lung cancer mortality in the United States: 1985—2025. *Journal of the National Cancer Institute, 80,* 43–51.

Brownell, K. et al. (1986). Understanding and preventing relapse. *American Psychologist, 41,* 765–782.

Buchner, D., & Wagner, E. (1992). Preventing frail health. *Clinical Geriatric Medicine, 8*(1), 1–17.

Buchowski, M., & Sun, M. (1996). Energy expenditure, television viewing and obesity. *International Journal of Obesity, 20,* 236–245.

Building immunity. (1997, September). *Nutrition Action Healthletter,* pp. 4–7.

Burack, R., & Liang, J. (1989). Acceptance and completion of mammography by older black women. *American Journal of Public Health, 79,* 721–726.

Burack, R., &. Liang, J. (1987). The early detection of cancer in the primary care setting: Factors associated with the acceptance and completion of recommended procedures. *Preventive Medicine, 16,* 739–751.

Burns, D. (1980). *Feeling good: The new mood therapy.* New York: William Morrow.

Butler, R. (1995). Foreword: The life review. In B. Haight & J. Webster (Eds.), *The art and science of reminiscing* (pp. xvii–xxi). Washington, DC: Taylor and Francis.

Butler, R. (1974). Successful aging and the role of the life review. *Journal of the American Geriatrics Society, 22,* 529–535.

Butler, R. et al. (1998). *Aging and mental health: Positive psychosocial and biomedical approaches* (5th ed.). Needham Heights, MA: Allyn & Bacon.

Butler, R. et al. (1991). *Aging and mental health: Positive psychosocial and biomedical approaches.* Columbus, OH: Charles E. Merrill.

Caggiula, A. et al. (1987). The multiple risk intervention trial (MRFIT). IV. Intervention on blood lipids. *Preventive Medicine, 10,* 443–475.

Cahalin, L. et al. (2002). Eficacy of diaphragmatic breathing in persons with chronic obstructive pulmonary disease: A review of the literature. *Journal of Cardiopulmonary Rehabilitation, 22,* 7–21.

Caine, E. et al. (1996). Diagnosis of late-life depression: Preliminary studies in primary care settings. *American Journal of Geriatric Psychiatry, 4,* S45–S50.

Calcium and vitamin D. (1996, June). *Mayo Clinic Health Letter,* Medical essay supplement, pp. 4–5.

Calfas, K. et al. (1996). A controlled trial of physician counseling to promote the adoption of physical activity. *Preventive Medicine, 25,* 225–233.

California cigarette sales fall due to stiff new tax. (1999, September 27). *American Medical News,* p. 9.

Callahan, D. (2000). *Promoting healthy behavior: How much freedom? Whose responsibility?* Washington, DC: Georgetown University Press.

Callahan, D. et al. (1995). Documentation and evaluation of cognitive impairment in elderly primary care patients. *Annals of Internal Medicine, 122,* 422–429.

Callahan, E. et al. (2000). The influence of patient age on primary care resident physician-patient interaction. *Journal of the American Geriatrics Society, 48,* 30–35.

Calle, E. et al. (2003). Overweight, obesity, and mortality from cancer in a prospectively studied cohort of U.S. adults. *New England Journal of Medicine, 348,* 1625–1638.

Calle, E. et al. (1999). Body-mass index and mortality in a prospective cohort of U.S. adults. *New England Journal of Medicine, 341,* 1097–1105.

Campanelli, L. (1990). Promoting healthy aging. *Educational Gerontology, 16,* 517–518.

Campbell, A. et al. (1997). Randomized controlled trial of a general practice programme of home based exercise to prevent falls in elderly women. *British Medical Journal, 315,* 1065–1069.

Cardenas, L. et al. (1987). Adult onset diabetes mellitus: Glycemic control and family function. *American Journal of the Medical Sciences, 293,* 28–33.

Cardinal, B., & Engels, H. (2001). Ginseng does not enhance psychological well-being in healthy, young adults: Results of a double-blind, placebo-controlled, randomized clinical trial. *Journal of American Dietetic Association, 101,* 655–660.

Carlston, M. et al. (1997). Alternative medicine instruction in medical schools and family practice residency programs. *Family Medicine, 29,* 559–562.

Caro, F., & Morris, R. (2001). Maximizing the contributions of older people as volunteers. In S. Levkoff et al. (Eds.), *Aging in good health* (pp. 341–356). New York: Springer.

Cassel, C. (2002). Use it or lose it. *Journal of the American Medical Association, 288,* 2333–2335.

Castillo-Richmond, A. et al. (2000). Effcts of stress reduction on carotid atherosclerosis in hypertensive African Americans. *Stroke, 31,* 568–573.

Caterson, I. (1990). Management strategies for weight control: Eating, exercise and behavior. *Drugs, 39*(Suppl. 3), 20–32.

Centers for Disease Control and Prevention. (2002). Prevalence of health-care providers asking older adults about their physical activity levels—United States, 1998. *Morbidity and Mortality Weekly Report, 51,* 412–414.

Centers for Disease Control and Prevention. (1999). *Suicide deaths and rates per 100,000.* Available online at www.cdc.gov/ncipc/data/us9794/suic.htm.

Centers for Disease Control and Prevention. (1992). Cigarette smoking among adults, United States, 1990: Effectiveness of smoking-control strategies—United States. *MMWR, 41,* 354–355, 361–362, 645–647, 653.

Chandra, R. (2001). Effect of vitamin and trace-element supplementation on cognitive function in elderly subjects. *Nutrition, 17,* 709–712.

Chandra, R. (1997). Graying of the immune system: Can nutrient supplements improve immunity in the elderly? *Journal of the American Medical Association, 277,* 1398–1399.

Chandra, R. (1992). Effect of vitamin and trace-element supplementation on immune responses and infection in elderly subjects. *Lancet, 340,* 1124–1127.

Chang, P. et al. (2002). Anger in young men and subsequent premature cardiovascular disease: The precursors study. *Archives of Internal Medicine, 162,* 901–906.

Chao, D. et al. (1999). Naloxone reverses inhibitory effect of electroacupuncture on sympathetic cardiovascular reflex responses. *American Journal of Physiology, 276*(6 pt. 2), H2127–2134.

Chen, C. et al. (2002). Hormone replacement therapy in relation to breast cancer. *Journal of the American Medical Association, 287,* 734–741.

Cherkin, D. et al. (2001). Randomized trial comparing traditional Chinese medical acupuncture, therapeutic massage, and self-care education for chronic low back pain. *Archives of Internal Medicine, 161,* 1081–1088.

Cherry, R. et al. (1995). Service directories: Reinvigorating a community resource for self-care. *Gerontologist, 35,* 560–563.

Chin, T. (2002a, September 9). Information driveway. *American Medical News,* p. 19.

Chin, T. (2002b, September 2). Americans trail much of Europe in adopting EMRs. *American Medical News.*

Chiriboga, D. (1992). Paradise lost: Stress in the modern age. In M. Wykle et al. (Eds.), *Stress and health among the elderly* (pp. 35–71). New York: Springer.

Chobanian, A. (2001). Control of hypertension—An important national priority. *New England Journal of Medicine, 345,* 534–535.

Cholesterol-lowering drugs less effective than in studies. (2001, November 12). *The Star Press,* p. 8C.

Christensen, A., & Rankin, D. (1979). *Easy does it yoga for older people.* San Francisco: Harper & Row.

Chung, M., & Barfield, J. (2002). Knowledge of prescription medications among elderly emergency department patients. *Annals of Emergency Medicine, 39,* 605–608.

Clark, A. et al. (2001). Inverse association between sense of humor and coronary heart disease. *International Journal of Cardiology, 80,* 87–88.

Cohen, C. et al. (2002). Positive aspects of caregiving: Rounding out the caregiver experience. *International Journal of Geriatric Psychiatry, 17,* 184–188.

Cohen, R. et al. (2002). Complementary and alternative medicine (CAM) use by older adults: A comparison of self-report and physician chart documentation. *Journal of Gerontology: Medical Sciences, 57A,* M223–M227.

Cohen, S. et al. (1997). Social ties and susceptibility to the common cold. *Journal of the American Medical Association, 277,* 1940–1944.

Cohen, S. et al. (1990). Debunking myths about self-quitting: Evidence from 10 prospective studies of persons who attempt to quit smoking by themselves. *American Psychologist, 44,* 1355–1365.

Cohen, S. et al. (1989). Encouraging primary care physicians to help smokers quit. *Annals of Internal Medicine, 110,* 648–652.

Colangelo, R. et al. (1997). The role of exercise in rehabilitation patients with end-stage renal disease. *Rehabilitation Nursing, 22,* 288–292, 302.

Colcombe, S. et al. (2003). Aerobic fitness reduces brain tissue loss in aging humans. *Journal of Gerontology: Series A, 58,* 176–180.

Colditz, G. (1999). Economic costs of obesity and inactivity. *Medicine & Science in Sports & Exercise, 31,* S663–S667.

Collacott, E. et al. (2000). Bipolar permanent magnets for the treatment of chronic low back pain: A pilot study. *Journal of the American Medical Association, 283,* 1322–1325.

Collins, H., & Pancoast, D. (1976). *Natural helping networks: A strategy for prevention.* Washington, DC: National Association of Social Workers.

Comfort, A. (1972). *The joy of sex.* New York: Simon & Schuster.

Complementary curriculum. (2000, January 17). *American Medical News,* pp. 7–8.

Connolly, C. (2001, May 17). Living Longer, Independently: A new study shows that more older Americans are avoiding chronic impairment. *Washington Post,* p. D1.

Connolly, H. et al. (1997). Vavular heart disease associated with fenfluramine-phentermine. *New England Journal of Medicine, 337,* 581–584.

Constantino, R. (1988). Comparison of two group interventions for the bereaved. *Image: The Journal of Nursing Scholarship, 20,* 83–87.

*Consumer Reports.* (1993, June). Losing weight: What works. What doesn't, pp. 347–357.

*Consumer Reports on Health.* (2001, October). Should you take a vitamin E supplement? p. 5.

Controversial cases: You decide. (2002). *Consumer Reports on Health, 14*(4), p. 6.

Cook, J. et al. (2002). Suicidality in older African Americans: Findings from the EPOCH study. *American Journal of Geriatric Psychiatry, 10,* 437–446.

Cooper, K. (1994). *Dr. Kenneth H. Cooper's antioxidant revolution.* Nashville, TN: Thomas Nelson.

Cooper-Patrick, L. et al. (1999). Race, gender, and partnership in the patient-physician relationship. *Journal of the American Medical Association, 282,* 583–589.

Costamagna, G. et al. (2002). A prospective trial comparing small bowel radiographs and video capsule endoscopy for suspected small bowel disease. *Gastroenterology, 123,* 999–1005.

Cottreau, C. et al. (2000). Physical activity and reduced risk of ovarian cancer. *Obstetrics and Gynecology, 96,* 609–614.

Counting on food labels. (2000, January 10). *Washington Post National Weekly,* p. 32.

Coward, R., & Lee, G. (1985). *The elderly in rural society.* New York: Springer.

Coyne, A. et al. (1993). The relationship between dementia and elder abuse. *American Journal of Psychiatry, 150,* 643–646.

Crossette, B. (2000, June 5). U.S. ranks far down on 'healthy life' list. *The New York Times,* pp. 1A, 9A.

Crowe, R. et al. (1997). The utility of the brief MAST and the CAGE in identifying alcohol problems. *Archives of Family Medicine, 6,* 447–483.

Curb, D. et al. (2000). Serum lipid effects of a high-monounsaturated fat diet based on macadamia nuts. *Archives of Internal Medicine, 160,* 1154–1158.

Curfman, G. (1997). Diet pills redux. *New England Journal of Medicine, 337,* 629–630.

Curtis, J. et al. (1989). Characteristics, diagnosis and treatment of alcoholism in elderly patients. *Journal of American Geriatrics Society, 37,* 310.

Cys, J. (2000, November 13). Clinical practice figures into Medicare coverage decision. *American Medical News,* p. 12.

Danner, D. et al. (2001). Positive emotions in early life and longevity: Findings from the nun study. *Journal of Personality and Social Psychology, 80,* 804–813.

Dass, R. (2000). *Still here: Embracing aging, changing and dying.* New York: Riverhead Books.

Davis, M. et al. (1995). *The relaxation and stress reduction workbook.* Oakland, CA: New Harbinger.

Davis, M. et al. (1985). Living arrangements and dietary patterns of older adults in the U.S. *Journal of Gerontology, 40,* 434–442.

Davis, R. et al. (1994). The urban church and cancer control: A source of social influence in minority communities. *Public Health Reports, 109,* 500–560.

Davis, R. (1988). Uniting physicians against smoking: The need for a coordinated national strategy. *Journal of the American Medical Association, 259,* 2900–2901.

Davison, K. et al. (2000). Who talks? The social psychology of illness support groups. *American Psychologist, 55,* 205–217.

Dawson, D. et al. (1987). Trends in routine screening examinations. *American Journal of Public Health, 77,* 1004–1005.

Dawson-Hughes, B. et al. (2000). Effect of withdrawal of calcium and vitamin D supplements on bone mass in elderly men and women. *American Journal of Clinical Nutrition, 72,* 745–750.

Day, A. (1992). *Remarkable survivors: Insights into successful aging among women.* Washington, DC: Urban Institute Press.

Day, L. et al. (2002). Randomised factorial trail of falls prevention among older people living in their own homes. *British Medical Journal, 325,* 128–131.

Dean, A. et al. (1990). Effects of social support from various sources on depression in elderly persons. *Journal of Health and Social Behavior, 31,* 148–161.

DeBusk, R. et al. (1990). Training effects of long versus short bouts of exercise in healthy subjects. *American Journal of Cardiology, 65,* 1010–1013.

DeGroen, P. et al. (1996). Esophagitis associated with the use of Alendroate. *New England Journal of Medicine, 335,* 1016–1021.

DeGuire, S. et al. (1996). Breathing retraining: A three-year follow-up study of treatment for hyperventilation syndrome and associated functional cardiac symptoms. *Biofeedback Self-Regulation, 21,* 191–198.

Delany, S. et al. (1993). *Having our say: The Delany sisters' first 100 years.* New York: Kodansha International.

de Lorgeril, M. et al. (1999). Mediterranean diet, traditional risk factors, and the rate of cardiovascular complications after myocardial infarction: Final report of the Lyon Diet Heart Study. *Circulation, 99,* 779–785.

Del Ser, T. et al. (1999). An autopsy-verified study of the effect of education on degenerative dementia. *Brain, 122,* 2309–2319.

Demling, R. (1999). Growth hormone therapy in critically ill patients. *New England Journal of Medicine, 341,* 837–839.

Devine, A. et al. (1995). A longitudinal study of the effect of sodium and calcium intakes on regional bone density in postmenopausal women. *American Journal of Clinical Nutrition, 62,* 740–745.

Diet & health: Ten megatrends. (2001, January/February). *Nutrition Action Healthletter,* pp. 3–12.

Dietary fat makes a comeback. (2001, July). *Tufts University Health & Nutrition Letter,* p. 4–5.

Dieting. (2002, June). *Consumer Reports, 67*(6), 26–31.

Dirx, M. et al. (2001). Baseline recreational physical activity, history of sports participation, and postmenopausal breast carcinoma risk in the Netherlands Cohort Study. *Cancer, 92,* 1638–1649.

Dishman, R. et al. (1985). The determinants of physical activity and exercise. *Public Health Reports, 100,* 158–171.

Dobkin, L. (2002). Senior wellness project secures health care dollars. *Innovations, 2,* 16–20.

Dorfman, S. (1991). *Health promotion for older minority adults.* Washington, DC: AARP National Resource Center on Health Promotion and Aging.

Dr Koop to cease operation. (2002, January 14). *American Medical News,* p. 12.

Duan, N. et al. (2000). Maintaining mammography adherence through telephone counseling in a church-based trial. *American Journal of Public Health, 90,* 1468–1471.

Duenwald, M. (2002, May 7). Religion and health: New research revives an old debate. *The New York Times,* pp. D1–D4.

Duffy, J. et al. (2002). Peak of circadian melatonin rhythm occurs later within the sleep of older subjects. *American Journal of Physiology—Endocrinology and Metabolism, 282,* E297–E303.

Duffy, M., & MacDonald, E. (1990). Determinants of functional health of older persons. *Gerontologist, 30,* 503–509.

Duffy, S. et al. (2002a). The mammographic screening trials: Commentary on the recent work by Olsen and Gotzsche. *Cancer, 52,* 68–71.

Duffy, S. et al. (2002b). Impact of organized mammography service screening on breast carcinoma mortality in seven Swedish counties. *Cancer, 93,* 458–469.

Dufour, M. et al. (1992). Alcohol and the elderly. In G. Omenn (Ed.), *Clinics in geriatric medicine* (pp. 127–141). Philadelphia: W. B. Saunders.

Duncan, J. (1996). *Exercise intensity.* Unpublished manuscript from the Cooper Institute, Dallas, TX.

Duncan, P. et al. (1998). A randomized, controlled pilot study of a home-based exercise program for individuals with mild and moderate stroke. *Stroke, 29,* 2055–2060.

Dunstan, D. et al. (2002). High-intensity resistance training improves glycemic control in older patients with Type 2 Diabetes. *Diabetes Care, 25,* 1729–1736.

Dustman, R. (1996, March/April). Think fast. *Health,* pp. 44–46.

Ebersole, P., & Hess, P. (1990). *Toward healthy aging: Human needs and nursing response.* St. Louis, MO: C.V. Mosby.

Ebrahim, S. (2002). The medicalization of old age. *British Medical Journal, 324,* 861–863.

Edinger, J. et al. (2001). Cognitive behavioral therapy for treatment of chronic primary insomnia: A randomized controlled trial. *Journal of the American Medical Association, 285,* 1856–1864.

Ehman, J. et al. (1999). Do patients want physician to inquire about their spiritual or religious beliefs if they become gravely ill? *Archives of Internal Medicine, 159,* 1803–1806.

Eisenberg, A. (2002, April 18). Such a comfort to grandma, and he runs on double-A's. *The New York Times,* pp. D1, D4.

Eisenberg, D. et al. (1998). Trends in alternative medicine use in the United States. 1990–1997. Results of a follow-up national survey. *Journal of the American Medical Association, 280,* 1569–1575.

Eisenberg, D. et al. (1993). Unconventional medicine in the United States: Prevalence, costs and patterns of use. *New England Journal of Medicine, 328,* 246–252.

Eisner, M. et al. (1998). Bartenders' respiratory health after establishment of smoke-free bars and taverns. *Journal of the American Medical Association, 280,* 1909–1914.

Elder, J. et al. (1995). Longitudinal effects of preventive services on health behaviors among an elderly cohort. *American Journal of Preventive Medicine, 11,* 354–359.

Elliot, P. et al. (1996). Intersalt revisited. *British Medical Journal, 312,* 1249–1253.

Elliott, V. (2002, October 21). Aftermath of HRT study: Patient-by-patient re-evaluation. *American Medical News,* p. 35.

Elliott, V. (2001, December 10). Statins found to work better in studies than in practice. *American Medical News,* pp. 1–2.

Elliot, V. (2001b, Sepember). Health of rural, urban residents lags behind suburbanites. *American Medical News,* p. 39.

Elliott, V. (2000, November 6). Poor patients do poorly after heart surgery. *American Medical News,* p. 41.

Ellis, A. (1975). *A new guide to rational living.* North Hollywood, CA: Wilshire Books.

Elmore, J. et al. (1998). Ten-year risk of false positive screening mammograms and clinical breast examinations. *The New England Journal of Medicine, 338,* 1089–1096.

Elward, K., & Larson, E. (1992). Benefits of exercise for older adults. In G. Omenn (Ed.), *Clinics in Geriatric Medicine* (pp. 35–50). Philadelphia: W. B. Saunders.

End of debate: Fiber's great. (1996, July/August). *Health,* p. 16.

Eng, E., & Young, R. (1992). Lay health advisors as community change agents. *Family and Community Health, 15,* 24–40.

Eng, P. et al. (2002). Social ties and change in social ties in relation to subsequent total and cause-specific mortality and coronary heart disease incidents in men. *American Journal of Epidemiology, 155,* 700–709.

Engelhart, J. et al. (2002). Dietary intake of antioxidants and risk of Alzheimer disease. *Journal of the American Medical Association, 287,* 3223–3229.

Engels, H., & Wirth, J. (1997). No ergogenic effects of ginseng during graded maximal aerobic exercise. *Journal of American Dietary Association, 97,* 1110–1115.

Ephedrine's deadly edge. (1997, July 7). *U.S. News and World Report,* pp. 79–80.

Erikson, E. et al. (1987). *Vital involvement in old age.* New York: W. W. Norton.

Eskin, S. (2001). Dietary supplements and older consumers. *AARP Public Policy Institute, Data Digest, 66,* 1–8.

Ettinger, R. (2001). Oral health. In E. Swanson et al. (Eds.), *Health promotion and disease prevention in the older adult.* New York: Springer.

Ettinger, W. et al. (1997). A randomized trial comparing aerobic exercise and resistance exercise with a health education program in older adults with knee osteoarthritis. *Journal of the American Medical Association, 277,* 25–31.

Ettinger, W. et al. (1992). Lipoprotein lipids in older people: Results from the Cardiovascular Heart Study. *Circulation. 86,* 858–869.

Etzioni, R. et al. (2002). Overdiagnosis due to prostate-specific antigen screening: Lessons from U. S. prostate cancer incidence trends. *Journal of National Cancer Institute, 94,* 981–990.

Evans, D. et al. (1989). Prevalence of Alzheimer's disease in a community population of older persons. Higher than previously reported. *Journal of the American Medical Association, 262,* 2551–2556.

Evans, L., & Strumpf, N. (1989). Tying down the elderly: A review of the literature on physical restraint. *Journal of American Geriatrics Society, 37,* 65.

Evans, W. et al. (1991). *Biomarkers: The 10 determinants of aging you can control.* New York: Simon and Schuster.

Expert Panel on Detection, Evaluation, and Treatment of Health Blood Cholesterol in Adults. (2001). Executive summary of the third report of The National Cholesterol Education Program (NCEP) Expert Panel on Detection, Evaluation, and Treatment of High Blood Cholesterol in Adults (Adult Treatment Panel III). *Journal of the American Medical Association, 285,* 2486–2497.

Fawzy, F. et al. (1995). Critical review of psychosocial interventions in cancer care. *Archive of General Psychiatry, 52,* 100–113.

Fedder, D. et al. (2002). New National Cholesterol Education Program III Guidelines for primary prevention lipid-lowering drug therapy. *Circulation, 105,* 152–156.

Federal Interagency Forum on Aging-Related Statistics. (2000). Older Americans 2000: Key indicators of well-being. *Indicator 29: Use of Health Care Services,* p. 44. Hyattsville, MD: Federal Interagency Forum on Aging-Related Statistics.

Fenlon, H. et al. (1999). A comparison of virtual and conventional colonoscopy for the detection of colorectal polyps. *New England Journal of Medicine, 341,* 1496–1503.

Ferraro, K., & Koch, J. (1994). Religion and health among black and white adults: Examining social support and consolation. *Journal for the Scientific Study of Religion, 33,* 362–375.

Ferrini, A., & Ferrini, R. (1989). *Health in the later years.* Dubuque, IA: William C. Brown.

Ferry, L. et al. (1999). Tobacco dependence curricula in US undergraduate medical education. *Journal of the American Medical Association, 282,* 825–829.

Feskanich, D. et al. (2002a). Walking and leisure-time activity and risk of hip fracture in postmenopausal women. *Journal of the American Medical Association, 288,* 2300–2306.

Feskanich, D. et al. (2002b). Vitamin A intake and hip fractures among post menopausal women. *Journal of the American Medical Association, 287,* 47–54.

Fiatarone, M. et al. (1990). High-intensity strength training in nonagenarians: Effects on skeletal muscle. *Journal of the American Medical Association, 263,* 3029–3034.

Fichtenberg, C., & Glantz, S. (2000). Association of the California Tobacco Control Program with declines in cigarette consumption and mortality from heart disease. *New England Journal of Medicine, 343,* 1772–1777.

Field, L., & Steinhardt, M. (1992). The relationship of internally-directed behaviour to self-reinforcement, self-esteem, and expectancy values for exercise. *American Journal of Health Promotion, 7,* 21–26.

Finn, S. (1988, January). Nutrition: What's your ideal weight? *50 Plus Magazine,* pp. 31–33.

Finucane, T. (1988). Planning with elderly outpatients for contingencies of severe illness: A survey and clinical trial. *Journal of General Internal Medicine, 2,* 322.

Fiore, M. (1992). Trends in cigarette smoking in the United States: The epidemiology of tobacco use. *The Medical Clinics of North America, 76,* 289–303.

Fiore, M. et al. (1992). Tobacco dependence and the nicotine patch: Clinical guidelines for effective use. *Journal of the American Medical Association, 269,* 2687–2694.

Fiore, M. et al. (1990). Methods used to quit smoking in the United States: Do cessation programs help? *Journal of the American Medical Association, 263,* 2760–2765.

Firestone, A. (2000). Exercise stress testing for older persons starting an exercise program. *Journal of the American Medical Association, 284,* 2591–2592.

Firman, J., & Holmes, C. (1999). The consequences of untreated hearing loss in older persons. *Innovations in Aging, 1,* 21–25.

Fishbein, M., & Ajzen, I. (1975). *Belief, attitude, intention and behavior: An introduction to theory and research.* Reading, MA: Addison-Wesley.

Fishing for safe seafood. (1996, November). *Nutrition Action Healthletter,* pp. 3–5.

Fitzgerald, F. (1994). The tyranny of health. *New England Journal of Medicine, 331,* 196–198.

Flaherty, J. et al. (2001). Use of alternative therapies in older outpatients in the United States and Japan: Prevalence, reporting patterns, and perceived effectiveness. *Journal of Gerontology: Medical Sciences, 56A,* M650–M655.

Flegal, K. et al. (2002). Prevalence and trends in obesity among US adults. *Journal of the American Medical Association, 288,* 1723–1727.

Flegal, K. et al. (1995). The influence of smoking cessation on the prevalence of overweight in the United States. *New England Journal of Medicine, 333,* 1165–1170.

Fletcher, A. (1994). *Thin for life.* Boston: Houghton Mifflin.

Fletcher, G. et al. (1992). Statement on exercise: Benefits and recommendations for physical activity programs for all Americans: A statement for health professionals by the Committee on Exercise and Cardiac Rehabilitation of the Council on Clinical Cardiology, American Heart Association. *Circulation, 86,* 340–344.

Fletcher, R., & Fairfield, K. (2002). Vitamins for chronic disease prevention in adults: Clinical applications. *Journal of the American Medical Association, 287,* 3127–3129.

Fleming, M. et al. (2000). Benefit-cost analysis of brief physician advice with problem drinkers in primary care settings. *Medical Care, 38,* 7–18.

Flint, A. (1994). Epidemiology and comorbidity of anxiety disorders in the elderly. *American Journal of Psychiatry, 151,* 640–649.

Foley, D. et al. (2002). Driving life expectancy of persons aged 70 years and older in the United States. *American Journal of Public Health, 92,* 1284–1289.

*Food and Nutrition Research Briefs.* (1996). U.S. Department of Agriculture Research Service. Washington, DC. January, pp. 1–2.

Foote, J. et al. (2000). Older adults need guidance to meet nutritional recommendations. *Journal of American College of Nutrition, 19,* 628–640.

Forrest, K. et al. (1997). Driving patterns and medical conditions in older women. *Journal of American Geriatrics Society, 45,* 1214–1218.

Foster, G. et al. (2001). Evaluation of the Atkins Diet: A randomized controlled trial. *Obesity Research, 9*(Suppl. 3), 132.

Franse, L. et al. (2001). Type 2 diabetes in older well-functioning people: Who is undiagnosed? *Diabetes Care, 24,* 2065–2070.

Frasure-Smith, N. et al. (1995). Depression and 18-month prognosis after myocardial infarction. *Circulation, 91,* 999–1005.

Fratiglioni, L. et al. (2000). Influence of social network on occurrence of dementia: A community-based longitudinal study. *The Lancet, 355,* 1315–1319.

Frazao, E. (1999). America's eating habits: Changes and consequences. *Agriculture Information Bulletin, 750.* Economic Research Service, US Department of Agriculture, Washington, DC.

Freedman, D. et al. (2002). Trends and correlates of class 3 obesity in the United States from 1990 through 2000. *Journal of the American Medical Association, 288,* 1758–1761.

Freedman, M. (2002, March-April). Prime Time author answers his older critics on retirement. *Aging Today,* pp. 3, 6.

Freedman, M. (1999). *Prime time: How baby boomers will revolutionize retirement and transform America.* New York: Public Affairs.

Freudenheim, M. (2002, April 9). Mammogram centers facing rising costs and low reimbursements. *The New York Times,* p. D9.

Friedan, B. (1993). *The fountain of age.* New York: Simon and Schuster.

Friedland, R. et al. (2001). Patients with Alzheimer's disease have reduced activities in midlife compared with healthy control-group members. *Proceedings of the National Academy of Sciences, 98,* 3440–3445.

Friedmann, E. et al. (1980). Animal companions and one-year survival of patients after discharge from a coronary care unit. *Public Health Reports, 95,* 307–312.

Fries, J. (1989). *Aging well: A guide for successful seniors.* Reading, MA: Addison-Wesley.

Fries, J., & Crapo, M. (1986). The elimination of premature disease. In K. Dychtwald (Ed.), *Wellness and Health Promotion for the Elderly* (pp. 19–37). Rockville, MD: Aspen.

Fritsch, T. et al. (2001). Effects of educational attainment on the clinical expression of Alzheimer's disease: Results from a research registry. *American Journal of Alzheimer's Disease and Other Dementias, 16,* 369–376.

Fuhrman, B. et al. (2000). Ginger extract consumption reduces plasma cholesterol, inhibits LDL oxidation and attenuates development of atherosclerosis in atherosclerotic, apolipoprotein E-Deficient mice. *Journal of Nutrition, 130,* 1124–1131.

Gallagher, D. et al. (2000). Healthy percentage body fat ranges: An approach for developing guidelines based on body mass index. *American Journal of Clinical Nutrition, 72,* 694–701.

Gallagher-Thompson, D. et al. (1990). Maintenance of gains versus relapse following brief psychotherapy for depression. *Journal of Consulting and Clinical Psychology, 58,* 371–374.

Gallo, J. et al. (1999). Attitudes, knowledge, and behavior of family physicians regarding depression in late life. *Archives of Family Medicine, 8,* 249–256.

Gallo, J. et al. (1994). Age differences in the symptoms of depression: A latent trait analysis. *Journal of Gerontology, 49,* P251–P264.

Gallup. (1988). *Research to prevent blindness.* New York.

Gambert, S. (2002). The promise of statins. *Clinical Geriatrics, 10,* 15–16.

Gamble, E. et al. (1991). Knowledge, attitudes and behavior of elderly persons regarding living wills. *Archive Internal Medicine, 151,* 277.

Ganzini, L. et al. (2002). Experiences of Oregon nurses and social workers with hospice patients who requested assistance with suicide. *New England Journal of Medicine, 347,* 582–588.

Garfinkel, M. et al. (1998). Yoga-based intervention for carpal tunnel syndrome. *Journal of the American Medical Association, 280,* 1601–1603.

Garlic: Case unclosed. (2000, October). *Nutrition Action Healthletter,* pp. 8–9.

Gearon, C. (2000). Going online . . . for health. *AARP Bulletin, 41,* 5, pp. 4, 14–15.

Gehlbach, S. et al. (2002). Recognition of osteoporosis by primary care physicians. *American Journal of Public Health, 92,* 271–273.

Gemson et al. (1988). Differences in physician prevention practice patterns for white and minority patients. *Journal of Community Health, 13,* 53–64.

George, L. (1993, Winter/Spring). Depressive disorders and symptoms in later life. *Generations,* pp. 35–38.

George, L. (1986, Spring). Life satisfaction in later life. *Generations,* pp. 5–8.

Getting a boost from insurers. (1999, June 7). *American Medical News,* pp. 13–14.

Gielen, S. et al. (2001). Benefits of exercise training for patients with chronic heart failure. *Clinical Geriatrics, 9,* 32–45.

Giger, J. et al. (1997). Health promotion among ethnic minorities: The importance of cultural phenomena. *Rehabilitation Nursing, 22,* 303–308.

Gill, T. et al. (2000). Role of exercise stress testing and safety monitoring for older persons starting an exercise program. *Journal of the American Medical Association, 284,* 342–349.

Gill, T. et al. (1999). A population-based study of environmental hazards in the homes of older persons. *American Journal of Public Health, 89,* 553–556.

Glass, T. et al. (1999). Population based study of social and productive activities as predictors of survival among elderly Americans. *British Medical Journal, 319,* 478–483.

Glassheim, C. (1992). *Health Partners Program mimeograph.* Albuquerque, New Mexico: The University of New Mexico School of Medicine's Primary Care Curriculum.

Glynn, T. (1990). Methods of smoking cessation: Finally, some answers. *Journal of the American Medical Association, 263,* 2795–2796.

Goldsteen, R. et al. (1991, November). *Examining the relationship between health locus of control and use of medical services.* Paper presentation at the Annual Gerontological Society of America meeting, Minneapolis.

Goldstein, M. et al. (1999). Physician-based physical activity counseling for middle-aged and older adults: A randomized trial. *Annals of Behavioral Medicine, 21,* 40–47.

Goleman, D., & Gurin, J. (1993). *Mind body medicine: How to use your mind for better health.* Younkers, NY: Consumer Reports Books.

Goodwin, J. et al. (1987). The effect of marital status on stage, treatment, and survival of cancer patients. *Journal of the American Medical Association, 258,* 3125–3130.

Goodwin, P. et al. (2001). The effect of group psychosocial support on survival in metastatic breast cancer. *The New England Journal of Medicine, 345,* 1719–1726.

Gorman, K., &. Posner, J. (1988). Benefits of exercise in old age. *Clinics in Geriatric Medicine, 4,* 181–192.

Gottlieb, B. (1985). Social networks and social support: An overview of research, practice, and policy implication. *Health Education Quarterly, 12,* 5–22.

Gotzsche, P., & Olsen, O. (2000). Is screening for breast cancer with mammography justified? *Lancet, 355,* 129–134.

Gould, L. et al. (1995). Changes in myocardial perfusion abnormalities by positron emission tomography after long-term, intense risk factor modification. *Journal of the American Medical Association, 274,* 894–901.

Grady, D. (2002a). A 60-year-old woman trying to discontinue hormone replacement therapy. *Journal of the American Medical Association, 287,* 2130–2137.

Grady, D. (2002b, April 18). Scientists question hormone therapies for menopause ills. *The New York Times,* pp. 1,6.

Grady, D., & Cummings, S. (2001). Postmenopausal hormone therapy for prevention of fractures: How good is the evidence? *Journal of the American Medical Association, 285,* 2909–2910.

Grandi, A. et al. (2001). Left ventricular changes in isolated office hypertension: A blood pressure-matched comparison with normotension and sustained hypertension. *Archives of Internal Medicine, 161,* 2677–2681.

Grandjean, A. et al. (2000). The effect of caffeinated, non-caffeinated, caloric and non-caloric beverages on hydration. *Journal of American College of Nutrition, 19,* 591–600.

Grasso, P., & Haber, D. (1995). A leadership training program at a senior center. *Activities, Adaptation and Aging, 20,* 13–24.

Greeley, A. (1990, October). Nutrition and the elderly. *FDA Consumer,* pp. 25–28.

Green, L., & Kreuter, M. (1999). *Health promotion planning: An educational and ecological approach* (3rd ed.). Mountain View, CA: Mayfield.

Greene, M. (1991, July). *Determinants and outcomes of the physician-elderly patient initial medical encounter.* Final report for the AARP Andrus Foundation, Washington, DC.

Greene, M. et al. (1989). Concordance between physicians and their older and younger patients in the primary care medical encounter. *Gerontologist, 29,* 808–813.

Greene, M. et al. (1987). Psychosocial concerns in the medical encounter: A comparison of the interactions of doctors with their old and young patients. *Gerontologist, 27,* 164.

Greenwood, R. (2002a). The PACE program: Rooted in community-based organizations. *Innovations, 3,* 29–34.

Greenwood, R. (2002b). The PACE Model. *Center for Medicare Education, 2,* 1–8.

Greiner, K. et al. (2000). Medical student interest in alternative medicine. *The Journal of Alternative and Complementary Medicine, 6,* 231–234.

Gueyffier, F. et al. (1999). Antihypertensive drugs in very old people: A subgroup meta-analysis of randomized controlled trials. *The Lancet, 353,* 793–796.

Guralnik, J. (1991). Prospects for the Compression of Morbidity. *Journal of Aging and Health, 3,* 138–154.

Gurwitz, J et al. (2003). Incidence and preventability of adverse drug events among older persons in the ambulatory setting. *Journal of the American Medical Association, 289,* 1107–1116.

Haber, D. (2003). The gerontology program practicum: Evaluation of selected components. *Gerontology and Geriatrics, 23,* 3, 51–63.

Haber, D. (2002a). Health promotion and aging: Educational and clinical initiatives by the federal government. *Educational Gerontology, 28,* 1–11.

Haber, D. (2002b). Wellness General of the United States: A creative approach to promote family and community health. *Family and Community Health, 25,* 71–82.

Haber, D. (2001a). Medicare prevention: Movement toward research-based policy. *Journal of Aging and Social Policy, 13,* 1–14.

Haber, D. (2001b). Promoting readiness to change behavior through health assessments. *Clinical Gerontologist, 23,* 152–158.

Haber, D. (1999). Minority access to hospice. *The American Journal of Hospice and Palliative Care, 16,* 386–390.

Haber, D. (1996). Strategies to promote the health of older persons: An alternative to readiness stages. *Family and Community Health, 19,* 1–10.

Haber, D. (1993a). Guide to clinical preventive services: A challenge to physician resourcefulness. *Clinical Gerontologist, 12,* 17–29.

Haber, D. (1993b). Chronic illness, aging, and health promotion. *Illness, Crises and Loss, 2,* 2–5.

Haber, D. (1992a). Self-help groups and aging. In A. Katz et al. (Eds.), *Self-help: Concepts and applications* (pp. 295–298). Philadelphia: The Charles Press.

Haber, D. (1992b). An obstacle to physicians recommending medical screenings to older adults. *Academic Medicine, 67,* 107.

Haber, D. (1989). *Health care for an aging society: Cost conscious community care and self-care approaches.* New York: Hemisphere/Taylor and Francis Group.

Haber, D. (1988a). A health promotion program in ten nursing homes. *Activities, Adaptation and Aging, 2,* 73–82.

Haber, D. (1988b). The Interfaith Volunteer Caregivers Program. *Journal of Religion & Aging, 3,* 151–156.

Haber, D. (1986). Health promotion to reduce blood pressure level among older blacks. *The Gerontologist, 26,* 119–121.

Haber, D. (1984). Church-based programs for caregivers of non-institutionalized elders. *Journal of Gerontological Social Work, 7*(4), 43–55.

Haber, D. (l983a). Yoga as a preventive health care program. *The International Journal of Aging and Human Development, 17,* 169–176.

Haber, D. (1983b). Promoting mutual help groups among older persons. *The Gerontologist, 23,* 251–253.

Haber, D. (1979, November/December). Old age in China. *Aging,* pp. 7–9.

Haber, D., & Lacy, M., (1993). A socio-behavioral health promotion intervention with older adults. *Behavior, Health, and Aging, 3,* 73-85.

Haber, D., & Looney, C. (2003). Health promotion directory: Development, distribution, and utilization. *Health Promotion Practice, 4,* 72–77.

Haber, D., & Looney. C. (2000). Health contract calendars: A tool for health professionals with older adults. *The Gerontologist, 40,* 235–239.

Haber, D., & Wicht, J. (1987). Worksite wellness and aging. *Journal of Individual, Family, and Community Wellness, 4,* 31–34.

Haber, D., & George, J. (l98l-1982). A preventive health care program with hispanic elders. *The Journal of Minority Aging, 6,* 1–11.

Haber, D. et al. (2000). Impact of a health promotion course on inactive, overweight, or physically limited older adults. *Family and Community Health, 22,* 48–56.

Haber, D. et al. (1997). Impact of a geriatric health promotion elective on occupational and physical therapy students. *Gerontology & Geriatrics Education, 18,* 65–76.

Haight, B. et al. (1998). Life review: Preventing despair in newly relocated nursing home residents' short- and long-term effects. *International Journal of Aging and Human Development, 47,* 119–142.

Hakim, A. et al. (1999). Effects of walking on coronary heart disease in elderly men: The Honolulu Heart Program. *Circulation, 100,* 9–13.

Hall, K., & Luepker, R. (2000). Is hypercholesterolemia a risk factor and should it be treated in the elderly? *American Journal of Health Promotion, 14,* 347–356.

Haller, C., & Benowitz, N. (2000). Adverse cardiovascular and central nervous system events associated with dietary supplements containing ephedra alkaloids. *New England Journal of Medicine, 343,* 1833–1838.

Haney, D. (1999, November 25). The latest thing in fine dining: Food that is also medicine. *The Daily News,* Galveston, TX, p. A22.

Harnack, L. et al. (2000). Temporal trends in energy intake in the United States: An ecologic perspective. *American Journal of Clinical Nutrition, 71,* 1478–1484.

Harrington, C. et al. (2001). Does investor ownership of nursing homes compromise the quality of care? *American Journal of Public Health, 91,* 1452–1455.

Harris, L. et al. (1989). *The Prevention Index '89: Summary Report.* Emmaus, PA: Rodale Press.

Harris, W. et al. (1999). A randomized, controlled trial on the effects of remote, intercessory prayer on outcomes in patients admitted to the coronary care unit. *Archives of Internal Medicine, 159,* 2273–2278.

Haug, M. (1979). Doctor patient relationships and the older patient. *Journal of Gerontology, 34,* 852–860.

Haug, M., & Lavin, B. (1981). Practitioner or patient—Who's in charge? *Journal of Health and Social Behavior, 22,* 212–229.

Haupt, B. (1997, April 25). Characteristics of hospice care discharges: United States, 1993–1994. *Advance Data, 287,* 1–14.

Hays, J. et al. (2003). Effects of estrogen plus progestin on health-related quality of life. *New England Journal of Medicine, 348,* 1839–1854.

Hayward, R. et al. (1987). Who gets preventive care? Results from a new national survey. Paper presentation at Concurrent Symposium A, SREPCIM Abstracts, April 1.

Hazzard, W. (1992). Dyslipoproteinemia in the elderly: Should it be treated? In G. Omenn (Ed.), *Clinics in geriatric medicine* (pp. 89–102). Philadelphia: W. B. Saunders and Company.

Health. (1996, July 1). *American Medical News,* pp. 13–14.

Health and fitness. (1991, November 19). Special Section, *Newsweek.*

Health guides could raise premiums. (2001, May 17). *USA Today,* p. 1.

Health promotion inter-change. (1997, Fall). Texas Department of *Health newsletter, 1, 2,* p. 3.

Heaney, R. et al. (2002). Risendronate reduces the risk of first vertebral fracture in osteoporotic women. *Osteoporosis International, 13,* 501–505.

Heaney, R. (1993). Thinking straight about calcium. *New England Journal of Medicine, 328,* 503–505.

Heart Protection Study Collaborative Group. (2002). MRC/BHF Heart Protection Study of cholesterol lowering simvastatin in 20,536 high-risk individuals: A randomized placebo-controlled trial. *Lancet, 360,* 7–22.

Hedberg, K. et al. (2002). Legalized physician-assisted suicide in Oregon. *New England Journal of Medicine, 346,* 450–452.

Heinonen, O. et al. (1998). Prostate cancer and supplementation with alpha-Tocopherol and beta-Carotene: Incidence and mortality in a controlled trial. *Journal of the National Cancer Institute, 90,* 440–446.

Heinzelmann, F., & Bagley, R. (1970). Response of physical activity programs and their effects on health behavior. *Public Health Reports, 85,* 905–911.

Heller, H. et al. (2000). Pharmacokinetic and pharmacoodynamic comparison of two calcium supplements in post-menopausal women. *Journal of Clinical Pharmocology, 40,* 1237–1244.

Henderson, S. et al. (1992). Benefits of an exercise class for elderly women following hip surgery. *The Ulster Medical Journal, 61,* 144–150.

Herbal hype. (2000, August 21). *American Medical News,* pp. 27–28.

Herbert, R., & Gabriel, M. (2002). Effects of stretching before and after exercising on muscle soreness and risk of injury: Systematic review. *British Medical Journal, 325,* 468–470.

Hernandez, M. et al. (2000). Results of a home-based training program for patients with COPD. *Chest, 118,* 106–114.

Hernandez-Reif, M. (2001). Evidence-based medicine and massage. *Pediatrics, 108,* 1053.

Hernandez-Reif, M. et al. (2001). Lower back pain is reduced and range of motion increased after massage therapy. *Neuroscience, 106*, 131–145.

Hertzman-Miller, et al. (2002). Comparing the satisfaction of low back pain patients randomized to receive medical or chiropractic care. *American Journal of Public Health, 92*, 1628–1633.

Heshka, S. et al. (2003). weight loss with self-help compared with a structured commercial program. *Journal of the American Medical Association, 289*, 1792–1798.

Hesser, A. (2002, October 30). Big eaters, sure, but this is absurd. *The New York Times*, pp. D1, D5.

Hesson, J. (1995). *Weight training for life*. Englewood, CO: Morton Publishing Company.

High, K. (2001). Nutritional strategies to boost immunity and prevention infection in elderly individuals. *Clinical Infectious Disease, 33*, 1892–1900.

Hildreth, C., & Saunders, E. (1992). Heart disease, stroke and hypertension in blacks. In R. Braithwaite & S. Taylor (Eds.), *Health issues in the Black community* (pp. 90–105). San Francisco: Jossey-Bass.

Hill, D. et al. (1988). Self examination of the breast: Is it beneficial? *British Medical Journal, 297*, 271–275.

Himes, J. (2001). Prevalence of individuals with skin-folds too large to measure. *American Journal of Public Health, 91*, 154–155.

Himmelfarb, S., & Murrell, S. (1984). The prevalence and correlates of anxiety symptoms in older adults. *Journal of Psychology, 111*(2nd Half), 159–167.

Hinman, R. et al. (2002). Effects of static magnets on chronic knee pain and physical function: A double-blind study. *Alternative Therapies, 8*, 50–55.

Hodis, H. et al. (2002). Alpha-tocopherol supplementation in healthy individuals reduce low-density lipoprotein oxidation but not atherosclerosis: The Vitamin E Atherosclerosis Prevention Study. *Circulation, 106*, 1453–1459.

Hoeger, W., & Hoeger, S. (1997). *Principles and labs for fitness and wellness, 4th ed.* Colorado: Morton Publishing Company.

Hohl, C. et al. (2001). Polypharmacy, adverse drug-related events, and potential adverse drug interactions in elderly patients presenting to an emergency department. *Annals of Emergency Medicine, 38*, 666–671.

Hollowell, J. et al. (2002). Serum TSH, T4, and thyroid antibodies in the United States population (1988 to 1994): NHANES III. *Journal of Clinical Endocrinology Metabolism, 87*, 489–499.

Holmberg, L. et al. (2002). A randomized trial comparing radical prostatectomy with watchful waiting in early prostate cancer. *New England Journal of Medicine, 347*, 781–789.

Holmes, T., & Rahe, R. (1967). The social readjustment rating scale. *Journal of Psychosomatic Research, 11*, 213–218.

Hooyman, N., & Kiyak, H. (1999). *Social gerontology* (5th ed.). Boston: Allyn and Bacon.

Horowitz, A., & Nourjah, P. (1996). Patterns of screening oral cancer among US adults. *Journal of Public Health Dentistry, 56*, 331–335.

Horrocks, S. et al. (2002). Systematic review of whether nurse practitioners working in primary care can provide equivalent care to doctors. *British Medical Journal, 324*, 819–823.

Horton, J. (1986). Education programs on smoking prevention and smoking cessation for students and house staff in U.S. medical schools. *Cancer Detection and Prevention, 9*, 417–420.

Horwath, C. (1991). Nutrition goals for older adults: A review. *The Gerontologist, 31,* 811–821.

Horwarth, C. (1989). Marriage and diet in elderly Australians: Results from a large random survey. *Journal of Human Nutrition and Dietetics, 2,* 185–193.

House, J. et al. (1988). Social relationships and health. *Science, 241,* 540–545.

Howley, E., & Franks, B. (1997). *Health fitness instructor's handbook* (3rd ed.). IL: Human Kinetics.

How McNuggets changed the world. (2001, January 22). *U.S. News & World Report,* p. 54.

Hrobjartsson, A., & Gotzsche, P. (2001). Is the placebo powerless? An analysis of clinical trials comparing placebo with no treatment. *New England Journal of Medicine, 344,* 1594–1602.

HRSA. (2002). *Women's Health USA 2002,* Health Resources and Services Administration, USDHHS.

Hu, F. et al. (2001). Physical activity and risk for cardiovascular events in diabetic women. *Annals of Internal Medicine, 134,* 96–105.

Hu, F. et al. (1999). Walking compared with vigorous physical activity and risk of type 2 diabetes in women. *Journal of the American Medical Association, 282,* 1433–1439.

Hu, F. et al. (1997). Dietary fat intake and the risk of coronary heart disease in women. *New England Journal of Medicine, 337,* 1491–1499.

Huck, D., & Armer, J. (1995). Affectivity and mental health among elderly religious. *Issues in Mental Health Nursing, 16,* 447–459.

Humphrey, L. et al. (2002). Breast Cancer Screening: A summary of the evidence for the U.S. Preventive Services Task Force. *The Annals of Internal Medicine. 137*(5 Part 1), 347–360.

Hurley, J. (1992). *Nutrition and health.* Guilford, CT: Dushkin Publishing Co.

Hutchinson, S. (1998, January 12). The new case for patient education. *American Medical News,* p. 13.

Huusko, T. et al. (2000). Randomised, clinically controlled trial of intensive geriatric rehabilitation in patients with hip fracture: Subgroup analysis of patients with dementia. *British Medical Journal, 321,* 107–1111.

Hyman, D., & Pavlik, V. (2001). Characteristics of patients with uncontrolled hypertension in the United States. *New England Journal of Medicine, 345,* 479–486.

Hypericum Depression Trial Study Group. (2002). Effect of Hypericum perforatum (St John's wort) in major depressive disorder: A randomized controlled trial. *Journal of the American Medical Association, 287,* 1807–1814.

Hypertension Detection and Follow-Up Program Cooperative Group. (1988). Persistence of reduction in blood pressure and mortality of participants in the hypertension detection and follow-up program. *Journal of the American Medical Association, 259,* 2113–2122.

Idler, E. (1994). *Cohesiveness and coherence: Religion and the health of the elderly.* New York: Garland.

Idler, E., & Kasl, S. (1992). Religion, disability, depression, and the timing of death. *American Journal of Sociology, 97,* 1052–1079.

Institute of Medicine. (1990). *The second 50 years: Promoting health and preventing disability.* Washington, DC: National Academy Press.

Insull, W. et al. (1990). Results of a randomized feasibility study of a low-fat diet. *Archives of Internal Medicine, 150,* 421–427.

Is chocolate good for you? (2000, July). *Women's Health Advisor,* p. 8.

Israel, B. (1985). Social networks and social support: Implications for natural helper and community level interventions. *Health Education Quarterly, 12,* 65–80.

Israel, B., & Schurman, S. (1990). Social Support, Control, and the Stress Process. In K. Glanz et al. (Eds.), *Health behavior and health education: Theory, research and practice* (pp. 196–201). San Francisco: Jossey-Bass Publishers.

Is there a difference between natural and synthetic vitamin E? (2000, March). *Johns Hopkins Health After 50.*

Jackevicius, C. et al. (2002). Adherence with statin therapy in elderly patients with and without acute coronary syndromes. *Journal of the American Medical Association, 288,* 462–467.

Jackman, P. (1997, September 15). FTC Crackdowns on wellness infomercials. *Houston Chronicle,* Section C, p. 2.

Jacob. J. (2002, March). Wellness programs help companies save on health costs. *American Medical News,* pp. 32–33.

Jacob, J. (1998, September 21). Financial ratings of HMOs slide: Half lost money. *American Medical News,* p. 16.

Jacobson, M. (2000, December). Tax junk foods. *Nutrition Action Healthletter,* p. 2.

Jacobson, M., & Brownell, K. (2000). Small taxes on soft drinks and snack foods to promote health. *American Journal of Public Health, 90,* 854–857.

Jacoby, J. (1998, November 12). The bullies' next target: Junk food. *Boston Globe,* p. A25.

Jacoby, S. (1999, September–October). Great sex: What's age got to do with it? *Modern Maturity,* pp. 41–46.

Jacques, P. et al. (1997). Long-term vitamin C use and prevalence of early age-related lens opacities. *American Journal of Clinical Nutrition, 66,* 911–916.

Jakes, R. et al. (2001). Patterns of physical activity and ultrasound attenuation by heel bone among Norfolk cohort of European Prospective Investigation of Cancer. *British Medical Journal, 322,* 140–143.

Jakicic, J. et al. (1995). Prescription of exercise intensity for the obese patient: The relationship between heart rate, $Vo_2$ and perceived exertion. *International Journal of Obesity, 19,* 382–387.

JAMA. (1990). Report of the US Preventive Services Task Force. *Journal of the American Medical Association, 263,* 436–437.

Jampol, L. et al. (2001). Antioxidants, zinc and age-related macular degeneration: Results and recommendations. *Archives of Ophthalmology, 119,* 1533–1534.

Janson, C. et al. (2001). Effect of passive smoking on respiratory symptoms, bronchial responsiveness, lung function, and total serum IgE in the European Community Respiratory Health Survey: A cross-sectional study. *The Lancet, 358,* 2103–2109.

Janz, N. et al. (1984). Contingency contracting to enhance patient compliance: A review. *Patient education and Counseling, 5,* 165–178.

Jarrett, R. et al. (2001). Preventing recurrent depression using cognitive therapy with and without a continuation phase. *Archives of General Psychiatry, 58,* 381–388.

Jette, A. et al. (1999). Exercise—It's never too late: The Strong for Life program. *American Journal of Public Health, 89,* 66–72.

Jiang, W. et al. (1996). Mental stress-induced myocardial ischemia and cardiac events. *Journal of the American Medical Association, 275,* 1651–1656.

Jick, H. et al. (2000). Statins and the risk of dementia. *Lancet, 356,* 1627–1631.

*Johns Hopkins Medical Letter.* (1997). Health club membership rises.

Johnson, A. et al. (2001). Blood pressure is linked to salt intake and modulated by the angiotensinogen gene in normotensive and hypertensive elderly subjects. *Journal of Hypertension, 19,* 1053–1060.

Johnson, C. (1991). The status of health care among Black Americans. *Journal of the National Medical Association, 83,* 125–129.

Jonas, S. (2000). *Talking about health and wellness with patients.* New York: Springer.

Jones, J., & Jones, K. (1997, July). Promoting physical activity in the senior years. *Journal of Gerontological Nursing,* 41–48.

Jones, L. (1992, November 9). Physicians can do more to promote regular Pap tests. *American Medical News,* p. 6.

Jones, P., & Ross, R. (1999). Prevention of bladder cancer. *New England Journal of Medicine, 340,* 1424–1426.

Jorenby, D. et al. (1999). A controlled trial of sustained-release bupropion, a nicotine patch, or both for smoking cessation. *New England Journal of Medicine, 340,* 685–691.

Jorm, A. et al. (1987). The prevalence of dementia: A quantitative integration of the literature. *Acta Psychiatrica Scandinavica, 76,* 465–479.

Kampert, J. et al. (1996). Physical activity, physical fitness, and all-cause mortality: A prospective study of men and women. *Annuals of Epidemiology, 6,* 452–457.

Kane, R. (2001). Long-term care and a good quality of life: Bringing them closer to together. *Gerontologist, 41,* 293–304.

Kannus, P. et al. (2000). Prevention of hip fracture in elderly people with use of a hip protector. *New England Journal of Medicine, 343,* 1506–1513.

Kannus, P. et al. (1989). Sports injuries in elderly athletes: A three-year prospective controlled study. *Age and Ageing, 18,* 263.

Kant, A. (2000). Consumption of energy-dense, nutrient-poor foods by adult Americans: Nutritional and health implications. The third National Health and Nutrition Examination Survey, 1988–1994. *American Journal of Clinical Nutrition, 72,* 929–936.

Kaptchuk, et al. (1998). Chiropractic—Origins, controversies, and contributions. *Archives of Internal Medicine, 158,* 2215–2223.

Katon, W. et al. (1992). Adequacy and duration of antidepressant treatment in primary care. *Medical Care, 30,* 67–76.

Kawachi, I. et al. (1997). A prospective study of passive smoking and coronary heart disease. *Circulation, 95,* 2374–2379.

Kearney, S. (1998a). Barriers to physician providing health education in primary care settings. *The Health Education Monograph Series, 16,* 6–9.

Kearney, S. (1998b). Resistance training and bone mineral density in women. *American Journal of Physical Medicine Rehabilitation, 80,* 65–77.

Keim, N. (1995, April). Fates of fat. *Research Briefs.* U.S. Department of Agricultural Research Service. p. 2.

Keller, M. et al. (2000). A comparison of nefazodone, the cognitive behavioral-analysis system of psychotherapy, and their combination for the treatment of chronic depression. *New England Journal of Medicine, 342,* 1462–1470.

Keller, M. et al. (1989). Beliefs about aging and illness in a community sample. *Research in Nursing Health, 12,* 247–255.

Kelley, G. (2001). *Low-impact exercise can increase bone mass in women.* George Kelley, Massachusetts General Hospital Institute of Health Professions, American Public Association Annual Meeting, Atlanta, Georgia, October 22.

Kelley, G., & Kelley, K. (2000). Progressive resistance exercise and resting blood pressure: A meta-analysis of randomized controlled trials. *Hypertension, 35,* 838–843.

Kemper, D. et al. (1987). *Growing younger handbook.* Boise, ID: Healthwise.

Kemper, D. et al. (l985). *Pathways: A success guide for a healthy life.* Boise, ID: Healthwise.

Kenchaiah, S. et al. (2002). Obesity and the risk of heart failure. *New England Journal of Medicine, 347,* 305–313.

Kennelly, B. (2001). Suffering in deference: A focus group study of older cardiac patients' preferences for treatment and perceptions of risk. *Quality Health Care, 10*(Suppl. 1), i23–i28.

Kerlikowske, K. et al. (1999). Continuing screening mammography in women aged 70 to 79. *Journal of the American Medical Association, 282,* 2156–2163.

Khan, A. et al. (1991). Chronicity of depressive episode in relation to antidepressant-placebo response. *Neuropsychopharmacology, 4,* 125–130.

Khatri, P. et al. (2001). Effects of exercise training on cognitive functioning among depressed older men and women. *Journal of Aging and Physical Activity, 9,* 43–57.

Kiecolt-Glaser, J. et al. (1991). Spousal caregivers of dementia victims: Longitudinal changes in immunity and health. *Psychosomatic Medicine, 53,* 345–362.

Kiernat, J. (1991). *Occupational therapy and the older adult.* Gaithersburg, MD: Aspen.

Kim, K. et al. (1991). Development and evaluation of the Osteoporosis Health Belief Scale. *Research in Nursing and Health, 14,* 155–163.

King, A. et al. (2002). Effects of moderate-intensity exercise on physiological, behavioral, and emotional responses to family caregiving: A randomized controlled trial. *Journal of Gerontology: Medical Sciences, 57A,* M26–M36.

King, A. et al. (1997). Moderate-intensity exercise and self-rated quality of sleep in older adults. *Journal of the American Medical Association, 277,* 32–37.

Kinoshita, N. et al. (2000). Physiological profile of middle-aged and older climbers who ascended Gasherbrum II, an 8035-m Himalayan Peak. *Journal of Gerontology: Medical Sciences, 55A,* M630–M633.

Kirscht, J. (1988). The health belief model and predictions of health actions. In D. Gochman (Ed.), *Health behavior: Emerging research perspectives.* New York: Plenum Press.

Kizer, W. (1987). *The healthy workplace.* New York: John Wiley.

Klein, S. (1997). Personal communication with Sam Klein, The University of Texas Medical Branch, School of Medicine, Galveston, TX.

Klem, M. et al. (1997). A descriptive study of individual's successful at long-term maintenance of substantial weight loss. *American Journal of Clinical Nutrition, 66,* 239–246.

Kleyman, P. (1998, January/February). Using the Net for good health/Media's health role is growing. *Aging Today,* p. 18.

Kligman, E., & Pepin, E. (1992). Prescribing physical activity for older patients. *Geriatrics, 47,* 33–47.

Knight, B. et al. (1993). A meta-analytic review of interventions for caregiver distress: Recommendations for future research. *The Gerontologist, 33,* 240–248.

Knowler, W. et al. (2002). Reduction in the incidence of type 2 diabetes with lifestyle intervention or metformin. *New England Journal of Medicine, 346,* 393–403.

Koch, K. (1977). *I never told anybody.* New York: Random House.

Koenig, H. (2000). Religion, spirituality, and medicine: Application to clinical practice. *Journal of the American Medical Association, 284,* 1708.

Koenig, H. et al. (1999). Does religious attendance prolong survival? A six-year follow-up study of 3,968 older adults. *Journal of Gerontology: Biological and Medical Sciences, 54,* M370–M376.

Koenig, H. et al. (1997). Attendance at religious services, interleukin-6, and other biological parameters of immune function in older adults. *International Journal of Psychiatry in Medicine, 27,* 233–250.

Koepsell, T. et al. (2002). Crosswalk markings and the risk of pedestrian-motor vehicle collisions in older pedestrians. *Journal of the American Medical Association, 288,* 2136–2143.

Kofoed, L. et al. (1987). Treatment compliance of older alcoholics: An elderly-specific approach is superior to "mainstreaming." *Journal of Studies on Alcohol, 48,* 47–51.

Kolata, G. (1996, February 27). New era of robust elderly belies the fears of scientists. *The New York Times Science,* p. 1.

Kolata, G., & Moss, M. (2002, February 11). X-ray vision in hindsight: science, politics and the mammogram. *The New York Times,* p. A23.

Kotecki, J. et al. (2000). Health promotion beliefs and practices among pharmacists. *Journal of the American Pharmaceutical Association, 40,* 773–779.

Kottke, T. et al. (1988). Attributes of successful smoking cessation interventions in medical practice: A meta-analysis of 42 controlled trials. *Journal of the American Medical Association, 259,* 2883–2889.

Kramer, A. et al. (1999). Ageing, fitness and neurocognitive function. *Nature, 400,* 418–419.

Kraus, W. et al. (2002). Effects of the amount and intensity of exercise on plasma lipoproteins. *New England Journal of Medicine, 347,* 1483–1492.

Krause, N. (2002). Church-based social support and health in old age: Exploring variations by race. *Journal of Gerontology: Social Sciences, 57B,* S332–S347.

Krause, N., & Van Tran, T. (1989). Stress and religious involvement among older blacks. *Journal of Gerontology, 44,* 4–13.

Krause, N., & Wray, L. (1991, Fall). Psychosocial correlates of health and illness among minority elders. *Generations.*

Kreuzer, M. et al. (2000). Environmental tobacco smoke and lung cancer: A case-control study in Germany. *American Journal of Epidemiology, 151,* 241–250.

Kripke, D. et al. (2002). Mortality associated with sleep duration and insomnia. *Archives of General Psychiatry, 59,* 131–136.

Kritz-Silverstein, D. et al. (2001). Cross-sectional and prospective study of exercise and depressed mood in the elderly: The Rancho Bernardo Study. *American Journal of Epidemiology, 153,* 596–603.

Kruger, J. et al. (2002, May 17). Prevalence of health-care providers asking older adults about their physical activity levels—United States, 1998. *Morbidity and Mortality Weekly Report, 51,* 412–414.

Kumanyika, D. et al. (1992). Lose weight and win: A church-based weight loss program for blood pressure control among black women. *Patient Education and Counseling, 19,* 19–32.

Kupfer, D., & Frank, E. (2002). Placebo in clinical trials for depression: Complexity and necessity. *Journal of the American Medical Association, 287,* 1853–1854.

Kurlowicz, L. (1997). Nursing standard of practice protocol: Depression in elderly patients. *Geriatric Nursing, 18,* 192–200.

Kushi, L. et al. (1996). Dietary antioxidant vitamins and death from coronary heart disease in postmenopausal women. *New England Journal of Medicine, 334,* 1156–1162.

Kushner, R. (1995). Barriers to providing nutrition counseling by physicians: A survey of primary care practitioners. *Preventive Medicine, 24,* 546–552.

Lachman, M. (1986). Personal control in later life: Stability, change and cognitive correlates. In M. Baltes & P. Baltes (Eds.), *The psychology of control and aging.* Hillsdale, NJ: Erlbaum.

LaCroix, A. et al. (1996). Does walking decrease the risk of cardiovascular disease hospitalization and death in older adults? *Journal of American Geriatrics Society, 44,* 113–120.

LaCroix, A., & Omenn, G. (1992). Older adults and smoking. In G. Omenn (Ed.), *Clinics in Geriatric Medicine* (pp. 69–88). Philadelphia: W. B. Saunders.

Lagnado, L. (1996, October). Oxford to create alternative medicine network. *Wall Street Journal,* p. 1.

Lamy, P. (1988, Summer). Actions of alcohol and drugs in older people. *Generations,* pp. 9–13.

Lan, C. et al. (1999). The effect of Tai Chi on cardiorespiratory function in patients with coronary artery bypass surgery. *Medical Science Sports Exercise, 31,* 634–638.

Landa, A. (2002, September 2). Health care costs increasing. *American Medical News,* p. 5.

Landers, S. (2001, June 18). Beyond cholesterol: New uses for statins. *American Medical News,* pp. 32–33.

Landers, S. (2000, June 19). Medicare choices shrink as HMOs pull out. *American Medical News,* pp. 5, 7.

Lang, F. (2001). Regulation of social relationships in later adulthood. *Journal of Gerontology: Psychological Sciences, 56B,* P321–P326.

Langer, E., & Rodin, J. (1976). The effects of choice and enhanced personal responsibility for the aged: A field experiment in an institutional setting. *Journal of Personality and Social Psychology, 34,* 191–198.

Langlois, J. et al. (1997). Characteristics of older pedestrians who have difficulty crossing the street. *American Journal of Public Health, 87,* 393–397.

Lantz. M. (2002). Depression in the elderly: Recognition and treatment. *Clinical Geriatrics, 10,* 18–24.

Larson, D. (1995). Faith: The forgotten factor in healthcare. *American Journal of Natural Medicine, 2,* 10–15.

Latham, C., & Locke, E. (1991). Self-regulation through goal setting. *Organizational Behavior, 50,* 212–247.

Lau, R. (1988). Beliefs about control and health behavior. In D. Gochman (Ed.), *Health behavior: Emerging research perspectives* (pp. 43–63). New York: Plenum Press.

Laurence, L. (1997, May 14). Experts help consumers untangle web of health information on Net. *Houston Chronicle,* Section D, p.2.

Lawlor, D., & Hopker, S. (2001). The effectiveness of exercise as an intervention in the management of depression: Systematic review and meta-regression analysis of randomized controlled trials. *British Medical Journal, 322,* 763–767.

Lazarou, J. et al. (1998). Incidence of adverse drug reactions in hospitalized patients: A meta-analysis of prospective studies. *Journal of the American Medical Association, 279,* 1200–1205.

Lazarus, L., & Sadavoy, J. (1996). Individual psychotherapy. In J. Sadavoy (Ed.), *Comprehensive review of geriatric psychiatry* (2nd ed., pp. 819–826). Washington, DC: American Psychiatric Press.

Lazarus, R., & Folkman, S. (1984). *Stress, appraisal and coping.* New York: Springer.

Lazowski, D. et al. (1999). A randomized outcome evaluation of group exercise programs in long-term care institutions. *Journal of Gerontology: Medical Sciences, 54A,* M621–M628.

Leanse, J. (1986). The senior center as a wellness center. In K. Dychtwald (Ed.), *Wellness and health promotion for the elderly* (pp. 105–118). Rockville, MD: Aspen.

LeBars, P. et al. (1997). A placebo-controlled, double-blind, randomized trial of an extract of Ginkgo Biloba for dementia. *Journal of the American Medical Association, 278,* 1327–1332.

Lebowitz, B. (1995, Spring). Depression in older adults. *Aging and Vision News, 7,* p. 2.

Lee, C. et al. (1999). Cardiorespiratory fitness, body composition, and all-cause and cardiovascular disease mortality in men. *American Journal of Clinical Nutrition, 69,* 373–380.

Lee, G., & Cassidy, M. (1986). Family and kin relations of the rural elderly. In R. Coward & G. Lee (Eds.), *The elderly in rural society* (pp. 151–170). New York: Springer.

Lee, I. et al. (2003). Relative intensity of physical activity and risk of coronary heart disease. *Circulation, 107,* 1110–1116.

Lee, I. et al. (2000). Physical activity and coronary heart disease risk in men. *Circulation, 102,* 981–986.

Leeb, B. et al. (2000). A metaanalysis of chondroitin sulfate in the treatment of osteoarthritis. *Journal of Rheumatology, 27,* 205–211.

Leibel, R. et al. (1995). Changes in energy expenditure resulting from altered body weight. *New England Journal of Medicine, 332,* 621–628.

Leininger, L. et al. (1996). An office system for organizing preventive services. *Archives of Family Medicine, 5,* 108–115.

Lentzner, H. et al. (1992). Quality of life in the year before death. *American Journal of Public Health, 82,* 1093–1098.

Leslie, M., & Schuster, P.. (1991). The effect of contingency contracting on adherence and knowledge of exercise regimen. *Patient Education and Counseling, 18,* 231–241.

Leveille, S. et al. (1998). Preventing disability and managing chronic illness in frail older adults: A randomized trial of a community-based partnership with primary care. *Journal of American Geriatrics Society, 46,* 1191–1198.

Levin. R. (1987). *Wellness programs for older workers and retirees.* Washington, DC: Washington Business Group on Health.

Levine, J. et al. (1999). Role of nonexercise activity thermogenesis in resistance to fat gain in humans. *Science, 283,* 212–214.

Levine, M. et al. (1999). Criteria and recommendations for vitamin C intake. *JAMA, 281,* 1415–1423.

Levy, B. et al. (2002). Longevity increased by positive self-perceptions of aging. *Journal of Personality and Social Psychology, 83,* 261–270.

Lewis, C. (1988). Disease prevention and health promotion practices of primary care physicians in the United States. *American Journal of Preventive Medicine, 4*(4 suppl), 9–16.

Liberman, U. et al. (1995). Effect of oral alendronate on bone mineral density and the incidence of fractures in postmenopausal osteoporosis. *New England Journal of Medicine, 333,* 1437–1443.

Lieberman, D. et al., (2000). Use of colonoscopy to screen asymptomatic adults for colorectal cancer. *New England Journal of Medicine, 343,* 162–168.

Lieberman, M., & Borman, L. (1979). *Self-help groups for coping with crisis.* San Francisco, CA: Jossey-Bass Publishers.

Lieberman, M., & Videka-Sherman, L. (1986). The impact of self-help groups on the mental health of widows and widowers. *American Journal of Orthopyschiatry, 56,* 435–449.

Liebman, B. (1997, July/August). Carbo-Phobia: Zoning out on the new diet books. *Nutrition Action Healthletter,* pp. 3–5.

Liebman, B., & Hurley, J. (1996, November). One size doesn't fit all. *Nutrition Action Healthletter,* pp. 10–12

Light, E., & Lebowitz, B. (1991). *The elderly with chronic mental illness.* New York: Springer.

Lilly Issues Warning on Use of Prozac for Weight Loss. (1997, October 20). *American Medical News,* Health sub-section, p. 1.

Linden, W. et al. (2001). Individualized stress management for primary hypertension. *Archives of Internal Medicine, 161,* 1071–1080.

Lindsay, R. et al. (2002). Effect of lower doses of conjugated equine estrogens with and without medroxyprogesterone acetate on bone in early postmenopausal women. *Journal of the American Medical Association, 287,* 2668–2676.

Little, P. et al. (2002). Comparison of agreement between different measures of blood pressure in primary care and daytime ambulatory blood pressure. *British Medical Journal, 325,* p. 254.

Liu, S. et al. (2000). A prospective study of whole-grain intake and risk of type 2 diabetes mellitus in US women. *American Journal of Public Health, 90,* 1409–1415.

Logue, et al. (2000). Obesity management in primary care. Assessment of readiness to change among 284 family practice patients. *Journal of the American Board of Family Practice, 13,* 164–171.

Looney, C., & Haber, D. (2001).Interest in hosting an exercise program for older adults at African-American churches. *Journal of Religious Gerontology, 13,* 19–29.

Lopez, C., & Aguilera, E. (1991). *On the sidelines: Hispanic elderly and the continuum of care.* Washington, DC: National Council of La Raza.

Lorig, K. et al. (2001). Chronic disease self-management program. *Medical Care, 39,* 1217–1223.

Lorig, K. et al. (1999). Evidence suggesting that a chronic disease self-management program can improve health status while reducing hospitalization: A randomized trial. *Medical Care, 37,* 5–14.

Lorig, K. et al. (1996). *Outcome measures for health education and other health care interventions.* Thousand Oaks, CA: Sage.

Lorig, K. (1992). *Patient education: A practical approach.* St. Louis, MO: Mosby-Year Book.

Lorig, K. et al. (1989). Development and evaluation of a scale to measure perceived self-efficacy in people with arthritis. *Arthritis and Rheumatism, 32,* 37–44.

Lorig, K. et al. (1986). Outcomes of self-help education for patients with arthritis. *Arthritis and Rheumatism, 28,* 680–685.

Loss of Appetite. (1997, August). *Mayo Clinic Health Letter,* p. 7.

Lynne, J. (1997, July/August). Living wills: Tackle the hard stuff. *Health,* p. 30.

Madara, E., & Peterson, B. (1986). *Hospitals, churches, and self-help groups: Practical and promising relationships.* Unpublished manuscript, Denville, NJ.

Madison, P. et al. (2001). Do different dimensions of the metabolic syndrome change together over time? Evidence supporting obesity as the central feature. *Diabetes Care, 24,* 1758–1763.

Maheux, B. et al. (1989). Factors influencing physicians' preventive practices. *American Journal of Preventive Medicine, 5,* 201–206.

Maison, P. et al. (2001). Do different dimensions of the metabolic syndrome change together over time? Evidence supporting obesity as the central feature. *Diabetes Care, 10,* 1758–1763.

Maison, P. et al. (1998). Growth hormone as a risk for premature mortality in healthy subjects: Data from the Paris prospective study. *British Medical Journal, 316,* 1132–1133.

Malnutrition, food intake in elderly studied. (1995, November 6). *American Medical News,* p. 14.

Managed care cited for slowdown in spending. (1998, February 2). *American Medical News,* pp. 3, 8, 9.

Managed care strives to recover from '97 struggles. (1998, January 12). *American Medical News,* p. 25.

Mandelblatt, J. et al. (2002). Benefits and costs of using HPV testing to screen for cervical cancer. *Journal of the American Medical Association, 287,* 2372–2381.

Manson, J. et al. (2002). Walking compared with vigorous exercise for the prevention of cardiovascular events in women. *New England Journal of Medicine, 347,* 716–725.

Manson, J. et al. (1999). A prospective study of walking as compared with vigorous exercise in the prevention of coronary heart disease in women. *New England Journal of Medicine, 341,* 650–658.

Manton, K. et al. (1998). The dynamics of dimensions of age-related disability 1982-1994 in the U.S. elderly population. *Journal of Gerontology: Biological Sciences, 53A,* B59–B70.

Manton, K. et al. (1997). Chronic disability trends in elderly United State populations: 1982–1994. *Proceedings of the National Academy of Sciences, USA, 94,* 2593–2598.

Manton, K. et al. (1993). Forecasts of active life expectancy: Policy and fiscal implications. *Journal of Gerontology, 48*(Special Issue, September), 11–26.

Marcus, A., & Crane, L. (1987). *Current estimates of adult cigarette smoking by race/ethnicity.* Interagency Committee on Smoking and Health, invited paper, Washington, DC, March 31.

Marcus, B. et al. (1999). The efficacy of exercise as an aid for smoking cessation in women: A randomized controlled trial. *Archives of Internal Medicine, 159,* 1229–1234.

Marcus, M. (1997, August). Health and fitness: Women hit the weight room. *US News & World Report,* pp. 61–62.

Marcus, P. et al. (1996). Complete edentulism and denture use for elders in New England. *Journal of Prosthetic Dentistry, 76,* 260–266.

Mares-Perlman, J. et al. (2000). Vitamin supplement use and incident cataracts in a population-based study. *Archives of Ophthamology, 118,* 556–1563.

Margolin, A. et al. (2002). Acupuncture for the treatment of cocaine addiction: A randomized controlled trial. *Journal of the American Medical Association, 287,* 55–63.

Mark, E. et al. (1997). Fatal pulmonary hypertension associated with short-term use of fenfluramine and phentermine. *New England Journal of Medicine, 337,* 602–605.

Marks, G. et al., (1986). Role of health locus of control beliefs and expectations of treatment efficacy in adjustment to cancer. *Journal of Personality and Social Psychology, 51,* 443–450.

Marmar, C. et al. (1988). A controlled trial of brief psychotherapy and mutual-help group treatment of conjugal bereavement. *American Journal of Psychiatry, 145,* 203–209.

Marshall, T. et al. (2001). Inadequate nutrient intakes are common and are associated with low diet variety in rural, community-dwelling elderly. *Journal of Nutrition, 131,* 2192–2196.

Marshall, T. (2000). Exploring a fiscal food policy: The case of diet and ischaemic heart disease. *British Medical Journal, 320,* 301–305.

Marston, W. (1996a, March/April). How much is too much? *Health,* pp. 38, 40.

Marston, W. (1996b, September). High protein diets really do make you lose fat: That's where the problems start. *Health,* pp. 99–102.

Martel, G. et al. (1999). Strength training normalizes resting blood pressure in 65- to 73-year-old men and women with high normal blood pressure. *Journal of American Geriatrics Society, 47,* 1215–1221.

Martinez, M. et al. (1999). Physical activity body mass index, and prostaglandin E2 levels in rectal mucosa. *Journal of National Cancer Institute, 91,* 950–953.

Maruta, T. et al. (2000). Optimists vs. pessimists: Survival rate among medical patients over a 30-year period. *Mayo Clinic Proceedings, 75,* 140–143.

Mason, D. (2001). Editorial: An apple a day. *American Journal of Nursing, 101,* p. 7.

Materson, B. et al. (1993). Single-drug therapy for hypertension in men. A comparison of antihypertensive agents with placebo. *New England Journal of Medicine, 328,* 914–921.

Mattimore, T. et al. (1997). Surrogate and physician understanding of patients' preferences for living permanently in a nursing home. *Journal of the American Geriatrics Society, 45,* 818–824.

*Mayo Clinic Health Letter.* (1997, July). Coffee. p. 7.

Mazieres, B. et al. (2001). Chondroitin sulfate in osteoarthritis of the knee: A prospective, double blind, placebo controlled multicenter clinical study. *Journal of Rheumatology, 28,* 173–181.

McAlindon, T. et al. (2000). Glucosamine and chondroitin for treatment of osteoarthritis: A systematic quality assessment and meta-analysis. *Journal of the American Medical Association, 283,* 1469–1475.

McAuley, E. (1994). Physical activity and psychosocial outcomes. In C. Bouchard et al. (Eds.), *Physical activity, fitness, and health* (pp. 561–568). Illinois: Human Kinetics Publishers.

McAuley, E. (1993). Self-efficacy and the maintenance of exercise participation in older adults. *Journal of Behavioral Medicine, 16,* 103–113.

McAuley, E., & Courneya, K. (1993). Adherence to exercise and physical activity as health promoting behaviors: Attitudinal and self-efficacy influences. *Applied and Preventive Psychology, 2,* 65–77.

McAuley, E., & Rudolph, D. (1995). Physical activity, aging and psychological well-being. *Journal of Aging and Physical Activity, 3,* 67–96.

McCarthy, E. et al. (2000). Mammography use, breast cancer stage at diagnosis, and survival among older women. *Journal of the American Geriatrics Society, 48,* 1226–1233.

McCormack, G. et al. (1991). Culturally diverse elders. In J. Kiernat (Ed.), *Occupational therapy and the older adult* (pp. 11–25). Maryland: Aspen.

McCormick, W., & Inui, T. (1992). Geriatric preventive care: Counseling techniques in practice settings. In G. Omenn (Ed.), *Clinics in geriatric medicine.* Philadelphia: W. B. Saunders.

McDermott, M., & Burke, J. (1993). When the population is a congregation: The emerging role of the parish nurse. *Journal of Community Health Nursing, 10,* 179–190.

McDowell, I. et al. (1986). Comparison of three methods of recalling patients for influenza vaccination. *Canadian Medical Association Journal, 135,* 991.

McGinnis, J. (1992, Summer/Fall). Top leading cause of death. *The Interchange, 9,* p. 5, Texas Department of Health.

McGinnis, J., & Foege, W. (1993). Actual causes of death in the United States. *Journal of the American Medical Association, 270,* 2207–2212.

McGinnis, J. et al. (2002). The case for more active policy attention to health promotion. *Health Affairs, 21,* 78–93.

McGuire, L. et al. (2002). Depressive symptoms and lymphocyte proliferation in older adults. *Journal of Abnormal Psychology, 111,* 192–197.

McKinlay, J. (1975). Who is really ignorant—Physician or patient? *Journal of Health and Social Behavior, 16,* 3–11.

McMurray, J. (1990). Creative arts with older people. *Activities, Adaptation and Aging, 14,* 1/2, entire issue.

McNeil, J. et al. (1991). The effect of exercise on depressive symptoms in the moderately depressed elderly. *Psychology and Aging. 6,* 487–488.

McPherson, C. et al. (2002). The effects of mammographic detection and comorbidity on the survival of older women with breast cancer. *Journal of American Geriatrics Society, 50,* 1061–1068.

McTiernan, A. et al. (2002). Exercise and breast cancer rates. Presentation at the International Cancer Congress, July, Oslo.

McVea, K. et al. (2000). The organization and distribution of patient education materials in family medicine practices. *Journal of Family Practice, 49,* 319–326.

Meagher, E. et al. (2001). Effects of vitamin E on lipid peroxidation in healthy persons. *Journal of the American Medical Association, 285,* 1178–1182.

Measuring Alcohol's Effect on You. (1996, April). *Johns Hopkins Medical Letter: Health After 50, 8,* pp. 2–3.

Medicare patients skipping colon cancer tests. (2000, March 20). *American Medical News.*

Medicare screenings, vaccines underused. (2002, June 17). *American Medical News,* p. 7.

Meier, K., & Licari, M. (1997). The effect of cigarette taxes on cigarette consumption, 1955 through 1994. *American Journal of Public Health, 87,* 1126–1130.

Melchart, D. et al. (2000). Echinacea for preventing and treating the common cold. *Cochrane Database System Review, 2,* CD000530.

Mellin, L. et al. (1997). The Solution method: 2-year trends in weight, blood pressure, exercise, depression, and functioning of adults trained in development skills. *Journal of the American Dietetic Association, 97,* 1133–1138.

Mellinger, G., & Balter, M. (1983). *Collaborative Project* (GSMIRSB Report). Washington, DC: National Institute of Mental Health.

Melnikow, J. et al. (2000). Put prevention into practice: A controlled evaluation. *American Journal of Public Health, 90,* 1622–1625.

Mestel, R. (1997a,November/December). A safer estrogen. *Health,* pp. 73–75.

Mestel, R. (1997b, September). Sleeping lessons from recovered insomniacs. *Health,* pp. 108–115.

Mettler, M. (1997). Unpublished update on the Healthwise Handbook program, Healthwise, Inc., P.O. Box 1989, Boise, Idaho 83701.

Meydani, S. et al. (1997). Vitamin E supplementation and in vivo immune response in healthy elderly subjects. *Journal of the American Medical Association, 277,* 1380–1386.

Meyer, H. (1991, December 9). Shape up or shell out. *American Medical News,* p. 3.

Michael, Y. et al. (2001). Living arrangements, social integration, and change in function: Health status. *American Journal of Epidemiology, 153,* 123–131.

Michels, K. et al. (2000). Prospective study of fruit and vegetable consumption and incidence of colon and rectal cancers. *Journal of the National Cancer Institute, 92,* 1740–52.

Mieczkowski, T., & Wilson, S. (2002). Adult pneumococcal vaccination: A review of physician and patient barriers. *Vaccine, 20,* 1383–1392.

Miller, A. et al. (2002). The Canadian National Breast Screening Study. *The Annals of Internal Medicine, 137*(5 part I), 305–312.

Mittelman, M. et al. (1996). A family intervention to delay nursing home placement of patients with Alzheimer's disease. A randomized controlled trial. *Journal of the American Medical Association, 276,* 1725–1731.

Miyatake, N. et al. (1999). A new air displacement plethysmograph for the determination of Japanese body composition. *Diabetes, Obesity and Metabolism, 1,* 347–351.

Moberg, D. (1983). The ecological fallacy: Concerns for program planners. *Generations, 8,* 12–14.

Montamat, S., & Cusack, B. (1992). Overcoming problems with polypharmacy and drug misuse in the elderly. In G. Omenn (Ed.), *Clinics in geriatric medicine* (pp. 143–158), Philadelphia: W. B. Saunders.

Montgomery, P. (2002). Treatments for sleep problems in elderly people. *British Medical Journal, 325,* 1049.

Moore A. et al. (2002). Are there differences between older persons who screen positive on the CAGE questionnaire and the Short Michigan Alcoholism Screening Test—geriatric version? *Journal of the American Geriatrics Society, 50,* 858–862.

Moore, A. et al. (1999). Drinking habits among older persons: Findings from the NHANES I Epidemiological Followup Study (1982–1984). National Health and Nutrition Examination Survey. *Journal of the American Geriatrics Society, 47,* 412–416.

Moore, S., & Nagle, J. (1990). *Physician's guide to outpatient nutrition.* Kansas City, MO: American Academy of Family Physicians.

Morain, C. (1994, July 4). Still a long way to go, baby. *American Medical News,* pp. 11–14.

More people lifting weights—and getting injured. (2000). *Health & Nutrition Letter,* Tufts University, *18,* pp. 1, 8.

Morgan, D. (1993, May 24/31). The best prescription might be just taking time to care. *American Medical News,* p. 9.

Morin, C. et al. (1999). Behavioral and pharmacological therapies for late-life insomnia: A randomized controlled trial. *Journal of the American Medical Association, 281*, 991–999.

Morley, J. (2002). Drugs, aging and the future. *Journal of Gerontology: Medical Sciences, 57A*, M2–M6.

Morley, J. (2001). http://www.cyberrounds.com. Accessed June 21, 2001.

Morris, J. et al. (1999). Nursing rehabilitation and exercise strategies in the nursing home. *Journal of Gerontology: Medical Sciences, 54A*, M494–M500.

Morris, M. et al. (2002). Vitamin E and cognitive decline in older persons. *Archives of Neurology, 59*, 1125–1132.

Morrow-Howell, N. et al. (2003). Effects of volunteering on the well-being of older adults. *Journal of Gerontology, 58B*, S137–S145.

Morse, R., & Flavin, D. (1992). The definition of alcoholism. *The Journal of the American Medical Association, 268*, 1012–1014.

Mosca, L. et al. (2001). Hormone replacement therapy and cardiovascular disease. *Circulation, 104*, 499–503.

Moss, M. (2002, October 24). Senator says its time to upgrade standards. *The New York Times*, p. 12.

Most patients don't see excess weight as health danger. (1999, November 8). *American Medical News*, pp. 26–27.

Mozaffarian, D. et al. (2003). Cereal, fruit, and vegetable fiber intake and the risk of cardiovascular disease in elderly individuals. *Journal of the American Medical Association, 89*, 1659–1666.

Mukamal, K. et al. (2003). Roles of drinking pattern and type of alcohol consumed in coronary heart disease in men. *New England Journal of Medicine, 348*, 109–118.

Mukamal, K. et al. (2001). Prior alcohol consumption and mortality following acute myocardial infarction. *Journal of the American Medical Association, 285*, 1965–1970.

Mullan, F. (1992). Rewriting the social contract in health. In A. Katz et al. (Eds.), *Self-help: Concepts and applications* (pp. 61–67). Philadelphia: The Charles Press.

Murphy, J. et al. (1982). The long-term effects of spouse involvement upon weight loss and maintenance. *Behavior Therapy, 13*, 681–693.

Murphy, M. et al. (2002). Accumulating brisk walking for fitness, cardiovascular risk, and psychological health. *Medical Science & Sports Exercise, 34*, 1468–1474.

Murray, C., & Lopez, A. (1996). *Global burden of disease.* Cambridge, MA: Harvard University Press.

Myers, J. et al. (2002). Exercise capacity and mortality among men referred for exercise testing. *New England Journal of Medicine, 346*, 793–801.

Mynors-Wallis, L. et al. (1995). Randomized controlled trial comparing problem solving treatment with amitriptyline and placebo for major depression in primary care. *British Medical Journal, 310*, 441–445.

Naditch, M. (1984). The Staywell Program. In J. Matarazzo et al. (Eds.), *Behavioral health: A handbook of health enhancement and disease prevention.* New York: Wiley.

Napoli, M. (2001). Overdiagnosis and overtreatment. *American Journal of Nursing, 101*, 11.

Nathan, P. (1984). Johnson and Johnson's Live for Life: A comprehensive positive lifestyle change program. In J. Matarazzo et al. (Eds.), *Behavioral health: A handbook of health enhancement and disease prevention.* New York: Wiley.

National Center for Health Statistics. (1999). *Healthy People 2000 Review, 1998—1999.* Hyattsville, MD: USDHHS.

National Center for Health Statistics. (1990a). *Health, United States, 1989 and Prevention Profile.* DHHS Pub. No. (PHS) 90-1232. Hyattsville, MD: USDHHS.

National Center for Health Statistics. (1990b). *Healthy People 2000: National Health Promotion and Disease Prevention Objectives.* DHHS Publication No (PHS) 91-50213. Hyattsville, MD: USDHHS.

National Center for Health Statistics. (1988). *Vital and Health Statistics.* Series 10, No. 163. DHHS Pub. No. (PHS)88-1591. Washington, DC: USDHHS.

National Council on the Aging. (2002). American Perceptions of Aging in the 21st Century. Sampling, Interviewing and Data Preparation by Harris Interactive, Inc. www.ncoa.org.

National Health Interview Survey. (l985, November). Hyattsville, MD: U.S. Public Health Service. *Advance Data, 13.*

National Heart, Lung and Blood Institute. (1997). *Report of the Joint National Committee on Treatment of High Blood Pressure.* Washington, DC: USDHHS.

National Indian Council on Aging. (1984). Indians and Alaskan natives. In E. Palmore (Ed.), *Handbook on the aged in the United States.* Westport, CT: Greenwood Press.

National Institute on Aging. (1994). *NIH Consensus Statement on Optimal Calcium Intake, 12,* 1–31.

National Institutes of Health. (1992). Diagnosis and treatment of depression in late life. National Institutes of Health Consensus Development Panel on Depression in Late Life. *Journal of the American Medical Association, 268,* 1018–1024.

National Institutes of Health Consensus Development Panel on Acupuncture. (1998). Acupuncture. *Journal of the American Medical Association, 280,* 1518–1524.

Neale, A. et al. (1990). The use of behavioral contracting to increase exercise activity. *American Journal of Health Promotion, 4,* 441–447.

Neergaard, L. (1998, February 23). Dietary supplement users are advised to use caution. *Houston Chronicle,* p. 3.

Neighbors, H. et al. (1995). Health promotion and African-Americans: From personal empowerment to collective action. *American Journal of Health Promotion, 9,* 281–287.

Nelson, D. et al. (2002). State trends in health risk factors and receipt of clinical preventive services among US adults during the 1990s. *Journal of the American Medical Association, 287,* 2659–2667.

Nelson, H. et al. (2002). Screening for postmenopausal osteoporosis: A review of the evidence for the U.S. Preventive Services Task Force. *Annals of Internal Medicine, 137,* 529–541.

Nestle, M. (2002). *Food politics.* Los Angeles: University of California Press.

Neugarten, B. (1979). Policy for the 1980s: Age or need entitlement? In J. Hubbard (Ed.), *Aging: Agenda for the eighties* (pp. 48–52). Washington, DC: Government Research Corporation

Neville, K. (2000, March). Sugar: How do I disguise thee? *Environmental Nutrition, 23,* 3, p. 2.

Newcomer, J. et al. (1999). Decreased memory performance in healthy humans induced by stress-level cortisol treatment. *Archives of General Psychiatry, 56,* 527–533.

New diabetes screenings urged for older citizens. (2002, March 28). *Los Angeles Times.*

Nichol, K. et al. (2003). Influenza vaccination and reduction in hospitalizations for cardiac disease and stroke among the elderly. *New England Journal of Medicine, 348,* 1322–1332.

Nielsen, S., & B. Popkin. (2003). Patterns in trends in food portion sizes, 1977–1998. *Journal of the American Medical Association, 289,* 450–453.

Noble, H. (1999, September 5). Some say Koop sold out on Web by blurring line between ads, facts. *Houston Chronicle,* p. 16A.

Nordin, J. et al. (2001). Influenza vaccine effectiveness in preventing hospitalizations and deaths in persons 65 years or older in Minnesota, New York, and Oregon: Data from 3 health plans. *Journal of Infectious Diseases, 184,* 665–670.

Nutting, P. (1987). Community-oriented primary care: From principle to practice. In P. Nutting (Ed.), *Community-oriented primary care* (pp. xv–xxv). University of New Mexico Press.

Oberman, A., & Kreisberg, R. (2002). Lipid management in older patients. *Clinical Geriatrics, 10,* 41–50.

Oboler, S. et al. (2002). Public expectations and attitudes for annual physical examinations and testing. *Annals of Internal Medicine, 136,* 652–659.

Office on Smoking and Health. (1989). *Reducing the Health Consequences of Smoking: 25 Years of Progress. A Report of the Surgeon General.* DHHS Pub. No. (CDC)89-8411. Washington, DC: USDHHS.

Ohayon, M. et al. (1996). The elderly, sleep habits and use of psychotropic drugs by the French population. *Encephale, 22,* 337–350.

Oldridge, N., & Jones, N. (1983). Improving patient compliance in cardiac exercise rehabilitation: Effects of written agreement and self-monitoring. *Journal of Cardiac Rehabilitation, 3,* 257–262.

Oldridge, N. et al. (1988). Cardiac rehabilitation after myocardial infarction. *The Journal of the American Medical Association, 260,* 945–950.

O'Leary, A. (1985). Self-efficacy and health. *Behavioral Research and Therapy, 23,* 437–451.

Olestra-fried snacks fat-free, but not free of concerns. (1996, February). *American Medical News.*

Olfson, M. et al. (2002). National trends in the outpatient treatment of depression. *Journal of the American Medical Association, 287,* 203–209.

Oliveria, S. et al. (2002). Physician-related barriers to the effective management of uncontrolled hypertension. *Archives of Internal Medicine, 162,* 413–420.

Olsen, O., & Gotzsche, P. (2001). Cochrane review on screening for breast cancer with mammography. *Lancet, 358,* 1340–1342.

Olson, M. et al. (2000). Weight cycling and high-density lipoprotein cholesterol in women: Evidence of an adverse effect. *Journal of American College of Cardiology, 36,* 1565–1571.

Ornish, D. et al. (1998). Intensive lifestyle changes for reversal of coronary heart disease. *Journal of the American Medical Association, 280,* 2001–2007.

Ornish, D. (1992). *Dr. Dean Ornish's program for reversing heart disease.* New York: Ballantine Books.

Ornstein, R., & Sobel, D. (1989). *Healthy pleasures.* MA: Addison-Wesley.

Ostir, G. et al. (2002). Differential effects of premorbid physical and emotional health on recovery from acute events. *Journal of American Geriatrics Society, 50,* 713–718.

Ostir, G. et al. (2001). The association between emotional well-being and the incidence of stroke in older adults. *Psychosomatic Medicine, 63,* 210–215.

Ostir, G. et al. (2000). Emotional well-being predicts subsequent functional independence and survival. *Journal of the American Geriatrics Society, 48,* 473–478.

Palmore, E. (2000). Ageism in gerontological language. *The Gerontologist, 40,* 645.

Palombo, R. et al. (2002). *The Aging States Project: Promoting opportunities for collaboration between the public health aging networks.* Washington, DC: Association of State and Territorial Chronic Disease Program and the National Association of State Units on Aging.

Pargament, K. et al. (2001). Religious struggle as a predictor of mortality among medically ill elderly patients: A 2-year longitudinal study. *Annals of Internal Medicine, 161,* 1881–1885.

Pasternak, R. et al. (2002). ACC/AHA/NHLBI clinical advisory on the use and safety of statins. *Circulation, 106,* 1024–1028.

Pasternak, R. et al. (1997). The posttreatment illness course of depression in bereaved elders. High relapse/recurrence rates. *American Journal of Geriatric Psychiatry, 5,* 54–59.

Pate, R. et al. (1995). Physical activity and public health. *Journal of the American Medical Association, 273,* 402–407.

Paulson, R. et al. (2002). Pregnancy in the sixth decade of life: Obstetric outcomes in women of advanced reproductive age. *Journal of the American Medical Association, 288,* 2320–2323.

Pear, R. (2002, February 28). 9 in 10 nursing homes lack adequate staff, study finds. *The New York Times,* pp. A1, A11.

Pechacek, T. (2000, November 30). Centers for Disease Control and Prevention announcement by Dr. Terry Pechacek, CDC associate director for science and public health.

Peeters, A. et al. (2003). Obesity in adulthood and its consequences for life expectancy: A life-table analysis. *Annals of Internal Medicine, 138,* 24–32.

Pelletier, K. (1996). A review and analysis of the health and cost-effective outcome studies of comprehensive health promotion and disease prevention programs at the worksite: 1993–1995 update. *American Journal of Health Promotion, 10,* 380–388.

Pelletier, K. et al. (1999). Current trends in the integration and reimbursement of complementary and alternative medicine by managed care organizations and insurance providers: 1998 update and cohort analysis. *American Journal of Health Promotion, 14,* 125–133.

Penninx, B. (2000). A happy person, a healthy person? *Journal of the American Geriatrics Society, 48,* 590–592.

Penninx, B. et al. (2002). Exercise and depressive symptoms: A comparison of aerobic and resistance exercise effects on emotional and physical function in older persons with high and low depressive symptomatology. *Journal of Gerontology: Psychological Sciences, 57B,* P124–P132.

Penninx, B. et al. (2001). Physical exercise and the prevention of disability in activities of daily living in older persons with osteoarthritis. *Archives of Internal Medicine, 161,* 2309–2016.

Penninx, B. et al. (1998a). Depressive symptoms and physical decline in community-dwelling older persons. *Journal of the American Medical Association, 279,* 1720–1726.

Penninx, B. et al. (1998b). Chronically depressed mood and cancer risk in older persons. *Journal of the National Cancer Institute, 90,* 1888–1893.

Penrod, J. et al. (1995). Who cares? The size, scope, and composition of the caregiver support system. *Gerontologist, 35,* 489–497.

Peripheral vascular disease: What should you do if you have it? (2000, June). *Focus on Healthy Aging,* Mount Sinai School of Medicine, p. 7.

Persky, T. (1998). Overlooked and underserved: Elders in need of mental health care. *The Journal of the California Alliance for the Mentally Ill, 9,* 7–9.

Personal data on Web sites are vulnerable. (2000, February). *American Medical News.*

Pesticide exposure. (1997, June). *Nutrition Action Healthletter,* pp. 4–6.

Petersen, M. (2001, November 21). Increased spending on drugs is linked to more advertising. *The New York Times,* Business Section, p. B1.

Peterson, C., & Stunkard, A. (1989). Personal control and health promotion. *Social Science Medicine, 28,* 819–828.

Peterson, J. (1996). Acupuncture in the 1990s. *Archives of Family Medicine, 5,* 237–240.

Peto, R. et al. (1992). Mortality from tobacco in developed countries: Indirect estimates from national vital statistics. *The Lancet, 339,* 1268–1278.

Petrella, R., & Bartha, C. (2000). Home based exercise therapy for older patients with knee osteoarthritis: A randomized clinical trial. *Journal of Rheumatology, 27,* 2215–2221.

Petricoin, E. et al. (2002). Use of proteomic patterns in serum to identify ovarian cancer. *Lancet, 359,* 572–577.

Philipp, M. et al. (1999). Hypericum extract versus imipramine or placebo in patients with moderate depression: Randomized multicentre study of treatment for eight weeks. *British Medical Journal, 319,* 1534–1538.

Philipson, T. (2001). The worldwide growth in obesity: An economic research agenda. *Health Economist, 10,* 1–7.

Phipps, E. et al. (2000). Community water fluoridation, bone mineral density, and fractures: Prospective study of effects in older women. *British Medical Journal, 321,* 860–864.

Pickering, T. et al. (1988). How common is white coat hypertension? *Journal of the American Medical Association, 259,* 225.

Pignone, M. et al. (2002, May). *Screening for depression.* AHRQ Publication No. 02-S002. Rockville, MD: Agency for Healthcare Research and Quality.

Pinquart, M. (2001). Correlates of subjective health in older adults: A meta-analysis. *Psychology and Aging, 16,* 414–426.

Pitkala, K. et al. (2002). Inappropriate drug prescribing in home-dwelling elderly patients: A population-based survey. *Archives of Internal Medicine, 162,* 1707–1712.

Podolsky, D. (2000). Going the distance—The case for true colorectal-cancer screening. *New England Journal of Medicine, 343,* 207–208.

Pollock, B., & Mulsant, B. (1995). Antipsychotics in older patients. A safety perspective. *Drugs and Aging, 6,* 312–323.

Pontillo, D. et al. (2002). Management and treatment of anxiety disorders in the older patient. *Clinical Geriatrics, 10,* 38–49.

Porter, M. (2000). Resistance training recommendations for older adults. *Topics in Geriatric Rehabilitation, 15*(3), 60–69.

Potter, J., & Haigh, R. (1990). Benefits of antihypertensive therapy in the elderly. *British Medical Bulletin, 46,* 77–93.

Powell, P. et al. (2001). Randomised controlled trial of patient education to encourage graded exercise in chronic fatigue syndrome. *British Medical Journal, 322,* 387–390.

Prabhakaran, B. et al. (1999). Effect of 14 weeks of resistance training on lipid profile and body fat percentage in premenopausal women. *British Journal of Sports Medicine, 33,* 190–195.

Preserving your sight. (2002, February). *Consumer Reports on Health,* pp. 1, 4–5.

Prochaska, J. et al. (1993). Standardized, individualized, interactive, and personalized self-help programs for smoking cessation. *Health Psychology, 12,* 399–405.

Prochaska, J. et al. (1988). Measuring processes of change: Applications to the cessation of smoking. *Journal of Consulting Clinical Psychology, 56,* 520–528.

Prochaska, J., & Di Clemente, C. (1992). Stages of change in the modification of problem behaviors. In M. Herson et al. (Eds.), *Progress in behavior modification* (pp. 184–218). Thousand Oaks, CA: Sage.

Pronk, N. et al. (2000). Relationship between modifiable health risks and short-term health care charges. *Journal of the American Medical Association, 282,* 2235–2239.

Protecting yourself against prescription errors. (1996, January). *Johns Hopkins Medical Letter: Health After 50,* pp. 6–7.

Province, M. et al. (1995). The effects of exercise on falls in elderly patients: A pre-planned meta-analysis of the FICSIT Trials. *Journal of the American Medical Association, 273,* 1341–1347.

Pruchno, R., & McKenney, D. (2002). Psychological well-being of black and white grandmothers raising grandchildren: Examination of a two-factor model. *Journal of Gerontology, Psychological and Social Sciences, 57,* 444–451.

Putnam, R. (2000). *Bowling alone: The collapse and revival of American community.* New York: Simon & Schuster.

Pyke, S. et al. (1997). Change in coronary risk and coronary risk factor levels in couples following lifestyle intervention. *Archives of Famiy Medicine, 6,* 354–360.

Rabins, P. (1996). Barriers to diagnosis and treatment of depression in elderly patients. *American Journal of Geriatric Psychiatry, 4,* S79–S83.

Raina, P. et al. (1999). Influence of companion animals on the physical and psychological health of older people: An analysis of a one-year longitudinal study. *Journal of American Geriatrics Society, 47,* 323–329.

Rakowski, W. et al. (1991). Correlates of expected success at health habit change and its role as a predictor in health behavior research. *American Journal of Preventive Medicine, 7,* 89–94.

Rall, L. et al. (1996). The effect of progressive resistance training in rheumatoid arthritis. *Arthritis & Rheumatism, 39,* 415–426.

RAND. (2001). *Health risk appraisals and Medicare.* Baltimore: Centers for Medicare & Medicaid Services, Contract 500-98-0281.

Randsdell, L. (1995). Church-based health promotion: An untapped resource for women 65 and older. *American Journal of Health Promotion, 9,* 333–336

Rathore, S. et al. (2000). Mandated coverage for cancer-screening services: Whose guidelines do states follow? *American Journal of Preventive Medicine, 19,* 71–78.

Reddy, S. et al. (2002). Effect of low-carbohydrate high-protein diets on acid-base balance, stone-forming propensity, and calcium metabolism. *American Journal of Kidney Disease, 40,* 265–274.

Reger, B. et al. (2000). A comparison of different approaches to promote community-wide dietary change. *American Journal of Preventive Medicine, 18,* 271–275.

Regier, D. et al. (1988). One-month prevalence of mental disorders in the United States. *Archives of General Psychiatry, 45,* 977–986.

Reginster, J. et al. (2001). Long-term effects of glucosamine sulphate on osteoarthritis progression: A randomized, placebo-controlled clinical trial. *Lancet, 357,* 251–256.

Reid, I. et al. (2002). Intravenous zoledronic acid in postmenopausal women with low bone mineral density. *New England Journal of Medicine, 346,* 653–661.

Reid, M and P. Anderson (1997). Geriatric substance use disorders. *Medical Clinics of North America, 81,* 999–1016.

Report of the National Cholesterol Education Program. (1988). Evaluation, and treatment of high blood cholesterol in adults. *Archives of Internal Medicine, 148,* 1993–1997.

Report of the Special Committee on Aging. (1996). (1991). (1985). *Developments in aging, volume I.* U.S. Senate, Washington, DC: US Government Printing Office.

Report on Medical Guidelines. (1991). *Health and Sciences Communication,* 1909 Vermont Ave. NW, Suite 700, Washington, DC 20005.

Resnicow, K. et al. (2001). A motivational interviewing intervention to increase fruit and vegetable intake through black churches: Results of the Eat for Life Trial. *American Journal of Public Health, 91,* 1686–1693.

Retchin, S., &. Anapolle, J. (1993). An overview of the older driver. *Clinics in Geriatric Medicine, 9,* 279–296.

Revicki, D., & Mitchell, J. (1990). Strain, social support, and mental health in rural elderly individuals. *Journal of Gerontology, 45,* 267–274.

Rexrode, K. et al. (1997). A prospective study of body mass index, weight change, and risk of stroke in women. *Journal of the American Medical Association, 277,* 1539–1545.

Reynolds, C. et al. (1994). Treatment of consecutive episodes of major depression in the elderly. *American Journal of Psychiatry, 151,* 1740–1743.

Reynolds, R. et al. (2001). Discontinuation of postmenopausal hormone therapy in a Massachusets HMO. *Journal of Clinical Epidemiology, 54,* 1056–1064.

Rhodes, E. et al. (2000). Effects of one year of resistance training on the relation between muscular strength and bone density in elderly women. *British Journal of Sports Medicine, 34,* 18–22.

Rice, V., & Stead, L. (2002). Nursing interventions for smoking cessation. *The Cochrane Library,* issue 1, Oxford: Update Software.

Rich, J., & Black, W. (2000). When should we stop screening? *Effective Clinical Practice, 3,* 78–84.

Richards, M. et al. (2003). Cigarette smoking and cognitive decline in midlife. *American Journal of Public Health, 93,* 994–998.

Ricks, D. (2001, May 27). Study finds cholesterol drugs also cut risks of breast cancer. *Houston Chronicle,* p. 12A.

Ridker, P. et al. (2002). Comparison of C-reactive protein and low-density lipoprotein cholesterol levels in the prediction of first cardiovascular events. *New England Journal of Medicine, 347,* 1557–1565.

Rigaud, A., & Forette, B. (2001). Hypertension in older adults. *Journal of Gerontology: Medical Sciences, 56A,* M217–M225.

Rimer, B. (1988). Health Promotion and Aging: Smoking among Older Adults, In F. Abdellah & S. Moore (Eds.), *Surgeon general's workshop: Health promotion and aging background papers.* Washington, DC: DHHS, pp. I.1–I.20

Rimm, E. et al. (1996). Vegetable, fruit, and cereal fiber intake and risk of coronary heart disease among men. *Journal of the American Medical Association, 275,* 447–451.

Ritchie, K., & Kildea, D. (1995). Is senile dementia "age-related" or ageing-related"? Evidence from meta-analysis of dementia prevalence in the oldest old. *Lancet, 346,* 931–934.

Rivara, F. et al. (1997). Injury prevention: Part two. *New England Journal of Medicine, 337,* 613–614.

Roberts, S. et al. (1996). Effects of age on energy expenditure and susbtrate oxidation during experimental overfeeding and underfeeding in healthy men. *Journal of Gerontology, 51A,* B148–B166.

Robertson, M. et al. (2001). Effectiveness and economic evaluation of a nurse delivered home exercise programme to prevent falls: 1 and 2. *British Medical Journal, 322,* 697–704.

Robertson, N. (1988, February 21). The changing world of Alcoholics Anonymous. *The New York Times Magazine,* pp. 40–47, 57, 92.

Rockhill, B. et al. (1999). A prospective study of recreational physical activity and breast cancer risk. *Archives of Internal Medicine, 159,* 2290–2296.

Rockwood, K. et al. (2002). Use of lipid-lowering agents, indication bias, and the risk of dementia in community-dwelling elderly people. *Archives of Neurology, 59,* 223–227.

Rodin, J. (1986). Aging and health: Effects of the sense of control. *Science, 233,* 1271–1275.

Rodin, J., & Langer, E. (1977). Long-term effects of a control-relevant intervention with the institutionalized aged. *Journal of Personality and Social Psychology, 35,* 897–902.

Rodriguez, C. et al. (2001). Estrogen replacement therapy and ovarian cancer mortality in a large prospective study of US women. *Journal of the American Medical Association, 285,* 1460–1465.

Rolls, B. et al. (2002). Portion size of food affects energy intake in normal-weight and overweight men and women. *American Journal of Clinical Nutrition, 76,* 1207–1213.

Rosen, M. et al. (1984). Prevention and health promotion in primary care: Baseline results on physicians from the INSURE project on life cycle preventive health services. *Preventive Medicine, 13,* 535–548.

Rosendahl, E., & Kirschenbaum, P. (1992, November). Weight loss and mood among older adults. Paper presentation at the 45th Gerontological Society of America Annual Meeting, Washington, DC.

Rosenstock, I. (1990). The health belief model: Explaining health behavior through expectancies: Chapter 3. In K. Glanz et al. (Eds.), *Health behavior and health education: Theory, research, and practice* (pp. 39–61). San Francisco: Jossey-Bass Publishers.

Rost, K. (1990, October 1). *Introduction of the elderly patient's agenda in the medical visit.* Final report for AARP Andrus Foundation, Washington, DC.

Rotter, J. (1954). *Social learning and clinical psychology.* Englewood Cliffs, NJ: Prentice-Hall.

Rubenstein, L. et al. (2000). Effects of a group exercise program on strength, mobility, and falls among fall-prone elderly men. *Journal of Gerontology, 55,* M317–M321.

Rubenstein, L. et al. (1994). Falls in the nursing home. *Annals of Internal Medicine, 21,* 442–451.

Ruitenberg, A. et al. (2002). Alcohol consumption and risk of dementia. *Lancet, 359*, 282–286.

Russell, R. et al. (1999). Modified food guide pyramid for people over seventy years of age. *Journal of Nutrition, 129*, 751–753.

Rybarczyk, R. et al. (2002). Efficacy of two behavioral treatment programs for comorbid geriatric insomnia. *Psychology of Aging, 17*, 288–298.

Sacco, R. et al. (1999). The protective effect of moderate alcohol consumption on ischemic stroke. *Journal of the American Medical Association, 281*, 53–60.

Safron, E. et al. (2002). *Prescription drug coverage and seniors: How well are states closing the gap?* July 31 Internet report. www.kff.org.

Salon, I. (1997). Weight control and nutrition: Knowing when to intervene. *Geriatrics, 52*, 33–41.

Sandock, L. (2000). From rites of passage to last rights. *Journal of the American Medical Association, 284*, 3100–3102.

Sano, M. et al. (1997). A controlled trial of Selegilene, Alpha-Tocopherol, or both as treatment for Alzheimer's disease. *New England Journal of Medicine, 336*, 1216–1222.

Sapolsky, R. (1999). Glutocorticoids, stress, and their adverse neurological effects: Relevance to aging. *Experimental Gerontology, 34*, 721–732.

Sarafino, E. (1990). *Health psychology: Biopsychosocial interactions.* New York: John Wiley.

Saunders, C. (1977). Dying they live: St Christopher's Hospice. In H. Feifel (Ed.), *New meanings of death.* New York: McGraw-Hill.

Schachter-Shalomi, Z. (1995). *From age-ing to sage-ing.* New York: Warner Books, Inc.

Schaie, K. (1997, May). Exercising the mind. *Nutrition Action Healthletter*, p. 7.

Schardt, D. (2000a, October). Glucosamine & chondroitin: Joint relief? *Nutrition Action Healthletter*, p. 10.

Schardt, D. (2000b, September). Palmetto and the prostate. *Nutrition Action Healthletter*, p. 9.

Schatzkin, A. et al. (2000). Lack of effect of low-fat, high-fiber diet on the recurrence of colorectal adenomas. *New England Journal of Medicine, 342*, 1149–1155.

Schauffler, H. (2000). Politics trumps science: Rethinking state-mandated benefits. *American Journal of Preventive Medicine, 19*, 136–137.

Scheier, M. et al. (1999). Optimism and rehospitalization after coronary artery bypass graft surgery. *Archives of Internal Medicine, 159*, 829–835.

Schilling, L. et al. (2002). The third person in the room: Frequency, role, and influence of companions during primary care medical encounters. *Journal of Family Practice, 51*, 685–690.

Schillinger, D. et al. (2002). Association of health literacy with diabetes outcomes. *Journal of the American Medical Association, 288*, 475–482.

Schlenker, R. et al. (2002). Rural-urban home health care differences before the Balanced Budget Act of 1997. *Journal of Rural Health, 18*, 359–372.

Schlosser, E. (2001). *Fast food nation.* Boston: Houghton Mifflin.

Schmid, R. (2000, May 11). Study: Doctors often miss alcohol abuse symptoms. *Galveston Daily News*, p. 9.

Schmitt, C. (2002, September 30). Nursing home myth of old age. *U.S. News & World Report*, pp. 66–74.

Schneider, E. et al. (2002). Racial disparities in the quality of care for enrollees in Medicare managed care. *Journal of the American Medical Association, 287*, 1288–1294.

Schneider, E. et al. (2001). Racial disparity in influenza vaccination. *Journal of the American Medical Association, 286,* 1455–1460.

Schneider, L. (1996). Pharmacological considerations in the treatment of late life depression. *American Journal of Geriatric Psychiatry, 4,* S51–S65.

Schneider, L. (1995). Efficacy of clinical treatment for mental disorders among older persons. In M. Gatz (Ed.), *Emerging issues in mental health and aging* (pp. 19–71). Washington, DC: American Psychological Association.

Schneider, R. et al. (1995). A randomized controlled trial of stress reduction for hypertension in older African Americans. *Hypertension, 26,* 820–827.

Schonfeld, L. (1993, January/February). Research findings on a hidden population. *The Counselor,* pp. 20–26.

Schonfeld, L. et al. (1992). *Age-related differences in antecedents to substance abuse.* Paper presentation at Centennial meeting of the American Psychological Association, Washington, DC.

Schulz, R. (1976). Effects of control and predictability on the physical and psychological well-being of the institutionalized aged. *Journal of Personality and Social Psychology, 33,* 563–573.

Schwartz, J. (1997, September). Consumer health information. *Washington Post National Weekly Edition,* p.8.

Seals, D. et al. (2001). Blood pressure reductions with exercise and sodium restriction in postmenopausal women with elevated systolic pressure: role of arterial stiffness. *Journal of American College of Cardiology, 38,* 6–513.

Sears, B. (1997). *Mastering the zone.* New York: HarperCollins.

Sears, B. (1995). *Entering the zone.* New York: HarperCollins.

Sechrist, W. (1983). Causal attribution and personal responsibility for health and disease. *Health Education, 14,* 51–54.

Sellmeyer, D. et al. (2001). A high ratio of dietary animal to vegetable protein increases the rate of bone loss and the risk of fracture in postmenopausal women. *American Journal of Clinical Nutrition, 73,* 118–122.

Sennott-Miller, L., & Kligman, E. (1992). Healthier lifestyles: How to motivate older patients to change. *Geriatrics, 47,* 52–59.

Shamblin, G. (2000). *Rise above.* Franklin, TN: Weigh Down Workshop.

Shamblin, G. (1997). *The weigh down diet.* Franklin, TN: Weigh Down Workshop.

Sharp, D. (1997, November/December). The calcium problem. *Health,* pp. 103–107.

Shelton, D. (2000, April 10). Men avoid physician visits, often don't know whom to see. *American Medical News,* pp. 1, 33.

Shelton, D. (1999, April 12). Sleep problems are pervasive, poll finds. *American Medical News,* pp. 1–2.

Shelton, R. et al. (2001). Effectiveness of St. John's wort in major depression: A randomized controlled trial. *Journal of the American Medical Association, 285,* 1978–1986.

Shen, J. et al. (2000). Electroacupuncture for control of myeloablative chemotherapy-induced emesis: A randomized controlled trial. *Journal of the American Medical Association, 284,* 2755–2761.

Shlosser, E. (2001). *Fast food nation.* New York: Hougthon Mifflin.

Shmerling, R. et al. (1988). Discussing cardiopulmonary resuscitation: A study of elderly outpatients. *Journal of General Internal Medicine, 3,* 317.

Siegel, J. (1993). Companion animals: In sickness and in health. *Journal of Social Issues, 49,* 157–167.

Sierpina, V. (2001). *Integrative health care: Complementary and alternative therapies for the whole person.* PA: F. A. Davis.

Simon, G., & VonKorff, M. (1995). Recognition, management, and outcomes of depression in primary care. *Archives of Family Medicine, 4,* 99–105.

Simons, M. et al. (2001). Cholesterol and Alzheimer's disease. *Neurology, 57,* 1089–1093.

Sinaki, M. et al. (2002). Stronger back muscles reduce the incidence of vertebral fractures: A prospective 10 year follow-up of postmenopausal women. *Bone, 30,* 836–841.

Singh, N. et al. (2001). The efficacy of exercise as a long-term antidepressant in elderly subjects: A randomized, controlled trial. *Journal of Gerontology: Medical Sciences, 56A,* M497–M504.

Siris, E. et al. (2001). Identification and fracture outcomes of undiagnosed low bone mineral density in postmenopausal women: Results from the National Osteoporosis Risk Assessment. *Journal of the American Medical Association, 286,* 2815–2822.

Skinner, B. (1953). *Science and human behavior.* New York: MacMillan.

Slattery, M. et al. (1999). Lifestyle and colon cancer: An assessment of factors associated with risk. *American Journal of Epidemiology, 150,* 869–877.

Sloan, R. (1986). *Practical geriatric therapeutics.* New Jersey: Medical Economics Books.

Sloan, R., & Bagiella, E. (2002). Claims about religious involvement and health outcomes. *Annals of Behavioral Medicine, 24,* 14–21.

Small, G. (2002). What we need to know about age related memory loss. *British Medical Journal, 324,* 1502–1505.

Small, G., & Salzman, C. (1998). Treatment of depression with new and atypical antidepressants. In C. Salzman (Ed.), *Clinical geriatric psychopharmacology* (pp. 245–261). Baltimore: Williams & Wilkins.

Smith, E. et al. (1997). Church-based education: An outreach program for African Americans with hypertension. *Ethnicity & Health, 2,* 243–253.

Smyer, M., & Qualls, S. (1999). *Aging and mental health.* Malden, MA: Blackwell.

Smyth, J. et al. (1999). Effects of writing about stressful experiences on symptom reduction in patients with asthma or rheumatoid arthritis: A randomized trial. *Journal of the American Medical Association, 281,* 1304–1309.

Sneaker-clad army wins battle of the mall. (2001, August 28). *The New York Times,* pp. A1, A11.

Snowdon, D. et al. (2000). Linguistic ability in early life and the neuropathology of Alzheimer's disease and crebrovascular disease. Findings from the Nun Study. *Annals of New York Academy of Science, 903,* 34–38.

Snyder, P. (2001). Effects of age on testicular function and consequences of testosterone treatment. *Journal of Clinical Endocrinology Metabolism, 86,* 2369–2372.

Solomon, P. et al. (2002). Gingko for memory enhancement: A randomized controlled trial. *Journal of the American Medical Association, 288,* 835–840.

Sox, H. (1997, October). Expert questions call to expand prostate cancer screenings. *Aging Research & Training News,* p. 119.

Spake, A. (2002, January 21). Hormones on trail. *Health & Medicine,* pp. 1–4.

Speechley, M., & Tinetti, M. (1991). Falls and injuries in frail and vigorous community elderly persons. *Journal of American Geriatrics Society, 39,* 46.

Spiegel, D. (2001). Mind matters—Group therapy and survival in breast cancer. *New England Journal of Medicine, 345,* 1767–1768.

Spiegel, D. et al. (1989). Effect of psychosocial treatment on survival of patients with metastatic breast cancer. *The Lancet, 2,* 888–891.

Spiegel, D., & Bloom, J. (1983). Group therapy and hypnosis reduce metastatic breast cancer pain. *Psychosomatic Medicine, 45,* 333.

Spira, J. (2001). Comparison of St. John's wort and imipramine: Study design casts doubt on St. John's wort in treating depression. *British Medical Journal, 322,* 493–494.

Spirduso, W. (1995). *Physical dimensions of aging.* IL: Human Kinetics.

Spitzer, R. et al. (1999). Jet lag: Clinical features, validation of a new syndrome-specific scale, and lack of response to melatonin in a randomized, double-blind trial. *American Journal of Psychiatry, 156,* 1392–1396.

Squires, S. (2002, October 14–20). We're fat and getting fatter. *The Washington Post National Weekly Edition,* p. 34.

Staessen, J. et al. (1998). Subgroup and per-protocol analysis of the randomized European trial on isolated systolic hypertension in the elderly. *Archives of Internal Medicine, 158,* 1681–1691.

Stamler, J. et al. (1986). Is relationship between serum cholesterol and risk of premature death from coronary heart disease continuous and graded? Findings in 356,222 primary screenees of the Multiple Risk Factor Intervention Trial (MRFIT). *Journal of the American Medical Association, 256,* 2823–2828.

Starr, B. (1985). Sexuality and aging. In M. Lawton & G. Maddox (Eds.), *Annual review of gerontology and geriatrics, 5.* New York: Springer.

Starr, B., & Weiner, M. (1981). *Sex and sexuality in the mature years.* New York: McGraw-Hill.

State tobacco programs are effective. (2000, April). *The Nation's Health,* p. 6.

Statin drugs—Benefits beyond cholesterol lowering. (2001, June). *Tufts University Health & Nutrition Letter,* p. 6.

Stearns, S. et al. (2000). The economic implications of self-care: The effect of lifestyle, functional adaptations, and medical self-care among a national sample of Medicare beneficiaries. *American Journal of Public Health, 90,* 1608–1612.

Steffen-Batey, L. et al. (2000). Change in level of physical activity and risk of all-cause mortality or reinfarction: The Corpus Christi Heart Project. *Circulation, 102,* 2204–2209.

Stephens, N. et al. (1996). Randomised controlled trial of vitamin E in patients with coronary disease: Cambridge Heart Antioxidant Study (CHAOS). *Lancet, 347,* 781–786.

Steward, H. et al. (1998). *Sugar busters.* New York: Ballantine Books.

Stewart, K. et al. (2002). Exercise training for claudication. *New England Journal of Medicine, 347,* 1941–1951.

St. John's worts and all. (2000, September). *Nutrition Action Healthletter,* pp. 6–8.

Stokols, D. et al. (1995). Integration of medical care and worksite health promotion. *Journal of the American Medical Association, 273,* 1136–1142.

Stolberg, S. (2002). Minorities get inferior care, even if insured, study finds. *The New York Times,* pp. A1, A30.

Stores, G., & Crawford, C. (1998). Medical student education in sleep and its disorders. *Journal of Royal College Physicians, London, 32,* 149–153.

Strawbridge, W. et al. (2002). Physical activity reduces the risk of subsequent depression for older adults. *American Journal of Epidemiology, 156,* 328–334.

Strawbridge, W. et al. (1997). Frequent attendance at religious services and mortality over 28 years. *American Journal of Public Health, 87,* 957–961.

Strecher, V. et al. (1995). Goal setting as a strategy for health behavior change. *Health Education Quarterly, 22,* 190–200.

Strecher, V. et al. (1986). The role of self-efficacy in achieving health behavior change. *Health Education Quarterly, 13,* 73–91.

Stuart, R., & Davis, B. (1972). *Slim chance in a fat world.* Chicago: Research Press.

Studies suggest religious activities can improve health. (1996, March 4). *American Medical News.*

Study looks at patients' online use. (2002, May 6). *American Medical News,* p. 28.

Stunkard, A. (1987). Conservative treatments for obesity. *American Journal of Clinical Nutrition, 45,* 1142–1154.

Sulmasy, D., & Rahn, M. (2001). I was sick and you came to visit me: Time spent at the bedsides of seriously ill patients with poor prognoses. *American Journal of Medicine, 111,* 385–389.

Surwit, R. et al. (2002). Stress management improves long-term glycemic control in type 2 diabetes. *Diabetes Care, 25,* 30–34.

Sutton, S. (2001). Back to the drawing board? A review of applications of the transtheoretical model to substance use. *Addiction, 96,* 175–186.

Sutton, S., & Hallett, R. (1988). Understanding the effects of fear-arousing communications: The role of cognitive factors and the amount of fear aroused. *Journal of Behavioral Medicine, 11,* 353–360.

Swindle, R. et al. (2000). Responses to nervous breakdowns in America over a 40-year period. Mental health policy implications. *American Psychologist, 55,* 740–749.

Swoboda, F. (2001). Study challenges image of older drivers as dangerous. *Washington Post,* p. E01.

Szegedy-Maszak, M. (2001, August 6). The career of a celebrity pill. *U.S. News & World Report,* pp. 38–39.

Tabar, L. et al. (2001). Beyond randomized controlled trials. *Cancer, 91,* 1724–1731.

Take vitamin B-12, new study advises. (1998). *AARP Bulletin, 39,* 5, p. 3.

Tanaka, H. et al. (2001). Age-predicted maximal heart rate revisited. *Journal of American College of Cardiology, 37,* 153–156.

Tanasescu, J. et al. (2003). Physical activity in relation to cardiovascular disease and total mortality among men with type 2 diabetes. *Circulation,* April, epub ahead of print.

Tanasescu, M. et al. (2002). Exercise type and intensity in relation to coronary heart disease in men. *Journal of the American Medical Association, 288,* 1994–2000.

Tayback, M. et al. (1990). Body weight as a risk factor in the elderly. *Archives of Internal Medicine, 150,* 1065–1072.

Taylor, A. et al. (2002). Long-term intake of vitamins and carotenoids and odds of early age-related cortical and posterior subcapsular lens opacities. *American Journal of Clinical Nutrition, 75,* 540–549.

Taylor, D. et al. (2002). Benefits of smoking cessation for longevity. *American Journal of Public Health, 92,* 990–996.

Taylor, H., & Kagay, M. (1985). *Prevention in America III: Steps people take—or fail to take—for better health.* New York: Louis Harris.

Taylor, J. et al. (2002). Vitamin E supplementation and macular degeneration: Randomised controlled trial. *British Medical Journal, 325,* 11–14.

Taylor, R. et al. (1982). *Health promotion: Principles and clinical applications.* Connecticut: Appleton-Century-Crofts.

Taylor, S. et al. (1984). Attributions, beliefs about control, and adjustment to breast cancer. *Journal of Personality and Social Psychology, 46,* 489–502.

Teno, J. et al. (2002). Medical care inconsistent with patients' treatment goals: Association with 1-year Medicare resource use and survival. *Journal of American Geriatrics Society, 50,* 496–500.

Teri, L. et al. (1997). Behavioral treatment of depression in dementia patients: A controlled clinical trial. *Journals of Gerontology, Series B, 52,* 156–166.

Teri, L., & Gallagher-Thompson, D. (1991). Congitive-behavioral interventions for treatment of depression in Alzheimer's patients. *Gerontologist, 31,* 413–416.

The Heart Outcomes Prevention Evaluation Study Investigators. (2000). Vitamin E supplementation and cardiovascular events in high-risk patients. *The New England Journal of Medicine, 342,* 154–160.

The many benefits of fiber. (1996, September). *Johns Hopkins Medical Letter: Health After 50,* p. 4.

The new diet pill. (2000, March). *Berkeley Wellness Letter, 16,* 6, p. 2.

The power of the placebo effect. (2000, November 3). *Focus on Healthy Aging,* Mount Sinai School of Medicine, 11, pp. 1, 6.

The surprising power of placebos. (2000, February). *Self Healing,* pp. 2–3.

Theodosakis, J. (1997). *The arthritis cure.* New York: St. Martin's Press.

Thomas, D. et al. (2002). Randomized trial of breast self-examination in Shanghai: Final results. *Journal of National Cancer Institute, 94,* 1445–1457.

Thomas, K. et al. (2002). Home based exercise programme for knee pain and knee osteoarthritis: Randomised controlled trial. *British Medical Journal, 325,* p. 752.

Thomas, S. et al. (1994). The characteristics of northern black churches with community health outreach programs. *American Journal of Public Health. 84,* 575–579.

Thomas, W. (1996). *The eden alternative.* MA: VandenWyk and Burnham.

Thompson, R. et al. (1998). Orientation to community in a family medicine residency program. *Family Medicine, 30,* 22–26.

Thompson, R. et al. (1996). COPC in a family medicine residency program. *Family Medicine, 28,* 326–330.

Thorson, J. (2000). *Aging in a changing society.* New York: Taylor & Francis.

Thun, M. et al. (1997). Alcohol consumption and mortality among middle-aged and elderly U.S. adults. *New England Journal of Medicine, 337,* 1705–1714.

Time to deal with hearing loss? (2002). *Consumer Reports on Health, 14,* pp. 1, 4–6.

Tinetti, M. et al. (1994). Fear of falling and fall-related efficacy in relationship to functioning among community-living elders. *Journal of Gerontology, 49,* M140–M147.

Tinetti, M. et al. (1993). FICSIT: Risk factor abatement strategy for fall prevention. *Journal of American Geriatric Society, 41,* 315–320.

Tough anti-tobacco effort cited for 14% decline in lung cancer. (2000, December 1). *Houston Chronicle,* p. 9A.

Trafford, A. (2000, July 3). What will people do with the extra decade? *Houston Chronicle,* p. 3C.

Trans: The phantom fat. (1996, September). *Nutrition Action Healthletter,* pp. 10–11.

Trappe, S. et al. (2002). Maintenance of whole muscle strength and size following resistance training in older men. *The Journal of Gerontology: Biological Sciences, 57A,* B138–B143.

Trichopoulou, A. et al. (1999). Mediterranean diet and coronary heart disease: Are antioxidants critical? *Nutrition Reviews, 57,* 253–255.

Trivedi, D. et al. (2003). Effect of four monthly oral vitamin D3 (cholecalciferol) supplementation on fractures and mortality in men and women living in the community: Randomised double blind controlled trial. *British Medical Journal, 326,* p. 469.

Trumbo, P. et al. (2001). Dietary reference intakes. *Journal of the American Dietetic Association, 101,* 294–301.

Tucker, K. et al. (2000). Plasma vitamin B-12 concentrations relate to intake source in the Framingham Offspring Study. *American Journal of Clinical Nutrition, 71,* 514–522.

Tuomilehto, J. et al. (2001). Prevention of type 2 diabetes mellitus by changes in lifestyle among subjects with impaired glucose tolerance. *New England Journal of Medicine, 344,* 1343–1350.

Turkoski, B. et al. (1997). Clinical nursing judgment related to reducing the incidence of falls by elderly patients. *Rehabilitation Nursing, 22,* 124–130.

Tyler, Varro. (1999). *Tyler's honest herbal* (4th ed.). New York: Haworth Herbal Press.

UC Berkeley Wellness Letter. (2000, September). Is this the right way to test supplements? *UC Berkeley Wellness Letter, 16,* 12, pp. 1–2.

University of California at Berkeley Wellness Newsletter. (1995). *The New Wellness Encylcopedia.* Boston: Houghton Mifflin.

Unutzer, J. et al. (2003). Depression treatment in a sample of 1,801 depressed older adults in primary care. Journal of American Geriatric Society, 51, 505–514.

Urban obstacles to healthy living. (1996, March–April). *Health,* p. 35.

Uriri, J., & Thatcher-Winger, R. (1995). Health risk appraisal and the older adult. *Journal of Gerontological Nursing, 5,* 25–31.

U. S. Department of Agriculture. (1997, July). *Briefs.* Agricultural Research Service.

U. S. Department of Agriculture. (1990). *Nutrition and your health: Dietary guidelines for Americans* (3rd ed.). Washington, DC: U.S. Department of Health and Human Services.

U. S. Department of Labor. (1989, March 29). Thirty-eight million persons do volunteer work. Bureau of Labor Statistics' press release USDL 90–154.

USDHHS. (2000). *Healthy people 2010.* Washington, DC: USGPO.

USDHHS. (1998). *Clinician's handbook of preventive services* (2nd ed.). United States Department of Health and Human Services, Washington, DC: USGPO.

USDHHS. (1996). *Guide to clinical preventive services* (2nd ed.). United States Preventive Services Task Force. Baltimore, MD: Williams & Wilkins.

USDHHS. (1985, June). *A resource guide for injury control programs for older persons.* Washington, DC: USGPO.

USDHHS. (1979). *Healthy people: The surgeon general's report on health promotion and disease prevention.* Washington, DC: USGPO.

*US News & World Report.* (1998, March 9). Who is worried about health care and why? p. 48.

U. S. Preventive Services Task Force. (2000). Screening adults for lipid disorders: Recommendations and rationale. *American Journal of Preventive Medicine, 20,* 73–76.

U. S. Preventive Services Task Force. (1996). *Guide to clinical preventive services.* Baltimore: Williams and Wilkins.

U. S. Preventive Services Task Force. (1989). *Guide to clinical preventive services: An assessment of the effectiveness of 169 interventions.* Baltimore: Williams and Wilkins.

USPSTF. (2000). Colon cancer screening (USPSTF recommendation). *Journal of American Geriatrics Society, 48,* 333–335.

U.S. Public Health Service. (1988). *The surgeon general's report on nutrition and health.* DHHS (PHS) Pub. No. 88-50210. Washington, DC: USDHHS.

Vachon, M. et al. (1980). A controlled study of self-help intervention for widows. *American Journal of Psychiatry, 137,* 1380–1384.

Vaillant, G. (2002). *Aging well: Surprising guideposts to a happier life from the land-mark Harvard study of adult development.* Boston: Little, Brown.

Vaillant, G., & Western, R. (2001). Healthy aging among inner-city men. *International Psychogeriatrics, 13,* 425–437.

Valcour, V. et al. (2002). Self-reported driving, cognitive status, and physician awareness of cognitive impairment. *Journal of American Geriatric Society, 50,* 1265–1267.

Van Dongen, M. et al. (2000). The efficacy of ginkgo for elderly people with demen-tia and age-associated memory impairment: New results of a randomized clini-cal trial. *Journal of American Geriatrics Society, 48,* 1183–1194.

Van Duyn, M., & Pivonka, E. (2000). Overview of the health benefits of fruit and veg-etable consumption for the dietetic professional. *Journal of the American Dietetic Association, 100,* 1511–1521.

Vanishing inner-city grocery stores. (1996, February 12). *American Medical News,* p. 23.

Van Itallie, T., & Lew, E. (1990). Health implications of overweight in the elderly. *Progress in Clinical and Biological Research, 326,* 89–108.

Vasan, R. et al. (2002). Residual lifetime risk for developing hypertension in middle-aged women and men: The Framingham Heart Study. *Journal of the American Medical Association, 287,* 1003–1010.

Vasan, R. et al. (2001). Impact of high-normal blood pressure on the risk of cardio-vascular disease. *New England Journal of Medicine, 345,* 1291–1297.

Vincent, K., & Braith, R. (2002). Resistance exercise and bone turnover in elderly men and women. *Medicine & Science in Sports & Exercise, 34,* 17–23.

Vincent, K. et al. (2002). Resistance exercise and physical performance in adults aged 60 to 83. *Journal of the American Geriatrics Society, 50,* 1100–1107.

Vincent, K. et al. (2002). Improved cardiorespiratory endurance following 6 months of resistance exercise in elderly men and women. *Archives of Internal Medicine, 162,* 673–678.

Vitamin B-12. (1998, May). *Nutrition Action Healthletter,* p. 5.

Vitamin report. (1994, October). *University of California at Berkeley Wellness Letter,* Palm Coast, FL.

Vitiello, M. (1997). Sleep disorders and aging: Understanding the causes. *Journal of Gerontology: Medical Sciences, 52A,* M189–M191.

Von Faber, M. et al. (2001). Successful aging in the oldest old: Who can be character-ized as aged? *Archive of Internal Medicine, 161,* 2694–2700.

Voters allow hefty cigarette tax to stand. (2000, March 20). *American Medical News,* p. 4.

Wagner, E. et al. (1991). Factors associated with participation in a senior health pro-motion program. *The Gerontologist, 31,* 598–602.

Wakimoto, P., & Block, G. (2001). Dietary intake, dietary patterns, and changes with age: An epidemiological Perspective. *Journal of Gerontology: Series A, 56A* (Special Issue II), 65–80.

Wallechinsky, D., & Wallace, A. (1993). *The people's almanac presents the book of lists: The '90s edition.* New York: Little, Brown.

Wallerstein, N., & Bernstein, E. (1988). Empowerment education: Freier's ideas adapted to health education. *Health Education Quarterly, 15,* 379–394.

Wallston, K., & Wallston, B. (1982). Who is responsible for your health? The con-struct of health locus of control. In G. Saunders & J. Suls (Eds.), *Social psychol-ogy of health and illness.* Hillsdale, NJ: Erlbaum.

Wallston, B. et al. (1976). Development and validation of the health locus of control scale. *Journal of Consulting and Clinical Psychology, 44*, 58–585.

Walsh, B. et al. (1998). Effects of raloxifene on serum lipids and coagulation factors in healthy postmenopausal women. *Journal of the American Medical Association, 279*, 1445–1451.

Wannamethee, S. et al. (2001). Physical activity and risk of cancer in middle-aged men. *British Journal of Cancer, 85*, 1311–1316.

Wechsler, H. et al. (1996). The physician's role in promotion revisited: A survey of primary care practitioners. *New England Journal of Medicine, 334*, 996–998.

Wechsler, H. et al. (1983). The physician's role in health promotion: A survey of primary care practitioners. *The New England Journal of Medicine, 308*, 97–100.

Wei, M. et al. (2000). Low cardiorspiratory fitness and physical inactivity as predictors of mortality in men with type 2 diabetes. *Annals of Internal Medicine, 132*, 605–611.

Weight control: What works and why. (1994). *Mayo Clinic Health Letter Supplement*, pp. 1–8.

Weinberg, A., & Minaker, K. (1995). Dehydration: Evaluation and management in older adults. *Journal of the American Medical Association. 274*, 1552–1556.

Weininger, B., & Menkin, E. (1978). *Aging is a lifelong affair.* Los Angeles, CA: The Guild of Tutors Press.

WELCOA. (1997, April). Health risk appraisals. *Worksite Wellness Works, 13*, 2.

Westman, E. et al. (2002). Effect of 6-month adherence to a very low carbohydrate diet program. *American Journal of Medicine, 113*, 30–36.

Wetzel, M. et al. (1998). Courses involving complementary and alternative medicine at US medical schools. *Journal of the American Medical Association, 280*, 784–787.

Wheeler, F. et al. (1989). Health Promotion beliefs and attitudes of physicians: A survey of two communities in South Carolina. *Journal of South Carolina Medical Association, 1*, 121–134.

Wheeler, J. et al. (1998). The beneficial effects of volunteering for older volunteers and the people they serve: A meta-analysis. *International Journal of Aging and Human Development, 47*, 69–79.

White, E. et al. (1996). Physical activity in relation to colon cancer in middle-aged men and women. *American Journal of Epidemiology, 144*, 42–50.

White, G., & Madara, E. (2002). *American self-help clearinghouse online.* Denville, NJ: Mental Help Net, CenterSite, LLC.

Whitehead, M. (1997). Editorial: How useful is the 'stages of change' model? *Health Education Journal, 56*, 111–112.

Whole-body screening: Worth the trouble? (2002, June). *Consumer Reports on Health*, p. 6.

Whooley, M. et al. (1997). Case-finding instruments for depression: Two questions are as good as many. *Journal of General Internal Medicine, 12*, 439–445.

Williams, J. et al. (2002a). Rational clinical examination. Is this patient clinically depressed? *Journal of the American Medical Association, 287*, 1160–1167.

Williams, J. et al. (2002b). The association between trait anger and incident stroke risk: The ARIC Study. *Stroke, 33*, 13–20.

Williams, J. et al. (2001). Effects of an angry temperament on coronary heart disease risk. The Atherosclerosis Risk in Communities Study. *American Journal of Epidemiology, 154*, 230–235.

Williams, M. (1996). Increasing participation in health promotion among older African-Americans. *American Journal of Health Behaviors. 20,* 389–399.

Williams, P. (1997, September). *Health,* pp. 27–29.

Williams, R. et al. (1992). Prognostic importance of social and economic resources among medically treated patients with angiographically documented coronary artery disease. *Journal of the American Medical Association, 267,* 520–524.

Willis, D. (1997). Animal therapy. *Rehabilitation Nursing, 22,* 78–81.

Wilson, F. (1996). Patient education materials nurses use in community health. *Western Journal of Nursing Research, 18,* 195–205.

Wilson, R. et al. (2002). Participation in cognitively stimulating activities and risk of incident Alzheimer's disease. *Journal of the American Medical Association, 287,* 742–748.

Wilt, T. et al. (1998). Saw palmetto extracts for treatment of benign prostatic hyperplasia. *Journal of the American Medical Association, 280,* 1604–1609.

Wind, J. (1990). Striving for the fullness of life: The church's challenge in health. *Second Opinion, 13,* 8–73.

Wing, R., & Jeffery, R. (1999). Benefits of recruiting participants with friends and increasing social support for weight loss and maintenance. *Journal of Consulting Clinical Psychology, 67,* 132–138.

Wisconsin study describes rural obesity problem. (1996, April 1). *American Medical News,* p. 25.

Woelk, H. et al. (2000). Comparison of St. John's wort and imipramine for treating depression: Randomised controlled trial. *British Medical Journal, 321,* 536–539.

Wold, J., & Williams, A. (1996). Student/faculty practice and research in occupational health: Health promotion and outcome evaluation. *Journal of Nursing Education, 35,* 252–257.

Wolf, S. et al. (1996). Reducing frailty and falls in older persons: An investigation of Tai Chi and computerized balance training. *Journal of the American Geriatrics Society, 44,* 489–497.

Wolfson, L. et al. (1996). Balance and strength training in older adults: Intervention gains and Tai Chi maintenance. *Journal of Geriatrics Society, 44,* 498–506.

Wolk, A. et al. (1998). A prospective study of association of monounsaturated fat and other types of fat with risk of breast cancer. *Archives of Internal Medicine, 158,* 41–45.

Wood, P. et al. (1988). Changes in plasma lipids and lipoproteins in overweight men during weight loss through dieting as compared with exercise. *New England Journal of Medicine, 2319,* 1173–1179.

Woodward, N., & Wallston, B. (1987). Age and health care beliefs: Self-efficacy as a mediator of low desire for control. *Psychology and Aging, 2,* 3–8.

Woolf, S., & Johnson, R. (2000). A one-year audit of topics and domains in the *Journal of the American Medical Association* and the *New England Journal of Medicine. American Journal of Preventive Medicine, 19,* 79–86.

Wykle, M., & Musil, C. (1993, Winter/Spring). Mental health of older persons: Social and cultural factors. *Generations,* pp. 7–12.

Wykle, M., & Segal, M. (1991). A comparison of black and white family caregivers' experience with dementia. *Journal of the Black Nurses Association, 5,* 29–41.

Yaffe, K. et al. (2002). Serum lipoprotein levels, statin use, and cognitive function in older women. *Archives of Neurology, 59,* 378–384.

Yaffe, K. et al. (2001). A prospective study of physical activity and cognitive decline in elderly women: Women who walk. *Archives of Internal Medicine, 161,* 1703–1708.

Yancy, W. et al. (2001). A randomized controlled trial of a very-low carbohydrate diet with nutritional supplements versus a very-low-fat/low-calorie diet. *Obesity Research, 9*(Suppl 3), 17.

Yanovski, J. et al. (2000). A prospective study of holiday weight gain. *New England Journal of Medicine, 342,* 861–867.

Yarnall, K. et al. (2003). Primary care: Is there enough time for prevention? *American Journal of Public Health, 93,* 635–641.

Year end update: Quality of care. (1985). *Business and Health, 3*(2), p. 35.

Yee, B. (1990). *Variations in aging: Older minorities.* Galveston, TX: The University of Texas Medical Branch.

Young, R., & Kahana, E. (1989). Age, medical advice about cardiac risk reduction, and patient compliance. *Journal of Aging and Health, 1,* 121–134.

Young, T., & Gelskey, D. (1995). Is noncentral obesity metabolically benign? *Journal of the American Medical Association, 274,* 1939–1941.

Your elderly patients may be hungry or malnourished. (1993, December 6). *American Medical News,* p. 11.

Zajac, B. (1992, Fall). Put a patch on your smoking habit. *Discover Health,* pp. 2–4.

Zarit, S. et al. (1998). Stress reduction for family caregivers: Effects of adult day care use. *Journals of Gerontology, Series B, 53,* S267–S277.

Zeni, A. et al. (1996). Energy expenditure with indoor exercise machines. *Journal of the American Medical Association, 275,* 1424–1427.

Zhan, C. et al. (2001). Potentially inappropriate medication use in the community-dwelling elderly: Findings from the 1996 Medical Expenditure Panel Survey. *Journal of the American Medical Association, 286,* 2823–2829.

Zhu, S. et al. (2002). Evidence of real-world effectiveness of a telephone quitline for smokers. *New England Journal of Medicine, 347,* 1087–1093.

Zimmerman, R., & Connor, C. (1989). Health promotion in context: The effects of significant others on health behavior change. *Health Education Quarterly, 16,* 57–75.

# Index

# 𝕊 *Springer Publishing Company*

*From the Springer Series on Life Styles & Issues in Aging...*

# Successful Aging and Adaptation with Chronic Diseases

## Leonard W. Poon, PhD, D Phil, hc
## Sarah Hall Gueldner, DSN, FAAN
## Betsy M. Sprouse, PhD, Editors

For many people, growing old means facing one or more chronic diseases. SUCCESSFUL AGING reviews, coalesces, and expands what we know about how older adults successfully experience the aging process, and how they feel about and live with chronic illnesses. Questions considered include: How do older adults approach and deal with everyday life when affected by multiple health problems? What kind of impact do they feel diseases have on their successful aging? How do existent models and theories of coping address these issues?

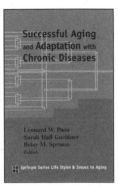

## Partial Contents:

- Self-Rated Successful Aging: Correlates and Predictors, *W.J. Strawbridge and M.I. Wallhagen*

- Successful Aging and Reciprocity Among Older Adults in Assisted Living Settings, *W. Rakowski, M.A. Clark, S.C. Miller, et al.*

- Successful Aging: Intended and Unintended Consequences of a Concept, *R.L. Kahn*

- Health Expectancy, Risk Factors, and Physical Functioning, *J. Penrod and P. Martin*

- What is Comorbidity? And What Do We Know About Older Adults Coping with Comorbidity? *L.W. Poon, L. Basford, C. Dowzer, et al.*

- The Efficacy of Coping Behaviors Used by Older Adults for Specific Chronic Health Conditions, *L. Basford, L.W. Poon, C. Dowzer, et al.*

- Coping with Multiple Chronic Health Conditions, *P. Martin*

- The Metanarratives Surrounding Successful Aging: The Medium Is the Message, *A.L. Whall and F.D. Hicks*

2003   280pp   0-8261-1975-1   hard

536 Broadway, New York, NY 10012 • (212) 431-4370 • Fax (212) 941-7842
Order Toll-Free: 877-687-7476 • Order on-line: www.springerpub.com

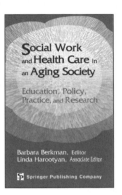